AF443112

eHEALTH: COMBINING HEALTH TELEMATICS, TELEMEDICINE, BIOMEDICAL ENGINEERING AND BIOINFORMATICS TO THE EDGE

Studies in Health Technology and Informatics

This book series was started in 1990 to promote research conducted under the auspices of the EC programmes' Advanced Informatics in Medicine (AIM) and Biomedical and Health Research (BHR) bioengineering branch. A driving aspect of international health informatics is that telecommunication technology, rehabilitative technology, intelligent home technology and many other components are moving together and form one integrated world of information and communication media. The complete series has been accepted in Medline. Volumes from 2005 onwards are available online.

Series Editors:
Dr. J.P. Christensen, Prof. G. de Moor, Prof. A. Famili, Prof. A. Hasman, Prof. L. Hunter,
Dr. I. Iakovidis, Dr. Z. Kolitsi, Mr. O. Le Dour, Dr. A. Lymberis, Prof. P.F. Niederer,
Prof. A. Pedotti, Prof. O. Rienhoff, Prof. F.H. Roger France, Dr. N. Rossing,
Prof. N. Saranummi, Dr. E.R. Siegel, Dr. P. Wilson, Prof. E.J.S. Hovenga,
Prof. M.A. Musen and Prof. J. Mantas

Volume 134

Recently published in this series

ISSN 0926-9630

eHealth: Combining Health Telematics, Telemedicine, Biomedical Engineering and Bioinformatics to the Edge

Global Experts Summit Textbook

Edited by

Bernd Blobel
University of Regensburg Medical Center, Germany

Peter Pharow
University of Regensburg Medical Center, Germany

and

Michael Nerlich
University of Regensburg Medical Center, Germany

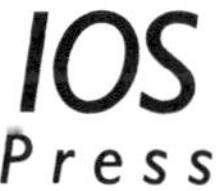

IOS Press

Amsterdam • Berlin • Oxford • Tokyo • Washington, DC

ISBN 978-1-58603-835-9
Library of Congress Control Number: 2008920797

Publisher
IOS Press
Nieuwe Hemweg 6B
1013 BG Amsterdam
Netherlands
fax: +31 20 687 0019
e-mail: order@iospress.nl

Distributor in the UK and Ireland
Gazelle Books Services Ltd.
White Cross Mills
Hightown
Lancaster LA1 4XS
United Kingdom
fax: +44 1524 63232
e-mail: sales@gazellebooks.co.uk

Distributor in the USA and Canada
IOS Press, Inc.
4502 Rachael Manor Drive
Fairfax, VA 22032
USA
fax: +1 703 323 3668
e-mail: iosbooks@iospress.com

eHealth: Combining Health Telematics, Telemedicine, Biomedical Engineering and
Bioinformatics to the Edge. Edited by B. Blobel, P. Pharow and M. Nerlich.
IOS Press, 2008

Foreword

Current demographic, economic and social conditions which developed countries are faced with require a paradigm change for delivering high quality and efficient health services. In that context, healthcare systems have to turn from organisation-centred to process-oriented and finally towards individualised patient care, also called personal care, based on eHealth platform services. Interoperability requirements for ubiquitous personalised health services reach beyond current concepts of health information integration among professional stakeholders and related Electronic Patient Records. Future personal health platforms have particularly to maintain semantic interoperability among systems using different modalities and technologies, different knowledge representation and domain experts' languages as well as different coding schemes and terminologies to include home care as well as personal and mobile systems. This development is not restricted to regions or countries, but appears globally, requiring a comprehensive international collaboration.

From December 2nd to 5th, 2007, the eHealth Competence Center (eHCC) supported by the International Center for Telemedicine (ICT) at the University of Regensburg Medical Center and several other organisations such as IMIA, EFMI, ISfTeH and the Czech Society of Biomedical Engineering and Medical Informatics, organised an International Conference on eHealth thereby aiming at uniquely combining Health Telematics, Telemedicine, Biomedical Engineering and Bioinformatics to the edge. This Global Experts Summit Textbook within the Series "Studies in Health Technology and Informatics" at IOS Press presents invited speeches from internationally leading experts representing all domains involved in eHealth. The International Conference has been completed through specific seminars, workshops and symposia addressing collaboration and potential projects between Europe and Latin America (ELAN), analysing cross-border activities between Germany, Austria, the Czech Republic, and Switzerland, promoting current eHealth achievements of MEDTEL (Prague, CZ), and presenting poster submissions to the conference concerning telematics and telemedical applications. Those results have been jointly published at IOS Press, Amsterdam, and Akademische Verlagsgesellschaft Aka GmbH, Berlin.

The editors would like to thank all the invited authors for their excellent contributions. Furthermore, they thank the Gold Sponsors Siemens AG Medical Solutions, InterComponentWare AG and InterSystems GmbH, and also HL7 Germany, AGFA HealthCare GmbH, ID-Berlin GmbH, ManaThea GmbH and SAP AG for their inevitable support.

Bernd Blobel
Regensburg, December 2007

Contents

New Sciences and Technologies

eHealth from Dream to Reality

National eHealth Strategies and Implementations

Multidisciplinary and Multilingual Semantic Interoperability

Combining the Domains

*eHealth: Combining Health Telematics, Telemedicine, Biomedical Engineering and
Bioinformatics to the Edge. Edited by B. Blobel, P. Pharow and M. Nerlich.
IOS Press, 2008*

Introduction into Advanced eHealth – The Personal Health Challenge

Bernd BLOBEL [1]
*eHealth Competence Center, University of Regensburg Medical Center, Regensburg,
Germany*

Abstract. For improving quality and efficiency of health delivery under the well-known burdens, the health service paradigm has to change from organization-centered over process-controlled to personal health. Established in connection to the already existing International Center for Telemedicine, the eHealth Competence Center in Regensburg has been dedicated to advance research, development, education and administration of comprehensive eHealth. In co-operation with internal and external partners, the Personal Health paradigm comprising of health telematics, telemedicine, biomedical engineering, bioinformatics and genomics is pushed ahead. The paper introduces the underlying paradigms, requirements, architectural framework and development processes for comprehensive service-oriented Personal Health interoperability chains.

Keywords. Personal health, system architecture, semantic interoperability, Generic Component Model, ubiquitous care

Introduction

Healthcare systems in industrialized countries, and increasingly those in countries in transition, are faced with the challenge of ensuring efficient and high quality care. This challenge must be realized despite demographic developments, the growth of multi-morbidity, demands for health services and expenditures for diagnostic and therapeutic procedures, and decreasing contributions to health insurance funds. To meet this challenge independently of time, location and local resources, utilizing advanced knowledge and technologies, the systems have been changing from an organization-centered towards a process-controlled care paradigm, which is also called shared care, managed care or disease management. This development is combined with extended cross-organizational communication and cooperation between all healthcare establishments directly or indirectly involved in patient's care. This process has to be supported by deploying advanced information and communication technologies (ICT) in health, connecting primary and secondary care. Regarding the need for prevention

---

[1] Corresponding Author. Bernd Blobel, PhD, Associate Professor, eHealth Competence Center, University of Regensburg Medical Center, Franz-Josef-Strauss-Allee 11, D-93053 Regensburg, Germany; Email. bernd.blobel@klinik.uni-regensburg.de; URL: http://www.ehealth-cc.de

and the integration of social care in an aging society (addressing citizens before becoming patients, and so moving the focus from healthcare to health) this process-controlled strategy is no longer sufficient. Health, nowadays provided by organizations such as hospitals, primary care offices, policlinics, or medical centers, has to move closer to the citizens' environment.

Observing the citizens' health status, context and conditions for providing person-centered (personalized) and dedicated health services imply the need for a new health paradigm: personal care, which completely integrates all principals involved in the care process. According to the definition of the Object Management Group (OMG), principals are any actors in the domain in question such as persons, organizations, systems, devices, applications, components, or even single objects. This does not mean that there will no longer be acute care and ambulant service, but such services will be tailored to relevant personal care needs.

Established in connection to the already existing International Center for Telemedicine at the University of Regensburg Medical Center, the eHealth Competence Center has been dedicated to advance research, development, education and administration of comprehensive eHealth. In co-operation with internal and external partners, the Personal Health paradigm comprising of health telematics, telemedicine, biomedical engineering, bioinformatics and genomics is pushed ahead.

The paper discusses requirements and solutions for advanced eHealth systems in the Personal Health context. This implies the semantic interoperability challenge, underlying architectural paradigms and multi-disciplinary settings.

1. Materials and Methods

In this section, the paradigms relevant for analyzing, designing, implementing and maintaining personal health information systems covering any type of principal and its components will be shortly discussed.

From a system-theoretical perspective, quality and efficiency of care delivery like any other process depend on the appropriate reflection of, and interrelations between, the environment and all actors related to a process on the one hand and on the optimal process design on the other. The first aspect is basically described through the information cycle model, the second concerns of workflows and interoperability chains. Following, both aspects are shortly discussed.

1.1 The Information Cycle

Conscious and intentional activities of human beings, organizations, and societies are based on observations of the environment and involved principals, simplified described or modeled in the context of the intended objectives. The model of, or the view on, the reality consisting of patient, health professionals, and related processes has to be provided in a way that guarantees the same understanding as well as coordination in performing actions. The first step provides the semantic aspect of interpreted information derived from an observation, the second deals with the pragmatic aspect of information in taking the right action. Both steps require knowledge of experts operating in the domains of interest. Such way of communication and co-operation is called semantic interoperability. Thereby, different domains and policies have to be linked to each other and combined forming a comprehensively operating system. Health-related domains are, e.g., medical, administrative, technological, or legal. A policy in the given context represents any legal, organizational, cultural, ethical, social, functional, and technical implication.

Meanwhile, our observations are no longer limited by our sensory performance. Diagnostic devices and investigation methodologies include universal and – importantly for medical practice – microscopic or even molecular dimensions. As observations have been enhanced by technology, also actions go meanwhile far beyond our natural power. The information cycle from the statistical approach to information through its semantic interpretation up to its pragmatic aspects is represented in different information definitions provided by C. E. Shannon, L.-M. Brillouin, and N. Wiener [1]. Modeling language and applied knowledge depend on the domain of interest and the observation means and methodologies applied. At different level of system composition such as populations, person/organ/tissue/micro structures or molecular structures (DNA; RNA; Protein, …), different informatics specialties are involved for managing the related information such as public health informatics, clinical informatics or bioinformatics, respectively, which are closely connected to the domains of interests such as the bunch of medical specialties, nursing, legal affairs, ethics, psychology, social sciences, biomedical engineering, technology, etc. The higher level of granularity leads to a greater amount of data observed and collected to be processed, requiring advanced methodologies like data mining and grid computing.

1.2. Interoperability Levels

Regarding the interoperability level, technical interoperability (technical plug&play, protocols), structural interoperability (simple EDI, envelopes), syntactic interoperability (messages, clinical documents), semantic interoperability (advanced messaging, common information model and terminology), and finally organizational/service interoperability (common business process) can be distinguished. As IEEE defines semantic interoperability "the ability of two or more systems or components to exchange information and to use the information that has been exchanged" [2] all projects and programs are looking for, the agreed behavior of collaborating applications requires the deployment of reference models, common terminologies and ontologies, and certified applications developed in a unified process. Interoperability levels reflect information cycle aspects. While communication focuses on exchange of meaningful and correctly interpreted messages, cooperation depends on the applications' behavior and functionality. The architecture of a system describes the system components, their functions and relationships. Therefore, application architectures define the achievable interoperability level. The assessment of systems regarding their interoperability has to be provided by analyzing their architecture and the completeness of the information cycle [3].

For a better understanding of the developed methodology, three definitions should be provided: models, concepts, and knowledge [4]. A model is a partial representation of reality, using appropriate grammars and being restricted to attributes the modeler is interested in. Defining the pragmatic aspect of a model, the interest depends upon the intended audience and the reason and the purpose for modeling the reality. The resulting model is used for a certain purpose and time as a proxy for reality. A purpose of models is to create knowledge. An outcome of developing mathematical models is that it helps model builders and decision makers to understand the relationships between important variables in a business situation. On the other hand, description and especially the interpretation of real systems are based on knowledge. Therefore, the model (which is the result of an interpretation) must be interpreted itself. Knowledge can be defined as a combination of instincts, ideas, rules and procedures that guide actions and decisions. It is used to transform data into information that is useful in a situation. Knowledge helps users to interpret, and act on, information. Eventually, a concept depicts, or corresponds to, a set of objects. It is represented by, or uses, knowledge representation languages for defining or designating the concept. Thus, it is part of a concept system. Domain expert knowledge is typically derived from general knowledge by constraining the underlying concepts and rules expressed in corresponding models, therefore named constraint models.

1.3. Technical Paradigms

To realize patient care at any location in an individualized way, three technological paradigms have to be managed: mobile computing, pervasive computing and autonomous computing (Figure 1). Mobile computing enables the permanent accessibility of the principals involved, providing, for example, teleconsultation services. Pervasive computing allows for location-independent service provision including any type of principals, established as telemedicine services. For providing personalized care, services have to be flexible and cannot be rigidly predefined. Such adaptive health information system design, towards a self-organizing environment, draws on current challenges in the research and development for autonomic computing.

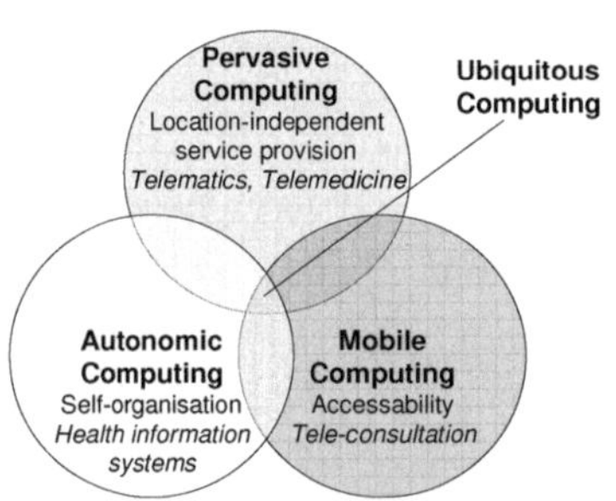

Figure 1. Computing paradigms deployed in the personal care context (after Kirn and Müller [5], changed)

Another aspect which is characteristic for personal health (pHealth) concerns the distance between the physical and the informational world. In the traditional ICT environment, this gap is mediated through human users. Introducing advanced technologies, this gap is getting closer to the real integration of the health subject (patient) in the health system, and even becoming a part of the information system environment (Figure 2).

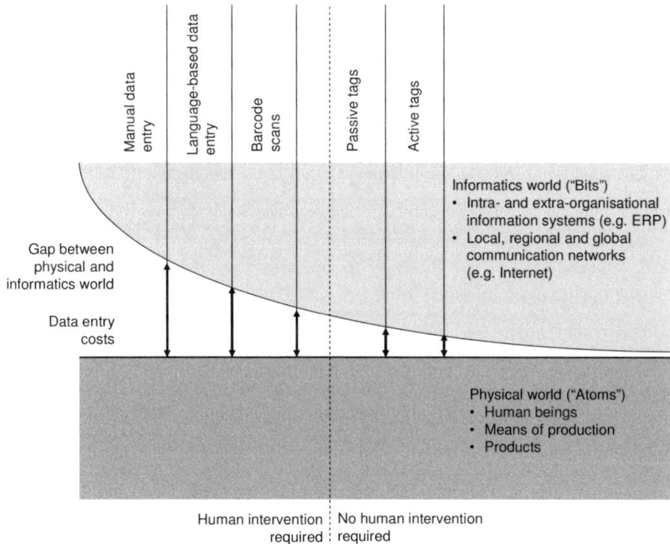

Figure 2. Closing the gap between physical and informational world (after Kirn and Müller[5], changed)

For designing and integrating component-oriented, distributed, and adaptive systems, a Reference Architecture and a Unified Development Framework are essential.

1.4. The Generic Component Model

For designing and implementing component-oriented, highly distributed, and adaptive personal health setting following the Ambient Intelligence paradigm, the simplification of systems through formal models can be provided in three dimensions according to the Generic Component Model (GCM) (Figure 3) [3], serving as a Reference Architecture. The first level of simplification concerns the restriction to the domain of interest. Examples for such domains are the medical domain, administrative domain, technical domain, legal domain, etc. Within this domain, the system considered can be decomposed or composed for analyzing or designing it. This results in different levels of granularity or complexity, respectively, using specialization or generalization relationships. In the Generic Component Model, the following granularity levels have been derived: business concepts, relations network, basic services/functions and basic concepts. The third dimension of generic system architecture touches different aspects of the system according to the ISO Reference Model – Open Distributed Processing [6]. Here, the business process is expressed by the Enterprise View, the informational expression of this process is expressed by the Information View and the functional aggregation of algorithms and services is expressed by the Computational View. The aforementioned views are described through platform independent models of the system expressing the system's logical content. Platform-specific implementation details are described by the Engineering View, and the Technology View represents technical and organizational implementation aspects. The system's architecture (i.e. the system's components, their functions and relationships) is characterized through the components' concepts and their aggregations. The representation of concepts and association rules is provided by constraint models, which are derived from reference models. All architectural elements (system's components, their functions and relationships) must be uniquely identified, certified, and registered. This includes any principal, which causes an identification challenge shortly discussed in Section 3.

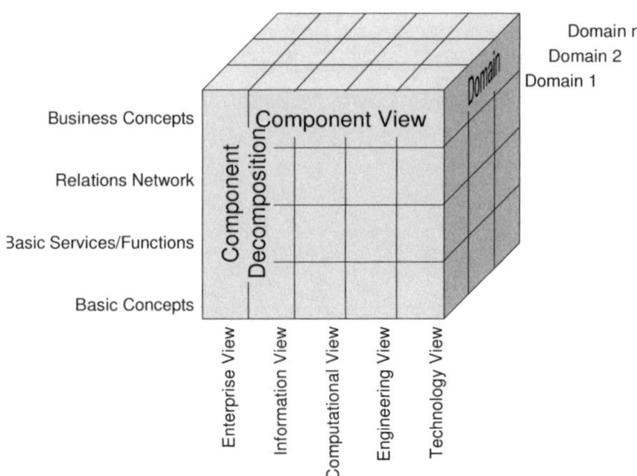

Figure 3. The Generic Component Model [7]

The resulting pHealth information system is characterized by openness, flexibility, scalability, portability, user friendliness and user acceptance, service orientation, distribution at Internet level, being based on standards, semantic interoperability, lawfulness and trustworthiness. Organizational, contextual, rule-related or other constraining aspects of the system and its components are expressed by binding policies to the components and by ruling the component aggregation by policies. Following the Generic Component Model approach, the pHealth information system architecture needs to combine the following paradigms: distribution; component-orientation; separation of platform-independent and platform-specific modeling, i.e. separation of logical and technological views; specification of reference and domain models at meta-level; interoperability at service level (concepts, contexts, knowledge); enterprise view driven process-controlled design; multi-tier architecture; appropriate multi-media GUIs; common terminology and ontology; unified design, development and deployment process; trustworthiness provided by appropriate security and privacy services, all as an integrated part of the design.

2. Results

2.1 Personal Health Systems Architecture

Architecture, i.e. the system's components, their functions and their interrelationships, has to be described by the representation of related concepts at corresponding level of granularity as well as their aggregations to another level. Deploying the definitions given in section 1, concepts are derived from reference models through constraint modeling. Because an object is represented by its concept and an appropriate designation, reference terminologies and ontologies are needed for assuring semantic interoperability. Also for the designation system, the Generic Component Model can be exploited. By harmonizing and integrating different systems with different modalities, from different business domains with different domain experts' languages, a consistent and coherent development framework for semantically interoperable health information systems is provided. This also includes component invocation as well as the instantiation of applications. For describing concepts, rules, and interrelations, meta-languages such as the Unified Modeling Language (UML) and its Object Constraint Language (OCL), or -with restriction to structural information- the eXtensible Markup Language (XML) family are used. Thereby, specializations have been developed such as the security and privacy related languages eXtensible Access Control Markup Language (XACML) and Security Assertion Markup Language (SAML) defined at OASIS [4], [8].

2.2. Integration of Biomedical Systems

The integration of biomedical devices for patient monitoring or patient care is typically done using the standard set CEN ISO/IEEE 11073 (derived from former ENV 13734/13735 "VITAL" und IEEE 1073-x) [9] as well as CLSI (ex NCCLS) POCT-1A [10]. Biomedical devices can be as scalable and flexibly designed and integrated as any other component system. This is especially true for future mobile, modular, personal systems for individual care of patients. Such systems can be implemented and used both in clinical settings and in persons'/patients' home, or they can follow the patient smoothing the transition between both environments.

In different development stages and accentuations, typical system concepts comprise the following basic components:

1. Highly integrated sensor and human-machine interface components (human interface) on the body on the one hand and intelligent, wireless sensors or wearable components on the other;

2. Components and infrastructure for the communication between those sub-systems and corresponding stationary systems and services including the transfer between primary and secondary care (Body Area Network, mobile phone, portable radio network, wireless in-house radio network, workstations with gateway functions in the patient's home including appropriate middleware);

3. Distributed functions for sensor signal processing, state recognition und control up to person-related and situation-specific activation of information and intervention offers (alert management, cumulative registration, processing and presentation of multiple parameters using PDAs or workstations);

4. Information and expert systems for recognition and treatment of emergency situations, for patient information as well as occasionally for decision support to health professionals (localization, access to reference information, person-specific support for data interpretation, secure access to sensitive patient information, Electronic Health Record or Personal Health Record).

The system functions planned also allow reasonable and meaningful escalation strategies. Thereby, the patient-related system components should be as self-reliant as possible to minimize communication, care efforts or power consumption but being ready to communicate occasionally with external system components (e.g. in the case of exceeding threshold values / recognizing exceptional situations, emergency or alerts, but also routine data transfer).

2.3. Standards for Semantically Interoperable Personal Health Systems

For enabling semantic interoperability by setting up a unified development process, the Rational Unified Process [11] or alternatively the HL7 Development Framework [12] can be exploited. For domain-related specifications, available domain-specific concept and process models such as HL7 Domain Information Models (D-MIMs) or even newer HL7 Domain Models (DIMs), HL7 Refined Message Information Models (R-MIMs), and Common Message Element Types (CMETs) but also GEHR/openEHR Archetypes [13] should be re-used. Other recent knowledge representation models might also be deployed, however [14]. The other domains related to a comprehensive eHealth/pHealth environment have to be represented in a standardized way. Initiated as HL7 work, the ISO TS 25720 "Health informatics – Genomic sequence variation markup language" [15] as well as biobank standards activities can be referenced here as practical examples. The standardization process for establishing semantically interoperable eHealth systems must comprises the entire development process and all aforementioned architectural paradigms such as modeling, formal languages, reference and domain models, knowledge representation tools, domain-specific terminologies and ontologies, security and privacy services, communication protocols, etc. [16].

2.4. Electronic Health Record and Personal Health Records

Future advanced and sustainable eHealth architectures for individualized care with regional or European dimensions are described in the eHealth Action Plan of the European Commission and the EU Member States. This challenging program defines the Electronic Health Record (EHR) as the core application for every eHealth platform. There are different approaches towards EHR system implementations in the various countries, however. The variant established are ranging from Medication Files in The Netherlands as well as in England over Sharable EHR as the Finnish solution up to the comprehensive EHR in Denmark. In the long term, all countries will approach a comprehensive EHR. Because of the individualized focus putting the person in the centre of the business and empowering him/her to play an important role in his/her health, the person will also contribute to the documentation of his/her status and processes applied. Therefore, EHR systems in Personal Health setting are also called Personal Health Records.

Beside the Electronic Health Record, the improvement of quality and safety of care through evidence-based medicine und decision support plays an extraordinary role. In this context, ePrescribing using decision support systems has been prioritized in Europe and in other eHealth regions as well.

2.5. Security and Privacy Services in Personal Health Settings

A comprehensive security infrastructure is a basic prerequisite for any distributed health information system or health network. Here, identification and authentication of principals involved as well as other security services such as comprehensive ID management, privilege management and access control, anonymization and pseudonymization, or audit have to be mentioned, which will be discussed in some more details in the next section. In that context security tokens (e.g. chip cards) are frequently used.

Such approach requires a completely different consideration of security and privacy services compared with the current practice. Security services can neither be predefined nor managed or administered at runtime by human administrators. They have to be formally modeled using meta-languages for allowing their management by systems and components deployed. As a basic requirement, all security services have to be ruled according to the actual status, ongoing processes as well as environmental and contextual conditions. Therefore, security and privacy services have to be policy-driven in a flexible and intelligent way. They must be built in as integrated architectural components. The diversity of use cases and inter-domain relationships cannot be completely regulated through legislations. Therefore, the implementation and application of ethical frameworks is getting increasing importance. This is combined with special administrative and educational challenges.

For integrating security and privacy services in Personal Health systems, those services have to be managed as any other system following all dimensions of the Generic Component Model. As a consequence, concepts for security services have to be formally expressed and must be bound to components representing other domains, by that way providing the aggregation of components within and between domains according to the Generic Component Model. Policy binding concerns all components such as actors, processes and target objects. For more information see, e.g., [17].

3. Identification Challenge in eHealth Settings

Communication and collaboration between systems truly depends of identification of systems and their components involved in the interoperability chain. There are two different approaches for identifying systems and components in a process: identification based on a managed identifier and identification based on pattern recognition.

As already mentioned in Section 1.4., identification and authentication of all architectural elements is a crucial challenge for highly distributed, component-based, self-organizing systems. This includes all principal types, but also information models, concepts, classes, etc., to always aggregating and using the right components. In that context, signatures are used for consistently identifying such components. A signature binding a special characteristic to an object is a very broad concept. Such a signature could be instantiated as a frequency in a spectrum identifying an astronomic object, an RFID (Radio Frequency Identification) chip labeling goods, a characteristic of a molecule in a solvent, an individual biometrics such as a fingerprint, or a footprint of an animal. It could represent the result of a process using an individual keys and related cryptographic algorithms, as performed in the digital signature context at different levels of trust. Signatures may relate to single components or to classes grouping them. Signatures are not only used for checking the identity and authenticity, but also the integrity of components, even including legal dimensions.

The challenge concerns the entire lifecycle of those components. Identification and authentication services facilitate security and privacy issues, but are also inevitable for reducing safety risks. Therefore, identification and authentication have to be logically and technically supported. In that context, identification and authentication tokens are playing an important role. Here, smartcards for identifying and authenticating persons and special individual (and persistent) properties (e.g., blood group) have to be mentioned, such as Health Professional Cards, electronic Health Insurance Cards, but also electronic passports. As information has to be identifiable, verifiable, and traceable, also goods labeled with an identifier can be authenticated and traced as well. Therefore, technologies such as RFID deployed in a globalizing environment are called "the Internet of goods".

Meanwhile, RFID is used for identifying and tracing medical devices, probes, patients, drugs, etc., as successfully demonstrated in Asklepios hospitals in Germany. FDA is looking for introducing a device identifier for tracing and maintaining medical devices. In Austria, pacemakers have been identified uniquely to be used in device management and to comparable and traceable analyze the device functions stored in a national cardiologic registry. Traceability of persons provides a privacy risk and might be restricted by legislations.

4. The Education Challenge

pHealth represents truly integrated care including many disciplines. Taking the lead in development and deployment of advanced pHealth requires broad and at the same time deep knowledge and proficiency about all involved domains, their concepts, methodologies, terminologies and ontologies, as well as appropriate means for formalizing and presenting them. Current educational programs do not meet those challenges. For overcoming this deficiency, the eHealth Competence Center at the University of Regensburg Medical Center in collaboration with renowned international partners from the USA, UK, The Netherlands and Belgium is preparing an international Master Course "International Master in eHealth". This course appropriately reflects the comprehensive eHealth concept presented in the paper. Such an educational program for aiming elite development establishes high challenges on the students admitted to this course. Therefore, special admission requirements, small classes, advanced infrastructures, appropriate practice partners and high qualifications of teaching staff are inevitable.

5. Discussion

Interoperability implies a number of different concepts, e.g. functional interoperability and internetworking, semantic interoperability and application gateways. Health information integration (eHealth) has established a demand for interoperability between clinical and healthcare-related stakeholders, systems and processes or workflows. Domain-specific communication and interoperability standards are well established, but have to be supplemented for trans-domain use. Interoperability concepts for medical devices and for personal or mobile systems need to involve all 7 ISO/OSI reference model layers, more properly advanced to the Generic Component Model, including terminology/coding aspects.

The advanced concept of pHealth extends eHealth by the inclusion of smart sensors, body-worn mobile systems and situation-specific activation of applications and human health professionals, thus providing personalized ubiquitous health services. Body Area Networks and micro-systems are building blocks of future personalized health telematics infrastructures, and extend existing interoperability concepts. Another important eHealth pillar is the field of bioinformatics and genomics. As personal health requires personalized process models for optimal care, the underlying diagnosis and therapy has also to be individualized. This can be achieved by developing and deploying advanced bioinformatics and genomics as mentioned earlier, which have to be integrated into the interoperability chain. Technologies and methodologies for gathering and managing personal molecular information at different granularity level from genomics through epigenetics, transcriptomics, posttranscriptomics up to proteomics have to be considered and enhanced. In that context, chips for investigating single nucleotid polymorphism as individual risk of illness indicators, arrays for detecting specific nucleic acids, micro-arrays for detecting antibodies or other genetic constituencies at different level of molecular granularity have to be mentioned. The result are collected and deployed in international genetic databases, e.g., PubMed and GenBank.

The transfer to pHealth information systems with process-controlled, service-oriented, context-sensitive, semantically-interoperable information and communication architectures requires open, highly flexible individually tailored application systems for the cared for and the caring parties. Such applications cannot be pre-manufactured any more, but must be dynamically created and adapted to the actual requirements and needs. In that way, besides the well-established technology paradigms of Mobile Computing for realizing accessibility (e.g. teleconsultation) and Pervasive Computing for realizing independency of location when providing services (e.g. telemedicine), the paradigm of Autonomous Computing for realizing self-organizing systems can be introduced. The combination of the aforementioned technology paradigms leads to Ubiquitous Computing, which is bound to other paradigms and trends such as health grids. Personal health also requires an adequate legal framework and the new orientation of traditional organizational patterns.

Acknowledgement

The author is indebted to the colleagues from HL7, ISO TC 215, CEN TC 251, IMIA, EFMI and many other institutions for kind support.

References

[1]   Blobel B. EPA-Modelle im Vergleich: openEHR, HL7 V3 Specs, EN/ISO 13606, CCR. In: Jäckel A (Hrsg.) Telemedizinführer Deutschland, Ausgabe 2008, Deutsches Medizin Forum, Minerva KG, Darmstadt.

[2]   IEEE Standard Computer Dictionary: A Compilation of IEEE Standard Computer Glossaries, IEEE, 1990

[3]   Blobel B: *Analysis, design and implementation of secure and interoperable distributed health information systems.* Stud Health Technol Inform Vol. 89, IOS Press, Amsterdam, 2002.

[4]   Blobel B: Concept Representation in Health Informatics for Enabling Intelligent Architectures. In: Hasman A, Haux R, van der Lei J, De Clercq E, Roger-France F (Edrs.) *Ubiquity: Technology for Better Health in Aging Societies,* pp. 285-291. Series Studies in Health Technology and Informatics, Vol. 124. IOS Press, Amsterdam, 2006.

[5]   Kirn S, Müller G. Ministudie zu den F&E-Perspektiven auf dem Gebiet der Gesundheitstelematik. Hohenheim, University of Hohenheim, 2005.

[6]   ISO/IEC 10746 "Information technology – Open Distributed Processing, Part 2 – Reference Model".

[7]   Blobel B. Advanced EHR architectures – promises or reality. *Methods Inf Med* 2006; 45: pp 95-101.

[8]   Organization for the Advancement of Structured Information Standards (OASIS): http://www.oasis-open.org (last accessed September 20, 2007)

[9]   http://www.ieee1073.org

[10] http://www.nccls.org or http://www.clsi.org

[11] IBM. Rational Unified Process. www.ibm.com/software/awdtools/rup/

[12] http://www.hl7.org

[13] CEN SSS-HIDE (2001). Health Informatics-Strategies for harmonisation and integration of device level and enterprise-wide methodologies for communication as applied to HL7, LOINC and ENV.

[14] Becks T, Dehm J. IMEX – A New Knowledge Platform for Microsystems in Medicine. http://www.vde-mikromedizin.de

[15] ISO TS 25720 "Health informatics – Genomic sequence variation markup language" International Organization for Standardization / TC 251 Medizinische Informatik http://www.iso.ch/tc215

[16] Engel K, Blobel B, Pharow P. Standards for Enabling Health Informatics Interoperability. In: Hasman A, Haux R, van der Lei J, De Clercq E, Roger-France F (Edrs.) *Ubiquity: Technology for Better Health in Aging Societies,* pp. 145-150. Series Studies in Health Technology and Informatics, Vol. 124. IOS Press, Amsterdam, 2006.

[17] Blobel B. EHR Architectures – Comparison and Trends. (in this volume)

eHealth: Combining Health Telematics, Telemedicine, Biomedical Engineering and Bioinformatics to the Edge. Edited by B. Blobel, P. Pharow and M. Nerlich.
IOS Press, 2008

eHealth and IMIA's Strategic Planning Process

IMIA Conference Introductory Address

Peter MURRAY [a,1], Reinhold HAUX [b] and Nancy LORENZI [c]
a CHIRAD, Nocton, UK
b Peter-Reichertz-Institute for Medical Informatics, TU Braunschweig, Germany
c Dept. of Biomedical Informatics, Vanderbilt University Medical Center, Nashville TN, USA

Abstract. The International Medical Informatics Association (IMIA) is the only organization in health and biomedical informatics which is fully international in scope, bridging the academic, health practice, education, and health industry worlds through conferences, working groups, special interest groups and publications. Authored by the IMIA Interim Vice President for Strategic Planning Implementation and co-authored by the current IMIA President and the IMIA Past-President, the intention of this paper is to introduce IMIA's current strategic planning process and to set this process in relation to 'eHealth: Combining Health Telematics, Telemedicine, Biomedical Engineering and Bioinformatics to the Edge', the theme of this conference. From the viewpoint of an international organization such as IMIA, an eHealth strategy needs to be considered in a comprehensive way, including broadly stimulating high-quality health and biomedical informatics research and education, as well as providing support to bridging outcomes towards a new practice of health care in a changing world.

Keywords. Medical informatics, health informatics, eHealth, strategic planning, IMIA

1. The International Medical Informatics Association

IMIA, the International Medical Informatics Association ([1]) has recently celebrated its 40th birthday. IMIA is the only organization in biomedical informatics which is fully international in scope, bridging the academic, health practice, education, and health industry worlds through conferences, working groups, special interest groups and publications.

IMIA started in 1967 as Technical Committee 4, Medicine, of the International Federation of Information Processing (IFIP). In the present version of the IMIA statutes, it is stated that the basic aims of IMIA shall be:

- "to promote informatics in health care and biomedical research;
- to advance international cooperation;
- to stimulate research, development and routine application;

---

[1] Corresponding Author: Peter J. Murray, MD, PhD, IMIA Interim Vice President for Strategic Planning Implementation, Centre for Health Information R@D CHIRAD, Coachman's Cottage, Nocton Hall, Nocton, Lincoln, United Kingdom; Email: peter@chirad.net

- to move informatics from theory into practice in a full range of settings, from physician's office to acute and long term care; and
- to further the dissemination and exchange of knowledge, information and technology."

Details on IMIA's development have been recently published in the IMIA Yearbook 2007 ([2], pp. 163-192). A comprehensive summary of IMIA publications from the recent past can be found in [3].

2. 'Towards IMIA 2015' - IMIA's Strategic Planning Process

2.1. Introduction

IMIA's General Assembly unanimously approved the IMIA Strategic Plan on August 18, 2007 when it met prior to Medinfo2007 in Brisbane, Australia. Titled 'Towards IMIA2015', this plan sets out a vision and strategic goals for IMIA ([4], [5]).

The IMIA Strategic Plan provides an agreed vision for IMIA, a set of guiding principles on which IMIA's future development will be based, and an Integrated Strategic Framework Model. The vision for IMIA sees its role as one of providing expertise and leadership in health and biomedical informatics to the multidisciplinary health focused community and to policy makers, in order to enable the transformation of health care in accordance with the world-wide vision of improving the health of the world population. IMIA therefore aims to be the informatics association through which the world's knowledge leaders come together to effectively and efficiently create, assemble, integrate, synthesize or assimilate intellectual knowledge, and to provide the informatics association that effectively and efficiently connects people and the nations of the world to be able to accomplish this purpose ([4]).

IMIA is now turning attention to the implementation of its Strategic Plan. A 'Transition Plan' is being developed; over the coming months and years, it will be further developed, supported by the continuing work of a planning team and lead by a new IMIA Vice President with specific responsibilities for implementation of the Strategic Plan.

In an editorial in *Methods of Information in Medicine*, one of IMIA's official journals, all members of the IMIA 'family', and all with interest in, and links to, our work, are invited to become involved in contributing to the implementation of the IMIA Strategic Plan [6].

2.2. Background

The concept of an IMIA Strategic Plan started in 2003. Following a world-wide survey conducted during 2003 and 2004, to assess what IMIA members would like to see IMIA do or become within the next 5 to 10 years, a strategic planning task force was appointed in 2004. Lead by the IMIA President Nancy Lorenzi, the task force members included Floyd Eisenberg (USA), HM Goh (Malaysia), Steven Huesing (Canada), Fernando Martin-Sanchez (Spain), Lincoln de Assis Moura, Jr. (Brazil), Peter Murray (UK), and Heather Strachan (UK), who represented the many parts of the IMIA family, i.e. national societies, working and special interest groups, and academic and corporate institutional members.

Over the three years from 2004 to 2007, the task force held physical meetings and virtual discussions, and consulted widely with all parts of the IMIA 'family'. By an iterative process of consultation addressing general principles and specific areas, we developed the components of the IMIA Strategic Plan. This culminated in a vision for how IMIA should be by 2015, and an Integrated Strategic Framework Model, underpinned by IMIA's Guiding Principles.

The Integrated Strategic Framework Model (also known as the IMIA 'rainbow umbrella') provides a multi-dimensional visual representation of the scope of IMIA's areas of legitimate interest and activity, connections and integration possibilities. From these arise a possible future structure for IMIA and its work to evolve. This multidimensional model comprises five concentric circle layers and six sectors to the overall circle. Each circle and each sector describes a component of IMIA.

Knowledge is the central core of IMIA, thus in the center of the model. All of IMIA's strategies, interactions and efforts emanate from this knowledge core. The second circle, directly touching the knowledge core, represents the science layer, portraying IMIA members' connection and integration with the science and discovery of informatics. The third circle represents the application of scientific discoveries, including the multiple questions and issues that are created and disseminated in informatics. The fourth circle represents IMIA's impact layer, referring to the potential impact that IMIA and its members can have on governments, nations, outcomes, health professionals, and all other stakeholders. The fifth, and outermost, circle represents the people layer, the level at which IMIA interacts with individuals, citizen organizations, personal health involvement, dissemination and acceptance, enabling personal responsibility, and public/personal health.

The second dimension of the Strategic Plan represents the various key sectors that IMIA as an international association must address. Superimposed on the five concentric circle layers of IMIA's integration and connection to others are six major sectors. Knowledge is at the center of each of the six sectors. At the top of the circles is the health sector; since the prime element of our vision is to improve health, this sector highlights our vision and the strategic goals supporting this sector. The other sectors are research/science (including how we understand and create evidence to support health); the behavioral responsibility (ethics) sector that refers to our ethical and social responsibility; education (including best practices in educating ourselves and others); the multiple types of relationships (communications and connections to build relationships among stakeholders); and finally the sixth sector is the reach (equity) of IMIA, our obligation to share, distribute and disseminate. It is not possible here to provide the full detail of the model, especially the detailed description of the components and the multi-color, multi-dimensional graphic representation; the current version can be downloaded for study and comment from the IMIA website ([1]).

The 2007 IMIA General Assembly unanimously approved this Strategic Plan and supported the recommendation to use up to US$50,000 of IMIA's reserve funds to nurture and encourage strategic efforts outlined in the plan that would enhance informatics around the world. The General Assembly recommended that the concept of a Vice President for Strategic Planning be developed and presented to the General Assembly meeting in Sweden in 2008.

For a more comprehensive summary on the background to the development of the IMIA Strategic Plan, the authors refer readers to [4] and to the recent and future IMIA Yearbooks of Medical Informatics.

2.3. Transition

We know from research into information system failures ([7]) and also from errors within hospitals that the time of "hand-offs", "hand-over's", "cut-over's", or other transition points, are the times when there is a higher probability for problems, issues, failures, and errors to occur. In order to avoid that phenomenon IMIA created a 'Transition Plan' as a bridge to the future.

3. IMIA's Approach in Contributing to International Stimulation of eHealth Initiatives

Transforming health care by significantly changing care processes and by appropriately using today's information technology is crucial for improving the quality of care. This can be seen to be true for all parts of our world, in particular as we consider the potential impacts on health care delivery of the many challenges facing our changing and aging societies. The potential interactions of new and emerging technologies with demographic and societal changes were considered by IMIA's Nursing Informatics Special Interest Group (IMIA-NI) at their NI2006 Post Congress Conference in Korea in June 2006. The resultant publication ([8]) recognized the role to be played by changing technologies in the ways in which we support and deliver care in the future, but also clearly demonstrated that technology is only one part of the equation, and that many other factors must be borne in mind.

IMIA contributed and contributes to this transition in many other ways. Its working groups are at the leading edge of developing and disseminating results on new information technologies and new organizational approaches. A new task force, which is exploring the potential application of Web 2.0 technologies within IMIA's activities and e-services ([9]), and wider implications for the health and biomedical informatics domains, is yet another example of IMIA recognizing the need to be fully engaged in all new developments that affect its areas of interest. In a variety of conferences, high-quality knowledge is shared among researchers and practitioners world wide, resulting in peer-reviewed publications. Transforming health care also needs well-educated health care professionals and specialists in health informatics and biomedical informatics. IMIA's member organizations, in particular its academic institutional members, continuously share, exchange and further develop educational approaches for health and biomedical informatics.

As an important component of IMIA's strategic planning initiatives and with relation to eHealth, IMIA's recent joint activities with the World Health Organization (WHO, [10]) provide as example of the need for organizations with common aims to work together.

WHO has identified information and communication technology as a significant factor for promoting its aims, with an important milestone in this development being the WHO eHealth Resolution of 2005 ([11], [12]). In 2006, WHO's Executive Board furthermore identified eight priority eHealth action areas: access to health information; eHealth norms and standards; legal and ethical issues; an observatory for eHealth; public-private partnerships for ICT research and development for health; ICT for health promotion; ICT for supporting human resources for health; and ICT for service delivery.

IMIA is a long-term non-governmental organization (NGO) of WHO. Recognizing the strategic dimension of this relationship, WHO and IMIA decided to intensify their collaboration, and announced during MedInfo 2007 in Brisbane steps to further strengthen their cooperation. In a communiqué, WHO and IMIA presented at MedInfo 2007, their most recent medical informatics world congress ([13]), three key areas of joint work for the next three years were identified:

- The Global Observatory for eHealth: To provide WHO Member States with strategic information and guidance on the application of ICT for health through a WHO coordinated country-based network.

- The use of ICT for the development of the health workforce: Human resources for health (HRH) are increasingly recognized as a crucial element in improving health systems and achieving the Millennium Development Goals. WHO's ICT for HRH initiative explores the use of eLearning and other ICT-mediated techniques in initial education and training, as well as for continuing professional development and support of health workers in developing countries.

- Sharing eHealth products and services related to intellectual property for development (SHIPD): Health systems are strengthened and health is improved in low and middle income countries by providing access to appropriate products and services protected by eHealth Intellectual Property Rights, through WHO.

Details on this collaboration can be found in [14].

4. Invitation to Collaborate

Irrespective of how exactly they view eHealth - and over 50 definitions have been identified ([15]) - the participants of this conference on 'eHealth: Combining Health Telematics, Telemedicine, Biomedical Engineering and Bioinformatics to the Edge' will probably agree that information technology helps to improve the quality of health care by disseminating and systematizing knowledge of diagnostic and therapeutic possibilities as well as the organization and management of care ([16], [17]). New information technologies, including unobtrusive, active, non-invasive technologies, such as wearable devices, now allow us to continuously monitor and respond to changes in the health of a patient. Such devices range from micro-sensors, integrated in textiles, through consumer electronics embedded in fashionable clothes, to belt-worn personal computers with head mounted displays ([18]).

These technologies will only be successful when appropriate organizational changes have been made in order to identify new, sustainable ways of managing care. These new ways promise to make it considerably easier for patients to maintain their good health while enjoying their life in their usual social setting, rather than having to spend much time at costly, dedicated health care facilities. This may prove to be essential for ensuring quality of life as well as health care for increasingly aging societies ([19]).

IMIA is devoted to contributing to these aims by the initiatives and activities mentioned. You may agree that we can be proud of having the good fortune of living today, in a world where the quality of health care and life expectancy is higher than ever before in the history of humankind. You may, however, also agree that there is an urgent need to reshape health care for our rapidly changing societies. We should be aware that we all, including IMIA and its member organizations, play an important role in successfully contributing to the development of good health in our societies. IMIA invites all institutions and individuals, devoted to these goals, to join in these efforts. While IMIA has many working groups dealing with aspects of eHealth, it may be that, as part of the implementation of the IMIA Strategic Plan, a specific new piece of work is needed to develop a dedicated eHealth plan or series of activities. We welcome discussion of these possibilities within this conference and beyond.

References

[1] http://www.IMIA.org. Last accessed October 13, 2007.

[2] IMIA Yearbook of Medical Informatics 2007: Biomedical Informatics for Sustainable Health Systems. *Methods Inf Med* 2007; 46 Suppl. 1.

[3] Peterson H, Hutter M. IMIA's publication history. IMIA Yearbook of Medical Informatics 2007. *Methods Inf Med* 2007; 46 Suppl 1: 192-96.

[4] Lorenzi N. Strategy in a fishbowl: an invitation to determine the shape of IMIA in 2015. Methods Inf Med 2006; 45: 235-9.

[5] Lorenzi N. Towards IMIA 2015 - the IMIA Strategic Plan. In: IMIA Yearbook of Medical Informatics 2007. *Methods Inf Med* 2007; 46 Suppl 1: 1-5.

[6] Murray P et al. Let a thousand flowers bloom: transition towards implementation of the IMIA Strategic Plan. To appear in: *Methods Inf Med*.

[7] Lorenzi NM, Riley RT. Managing change: an overview. *J Am Med Inform Assoc* 2000; 7:116-24.

[8] Murray PJ, Park H-A, Erdley WS and Kim J (Eds.) *Nursing Informatics 2020: Towards defining our own future*. Proceedings of NI2006 Post Congress Conference. Amsterdam: IOS Press; 2007.

[9] http://www.differance-engine.net/imia20. Last accessed October 13, 2007.

[10] http://www.WHO.int. Last accessed October 13, 2007.

[11] World Health Organization. eHealth Resolution. 58th World Health Assembly, Resolution 28. May 25, 2005. Geneva: WHO; 2005.
58th World Health Assembly's home page: http://www.who.int/gb/e/e_wha58.html.
English version: http://www.who.int/gb/ebwha/pdf_files/WHA58/WHA58_28-en.pdf.
Last accessed October 13, 2007.

[12] Healy JC. The WHO eHealth Resolution. eHealth for all by 2015? *Methods Inf Med* 2007; 46: 2-3.

[13] K.A. Kuhn, J.R. Warren and T.-Y. Leong (Edrs.) *MEDINFO 2007*. IOS Press, Amsterdam, 2007.

[14] Geissbuhler A et al. Towards health for all: WHO and IMIA intensify collaboration. Joint Communiqué during Medinfo 2007 in Brisbane. *Methods Inf Med* 2007; 46: 503-5.

[15] Oh H, Rizo C, Enkin M, Jadad A. What is eHealth (3): A systematic review of published definitions J Med Internet Res 2005;7(1):e1. http://www.jmir.org/2005/1/e1/ Last accessed October 13, 2007.

[16] Kuhn KA, Wurst SH, Bott OJ, Giuse DA. Expanding the scope of health information systems. Challenges and developments. IMIA Yearbook of Medical Informatics 2006. *Methods Inf Med* 2006; 45 Suppl 1:43-52.

[17] Maojo V, Kulikowski C. Medical informatics and bioinformatics: integration or evolution through scientific crises? *Methods Inf Med* 2006; 45: 474-82.

[18] Bott OJ et al. The challenge of ubiquitous computing in health care: technology, concepts and solutions. *Methods Inf Med* 2005; 44: 473-9.

[19] Haux R. Individualization, globalization and health - about sustainable information technologies and the aim of medical informatics. *Int J Med Inform* 2006; 75: 795-808.

*eHealth: Combining Health Telematics, Telemedicine, Biomedical Engineering and
Bioinformatics to the Edge. Edited by B. Blobel, P. Pharow and M. Nerlich.
IOS Press, 2008*

Analysis of Barriers in Implementation of Health Information Systems

EFMI Conference Introductory Address

George I. MIHALAS [1]
European Federation for Medical Informatics
Victor Babes University of Medicine and Pharmacy, Timisoara, Romania

Abstract. This paper tries to make an inventory and classification of several possible barriers, which can lead to unfulfillment in Health Information Systems implementation. The reports are compared and discussed within this context.

Keywords. Healthcare information systems, barriers, failure rate, implementation surveys, education

Introduction

The enthusiasm about the improvements brought by a new technology does usually make the innovators ignore the practical implementation potential difficulties or the side effects of their innovation. This is also the case of implementing information technology (IT) in Healthcare, often referred as healthcare information systems (HIS) or e-Health; the two terms have different definitions, but a substantial overlapping.

It is not a secret that, the success rate of HIS implementation was much below the expectations. Even it is difficult to collect real quantitative data, for various reasons, the failures are much rarely reported than successes, most often masked by mild terms („modest results") or even partially hidden.

1. Previous Studies

One of the best thorough reviews on "Factors affecting information systems success" was published in 1995 by Whyte and Bytheway [1]. More than ten studies have been presented, classified and analysed. The paper did not present cases but rather discussed the concept of success and failure in the provision of information systems under the viewpoint of service management. The analysis made by the authors is systematic but does not refer to implementations in a specific domain, the conclusions being rather general. We can cite here their list of the main causes of difficulty in implementation of information systems:

---

[1] Corresponding Author: George Mihalas, PhD, Professor, Victor Babes University of Medicine and Pharmacy, Eftimie Murgu Sq 2, Timisoara 300041, Romania; Email: mihalas@umft.ro.

- over optimistic estimates that subsequently lead to the system being delivered late and over budget
- ill-defined project objectives, mostly arising from uncertainty regarding the business needs to be satisfied
- poor communication between users and the development staff
- the technical limitations of a system and systems which are unfriendly and inflexible
- the use of inexperienced staff to develop systems.

The authors have used a repertory grid technique to collect the data (the perceptions about differences between the information system that they use), and made a statistical analysis (principal component analysis) in order to identify and classify or sort the major attributes (they have selected 21 attributes), which must be addressed to meet the users expectations.

We could notice that these surveys covered a large variety of information systems: industrial, financial, governmental, utilities, including healthcare; however, healthcare information systems were not specifically addressed.

Another well-documented study, with a comprehensive statistics on failure rates is presented by IT-Cortex [2]. Five surveys, carried out between 1995 and 2001 are referred. The figures show various unsuccessful rates, between 40% and 70% (table 1).

Table 1. List of surveys presented by IT-Cortex [2]

	Survey	Year	Country	Measure of failure	Unsuccessful (failure) Rate %	Size of survey	Area
1.	OASIG Study	1995	UK	• costs • delay	70%	45	
2.	Chaos report	1995	USA		31% cancelled 52% cost ~double only 16% complete (time and budget)	365	Banking, retail, healthcare, insurance
3.	KPMG Canada	1997	Canada	• costs delay	61	176	Public and private sector
4.	Confe-rence Board	2001	USA	• implement. costs • support costs • time to achieve results	40	117	Various companies
5.	Robbins -Gioia	2001	USA	Perception of respondents	51	232	Government, IT, industry, finance, communication, utilities, healthcare

The authors have also identified, by using several evaluation criteria, the major items associated with success or failure. We can cite here:
For failure:
- missed deadlines 75%
- exceeded budget 55%
- poor communications 40%
- inability to meet project requirements 37%

For success:

- meeting milestones 51%
- maintain the required quality levels 32%
- meeting the budget 31%

These surveys covered a large variety of information systems: industrial, financial, governmental, utilities, including healthcare; however, healthcare information systems were not specifically addressed.

Nevertheless, there are several studies targeted to healthcare information systems. Littlejohns [3] referred to a large project, which started in 1997 in the Limpopo Province South Africa. A well-designed evaluation program was used yielding a more extensive view than the traditional technical assessment of hardware and software. The evaluation revealed several problems, beside the inherent infrastructure problem:

- too many proposed functions to implement in one phase
- modules not created in time
- the advanced features of software caused delays
- a general poor organization of the implementation

Moreover, even in the hospitals that had the system installed, there were no significant differences in the quantitative outcome variables analyzed (time spent in outpatients, length of stay, bed occupancy, cost per case etc.). The authors made a careful analysis of the reasons for failure; we can cite here from their list: failure to take into account the social and professional cultures of healthcare organizations, neglect education of users, underestimation of the complexity of routine clinical and managerial processes, dissonance between the expectations of various parts involved, etc. The authors also mention some cases of HIS failures in UK (references 8 and 9 in [3]).

In 2003, BMJ published a series of comments and opinions on "Evaluating computerized health information systems" [4 and its "related articles"]. The authors expressed the view that the health professionals should be closely involved in the hospital information system implementation (Ladner J) but also that some lessons have been learnt (Longano BA).

2. Case Study

A project similar with the one in South Africa, HMIS – Healthcare Management Information System, started in Romania in 1997 with an initial credit of 16 M$. Even the World Bank expert has noticed some difficulties from the beginning [5], the project went on, exceeding the budget and reaching just a few of the goals [6]; several components have never been finalized. It was difficult to collect all relevant information. However, the report revealed several features, collected by the author in a study presented at the e-Health High Level Conference in Malaga [7].

We can mention here the major causes for this project failure:

- Lack of specialized personnel (most of the trained persons left the system),
- Change of legislation and regulations during the implementation (the national health insurance system was created immediately after the project started, yielding major changes in organizational structures); the modifications in the project were ad-hoc and failed to answer the new requirements; some components were too rigid and could not be adapted;

- The contract did not contain solutions for all possible cases that could occur (and did!);
- Lack of stability or political support – during the implementation, the project responsibility has been taken over by several high level persons in the ministry and the lead team has been changed several times;
- Inappropriate solutions and lack of interoperability – the Grenoble Hospital Information System has been proposed to be introduced in eight pilot Romanian hospitals, but the organizational system was so different and the programs could not be adapted; the translation was inaccurate and came late; finally, this solution has been abandoned;
- Surprisingly, the user acceptance was good at end-users in the healthcare settings of the pilot hospitals but much poorer at the staff level in the healthcare authorities and ministry offices. We can underline here the role of the pre-project preparation of the staff to be involved, which was successful in this case.

The authors have analysed also the "digital divide" within the healthcare systems, including in the analysis also the persons with decision positions, who, sometimes, failed to understand the real problems.

3. Recent Work

It became obvious from the previous work that the evaluation studies are essential for estimating the quality of health information systems. Both IMIA (International Medical Informatics Association) and EFMI (European Federation for Medical Informatics) have working groups on Qualitative Assessment of health information systems. A pilot Delphi study published by them [8] gives an excellent view over the factors influencing success and failure of health informatics systems, including also comments about defining "success" and "failure".

The journal Health Affairs is also hosting a collection of almost 80 articles on Health Information Technology, initiated in 2005. Kleinke [9], after remarking the US healthcare marketplace's continuing failure to adopt information technology, as a result of economic problems unique to healthcare, is even asking an aggressive governmental intervention, for creation of a national health IT system. This position was shared also by other authors of papers in the same issue (Taylor R, Frisse M, etc.)

Shay [10] and Hersch [11] have analysed another feature, which became quite common in the last years – the "legal" barriers associated with prevision of data confidentiality and privacy. The modern security technologies are not affordable in smaller practices or rural areas. Anderson [12] extends the view also over the social and ethical aspects.

The variety of barriers to be reported from all over the world made the MEDINFO 2007 Scientific Program Committee to organize a special section in the poster session, "Barriers to clinical system implementation", with 13 papers. [12] (P126-P138). The authors not only reported the barriers met in their implementation activities but also analysed the causes, proposed solutions and even revised the systems under the new view.

4. Discussion and Conclusions

The papers mentioned in the previous chapters represent just a part of the literature available on this topic. Most of these papers not only report the cases but also analyze the reasons and propose solutions. A natural question occurs then: "Why do we still have again similar situations?" Shortliffe [14] was rather optimistic by supposing that the "obvious" had already been perceived!

Maybe the analyses made up to now did not go deep enough to find the root – the "original" cause, if any. Another rhetoric question can arise: "Is the healthcare system prepared to accept and assimilate information technology? Why IT implementations went much smoother in industry or finance? We do not intend to speculate more on this feature.

Let us first notice that there were rarely technical problems; most of the times the product fulfilled the requirements. However, the implementation process and the service went wrong.

When one is trying to compare the discussions presented by various authors, he would easily find that one common thing in almost all reports concerned the user acceptance, most often connected with staff training and education.

It is, indeed, necessary to smooth the information transfer between different professionals involved in the information flow of the health information systems. As noticed before [7], there are gaps induced by the digital divide within the system, which reduces the real outcome at each step of transfer: the applications do not fully use the hardware and software performances, the direct users (healthcare managers) do not fully use or understand the applications performances while the end users (doctors, nurses) use even less.

Actually the importance of education and training has been recognized for a long while. The IMIA Working Group on Education and Training, chaired by Reinhold Haux, has elaborated in 1997 a set of Recommendations for Medical/Health Informatics Education [15]. A European Centre for Medical Informatics, Statistics and Epidemiology, chaired by Jana Zvarova, was created in Prague in 1999 [16]. EFMI has organized several events dedicated to educational aspects, the last one being a Special Topic Conference held in Athens in 2005 [17]. But the largest educational program started recently in USA, organized by American Medical Informatics Association, AMIA, called 10 x 10, aiming to train ten thousand clinical informaticians by 2010 [18].

We expect to have a visible increase of success rates of health information systems implementation when the number of health informatics professionals will increase. A thumb-rule estimates the needs of health informatics professionals as a ratio 1:6 to 1:8 to the number of physicians.

However, we must still be aware that there are also other causes: interoperability, which is a very hot topic (and beyond the purpose of this paper), but also organizational, managerial, legal or ethical issues, which still wait for appropriate solutions. Nevertheless, some solutions need a particular approach and have to be separately analyzed.

References

[1]   Whyte G, Bytheway A. Factors affecting information Systems success. 1995. www.smf-method.com /articles/Factors

[2]   www.it-cortex.com/Stat_Failure_Rate.htm, 2002. [last accessed in 5 Oct. 2007].

[3]   Littlejohns P, Wyatt JC, Garvican L. Evaluating computerized health information systems: hard lessons still to be learnt. *BMJ* 2003; 326: 860-863.

[4]   Evans MG. Evaluating computerized health information systems: We are still getting information technology wrong. *BMJ* 2003, 327: 163-164.

[5]   Neame R. Information Services for Healthcare in Romania. In: Richards B (Edr.) Tri-partite Bridges: Educators, Providers and Users. Seminar Proceedings, Tempus Project CME 0255-95, „Know-How Transfer from University to Industry", Sinaia 1998: 119-34.

[6]   Mihalas GI, Bazavan M, Farcas DD. Implementation of Health Information Systems in Romania. *Methods Inf Med* 2006; 45: 121-4.

[7]   Mihalas GI. Objective and Subjective Barriers in Healthcare Information Systems Implementation. e-Health 2006 High Level Conference, Malaga, Spain. www.ehealthconference2006.org/pdf/mihalas.pdf

[8]   Brender J, Ammenwerth E, Nykkanen P, Talmon J. Factors Influencing Success and Failure of Health Informatics Systems. *Methods Inf Med* 2006; 45: 125-36.

[9]   Kleinke JD. Dot-Gov: Market Failure and the Creation of a National Health Information Technology System. *Health Affairs,* 2005; 24(5): 1246-1262.

[10]   Shay EF. Legal barriers to electronic health records. 2005; http://physiciansnews.com/ law/505.html

[11]   Hersh W R. Health IT. Solutions to Conquering Systemic Barriers. *Physician's Weekly.* 2007; XXIV (26), www.physiciansweekly.com

[12]   Anderson J. Social, ethical and legal barriers to E-health. *Intl J Med Inf* 2006; 76 (5-6): 480-483

[13]   Kuhn K A, Warren J R, Leong T Y (Edrs.) *MEDINFO 2007.* Proceedings of the 12th World Congress in Health (Medical) Informatics. IOS Press, Amsterdam, 2007.

[14]   Shortliffe EH. Strategic Action in Health Information Technology: Why the Obvious Has Taken So Long. *Health Affairs,* 2005; 24(5): 1222-1233.

[15]   www.imia.org/edu/recommendations.html

[16]   www.euromise.org/education

[17]   Hasman A, Mantas J (Edrs.) *Health and Medical Informatics Applications.* Akademische Verlagsgesellschaft Aka Gmbh, Berlin, 2005.

[18]   Hersh W, Williamson J. Educating 10,000 informaticians by 2010: the AMIA 10 x 10 program. *Int J Med Inf* 2007; 76: 977-982.

Education in Biomedical Informatics and *e*Health

Jana ZVÁROVÁ [1]
European Center for Medical Informatics, Statistics and Epidemiology of Charles
University in Prague and Academy of Sciences of the Czech Republic,

Abstract. The long-term effect of education in the field of biomedical informatics and eHealth on efficiency and quality of healthcare is discussed. Selected educational methods and tools are presented and their applications are shown.

Keywords. Education, biomedical informatics, eHealth, knowledge society

Introduction

We are approaching to a knowledge society in healthcare, where knowledge is one of the decisive keys to success. Almost daily we learn about new technologies and technical devices, new drugs, as well as a spread of new diseases. To make the most of the advantages of new technologies and to prevent the potential dangers, we have to have access to and be able to work with the newest information, and use new technologies efficiently as quickly as they appear. Health professionals cannot rely, throughout their lifelong careers, only on the skills and knowledge acquired during their full-time education. Life-long learning and continuing education have become a necessity in our everyday reality. Flexible means enabling the acquisition of new knowledge even by health professionals in full-time employment need to be offered. Books, the traditional tool for self-study, should be complemented by *e*Learning tools using an electronic technology and media in support of learning.

Educational programs in the area that we nowadays refer to as biomedical informatics are covering topics from the field of medical informatics, health informatics and bioinformatics. The conceptual roots of such programs lead back more than thirty years and the programs are well established in many countries. The leading role in promoting activities concerning education in biomedical informatics has been given by the International Medical Informatics Association (IMIA) at MEDINFO congresses, special topics conferences and activities of the IMIA working group on Health and Medical Informatics Education. This working group initiated the development of IMIA Recommendations on Education in Health and Medical Informatics [1] translated till now into Spanish, Chinese, Italian, Turkish, Czech and Japanese languages. Let us mention at least the IMIA conference on medical informatics education held in Prague 1990. It brought together participants from 18 countries and the „Knowledge, Information and Medical Education" proceedings [2]

[1] Corresponding Author: Jana Zvarova, PhD, Professor, Institute of Computer Science AS CR, v.v.i., Pod Vodarenskou vezi 2, 182 07 Prague 8, Czech Republic; Email: zvarova@euromise.cz

contained more than 60 selected contributions and covered the role of informatics in the medical curriculum and experiences existing in many medical faculties all over the world. During the 58th World Health Assembly held in Geneva in May 2005, the Ministers of Health of the 192 member states of the United Nations approved the so called *e*Health Resolution [3] that officially recognizes the added value of the information and communication technologies for health purposes. *e*Health technologies opened the doorway to a new type of medical services where healthcare professionals are able to utilize them fully for prevention and management of diseases, lifelong learning and communication with colleagues and patients. Moreover, education and use of *e*Health technologies can help to change a passive attitude of patients against their diseases towards a proactive attitude of informed citizens for managing their own health. Further we will discuss different approaches to biomedical informatics and *e*Health education developed in the Czech Republic with the support of national and European projects.

1. EuroMISE Courses in English

University education is the basis for research and development. In Europe the curricula still differ in a content, structure and style. European programmes such as SOCRATES, ERASMUS and TEMPUS were created to assist in the transfer of knowledge among European countries. In the period 1993-1995 the Joint European Project "Education in the Methodology Field of Health Care" of the TEMPUS programme was running and giving the assistance of European Union countries to Central and Eastern European countries. The more detail information about the aims of the project was given in [4]. The project was running under the acronym EuroMISE (European education in Medical Informatics, Statistics and Epidemiology) with participation of eleven leading universities and research institutions from EU countries [5]. Training and education in EuroMISE consisted of three overlapping methodological branches: medical informatics, medical statistics and epidemiology. One of the main goals of the EuroMISE project was to create a teaching network for higher education in the multidisciplinary field of health care and to create basic conditions to multiply knowledge and skills received in the courses. During the year 1993 the EuroMISE courses in English were developed and in April 1994 the EuroMISE Center as the joint teaching and research centre of Charles University in Prague and the Academy of Sciences of the Czech Republic was set up. The teaching in the EuroMISE courses was given in the years 1994 and 1995 by university professors and senior researchers from EU universities and research institutions. More than 70 certificates were passed in the Charles University Aula Magna for successful completion of the European EuroMISE courses in 1994 and 1995 by participants from the Czech Republic and other Central and Eastern European countries (Bosnia and Herzegovina, Bulgaria, Croatia, Hungary, Poland, Romania, and Slovenia). Between 1996 and 1997 postgraduate and continuing education in the EuroMISE courses in English, which started in the frame of the European cooperation via the EuroMISE project, were further running with the great support of participating EU institutions (Erasmus University, Rotterdam and Limburg University, Maastricht, The Netherlands, Ruprecht-Karls University, Heidelberg, Phillips University, Marburg and MEDIS Institute, Neuherberg, Germany, University of Manchester, Institute of Science and Technology, United Kingdom). The support of the EU institutions made possible to run the EuroMISE courses free of charge for students from different European countries. More than 50 certificates were passed for successful completion of the EuroMISE courses in the years 1996 and 1997. The EuroMISE courses have opened the challenge to improve the training opportunities in the field of medical informatics, statistics and epidemiology in Central and Eastern European countries and contributed to positive changes in the health care sector.

2. *e*Learning Strategies

The main aim of the project of the 4th Framework Programme of EU countries IT EDUCTRA (Information Technologies EDUcation and TRAining) running during the years 1996-1998 was to contribute to the propagation of knowledge how to utilize information technologies in teaching and training in health care. The project associated 20 universities, research institutions and companies. One of the associated partners in the project was also the EuroMISE Centre of Charles University in Prague and the Academy of Sciences CR. To reach determined aims, the project firstly summarized knowledge gained in other European programmes, e.g. AIM, ERASMUS, DELTA or TEMPUS [6]. Consequently, the main directions for designing of teaching materials were proposed. Ten teaching topics were designed on bases of carried analyses of needs in teaching for healthcare. Suitable teaching aids, e.g. pictures, tables and graphs in an electronic form, examples with results of their solution or surveys of a contemporary state of problems in the world were created in the project. Teaching materials were developed firstly in English. Gradually their versions in German, French, Spanish, Czech and in other European languages were created [7]. The Handbook of Medical Informatics [8] and its Internet version opened new possibilities for European education in medical informatics. Different approaches how to teach medical informatics nurses, engineers, or other health professionals were developed, e.g. in [9], [10], [11]. Education provided by the EuroMISE center relied on above mentioned methods and tools but several new approaches were added for the Czech needs.

2.1. Electronic Books

Based on the experience in the European projects the EuroMISE Center has started to develop two editions named "Biomedical Informatics" and "Biomedical Statistics" of books in the Czech language. The books are published by the Carolinum Printing House of Charles University in Prague and their electronic versions are available for registered user on the web pages http://www.euromise.cz/. The books and their electronic versions are used in pre-graduate and doctoral studies at Charles University in Prague. First information on biomedical informatics doctoral studies and on the exploration of the electronic books in these studies was presented in [12].

2.2. System ExaMe

Since 1998 the ExaMe system for evaluation of a targeted knowledge has been developing [13]. The idea of the system is based on multiple-choice questions, but with no prior restrictions on the number of selected answers. The only restriction is that at least one answer is correct and at least one wrong. This new idea has led to new concepts of standardization of test results and also to new research problems in statistics. The ExaMe evaluation system is an important part of education and training in the EuroMISE Center. The ubiquity of the Internet and its World Wide Web applications made it possible to realize the new educational goals in an innovative and creative way. New features of the ExaMe evaluation system and statistical issues of evaluation were described in [14] in more details. The last version of the ExaMe program was issued with the support of the project of the European Structural Funds (ESF) in 2006.

2.3. eHealth Courses

In the years 2005-2007 the project titled "Network for education in health telematics and eHealth" coordinated by the MEDTEL organization and supported by ESF and the Czech Ministry of Social Affairs further contributed to eHealth education in the Czech Republic. The EuroMISE Center via the Department of Medical Informatics of the Institute of Computer Science AS CR, developed and provided five different types of courses in the Czech language covering topics of health telematics and *e*Health, e.g. information systems and electronic health record, telemedicine, bioinformatics and statistics, knowledge discovery and decision support systems, standards, interoperability, safety and security, evidence-based medicine and other. The total number of participants in these courses in the years 2006-2007 was 132, the number of successful graduates was 109. These courses highly used eLearning technologies, e.g. electronic books, ExaME program, multimedia presentations of lectures and different software tools developed in the EuroMISE Center for applications in education and health care. First, more detail presentation on education activities in the frame of the ESF project was given during the Med-e-Tel conference in Luxembourg 2006 [16].

3. Doctoral Degree – Ph.D. in Biomedical Informatics

Education can help with penetration of biomedical informatics methods and tools in biomedical research and health care. The agreement on cooperation of Charles University in Prague and the Academy of Sciences of the Czech Republic in postgraduate doctoral studies in biomedicine was signed on April 23rd, 1997. For this purpose the conceptually unified system for postgraduate doctoral studies has been established. There are now 19 boards of scientific disciplines in postgraduate doctoral studies in biomedicine, one of them is the scientific board of Biomedical Informatics accredited in the year 2002 for teaching in Czech and accredited in the year 2005 for teaching in English as well. Students enter studies in biomedical informatics as the doctoral students of Charles University in Prague, First Faculty of Medicine after they have passed the enter examination successfully (http://pdsb.avcr.cz/). The scientific board of Biomedical Informatics accepts about 10 new students each year and the first student graduated successfully in the Biomedical Informatics doctoral program in the year 2004. During their studies the doctoral students have to choose at least two courses from selected scientific disciplines connected with topics of their thesis. Selected courses prepared and given in the EuroMISE Center are based on the experience from above mentioned European cooperation.

4. Dissemination of Biomedical Informatics Knowledge

4.1. Workshops and Conferences

The EuroMISE Center has participated in dissemination and educational activities in many national and international meetings. Let use mention at least the *Tempus International Conference on Information, Health and Education* organized in 1995 [16] and the *International Joint Meeting EuroMISE 2004* that was composed of several scientific events. The IMIA working group on *Biomedical Statistics and Information Processing* organized the conference *Statistical Methodology in Bioinformatics and Clinical Trials* and focused strongly on new biomedical informatics developments. The working group on *Electronic Health Record* of EFMI organized the symposium *Electronic Health Record, Healthcare Registers and Telemedicine* that brought together researchers and health professionals to discuss different approaches to electronic health record development, to examine possibilities of current technologies for telemedicine and to examine healthcare registers as important sources for evidence-based medicine. The symposium *Biomedical Informatics and Biomedical Statistics Education* was held on the occasion of the 10th anniversary of the EuroMISE Centre foundation. The symposium *European Potential for Building Information Society in Healthcare* covered mainly lectures on this topic from Central and Eastern European countries. Selected papers of these events were published in [17], [18], [19] and [20]. The symposium on *Computerized Guidelines and Protocols* intended to identify use cases for guideline-base applications in healthcare, pressing issues and promising approaches for developing usable and maintainable vehicles for guideline delivery [21]. Finally, the workshop on the HL7 standard was held in the frame of the Prague meeting.

4.2. European Journal for Biomedical Informatics

In the year 2005 the EuroMISE Centre came with a new initiative to publish the European Journal for Biomedical Informatics on Internet (http://www.ejbi.org/). The journal gives the possibility to publish papers in original English versions with translations to other European languages simultaneously. The multilingual versions of papers help to solve problems with terminology and support semantic interoperability.

5. Conclusions

The ability to manage modern communication tools such as Internet services is one of the most important prerequisites for the development and use of e-education (especially in the area of lifelong education) and e-health applications. In medicine and health care the sound education and training plays a very important role to achieve the high quality and economy of healthcare. The research in the field of biomedical informatics can strengthen and accelerate the possibility to reach this goal. Everyone understands that the main source of wealth of any nation is information management and the efficient transformation of information into knowledge. There appear completely new decisive factors for the economics of the near future based on circulation and information exchange. It is clear that modern healthcare cannot be built without information and communication technologies. Telemedicine is largely based on an electronic health record and new methods and tools how to structure information, extract information from free medical texts and sharing knowledge is the main objective of many research projects.

Acknowledgments

The work was supported by the project 1ET200300413 of the grant agency of the Academy of Sciences of the Czech Republic.

References

[1] Haux R et al. Recommendations of the International Medical Informatics Association (IMIA) on Education in Health and Medical Informatics. *Methods Inf Med* 2000; 39: 267-77.

[2] Van Bemmel JH, Zvárová J. (Edrs.). *Knowledge, Information and Medical Education.* Elsevier, Amsterdam, 1991.

[3] Healy JC. The WHO eHealth Resolution, eHealth for All by 2015? *Methods Inf Med* 2007 (in print).

[4] Zvarova J. Education in the Methodology Field of Health Care – EuroMISE. *Methods Inf Med* 3, 33, 1994, 315 – 317.

[5] Zvarova J, Engelbrecht R, van Bemmel JH. Education in Medical Informatics, Statistics and Epidemiology, *Int J Med Inform* 45, 1/2, 1997, 3 – 8.

[6] Hasman A, Albert A, Wainwright P, Klar R and Sosa M (Edrs.) *Education and Training in Health Informatics in Europe.* IOS Press, Amsterdam, 1995.

[7] IT EDUCTRA CD. Commision of the European Communities, 1998.

[8] Van Bemmel JH, Musen MA. *Handbook of Medical Informatics.* Springer Verlag, Heidelberg-New York, 1997.

[9] Haux R, Leven FJ, Moehr JR, Protti DJ (eds). Health and Medical Informatics Education. Meth Inform Med 33, 3,1994, 246-331.

[10] Iakovidis I, Maglaveras N, Trakatellis A (eds). User Acceptance of Health Telematics Applications, Amsterdam, IOS Press 2000.

[11] Hovenga EJS, Mantas J. (eds). Globalization of Health Informatics Education. Studies in Health Technology and Informatics, Vol 109, IOS Press, Amsterdam, 2004.

[12] Zvarova J, Svacina S. New Czech Postgraduate Doctoral Program in Biomedical Informatics In: Surjan G, Engelbrecht R, McNair P (Edrs.) *Health Data in the Information Society.* Proceedings of MIE2002. IOS Press, Amsterdam, 2002, 766-769.

[13] Zvarova J, Zvara K. Evaluation of Knowledge Using ExaMe Program on the Internet. In: Iakovidis I, Maglaveras N, Trakatellis A (Edrs.) *User Acceptance of Health Telematics Applications.* IOS Press, Amsterdam, 2000, 145-151.

[14] Martinkova P, Zvara K jr., Zvarova J, Zvara K. The New Features of the ExaMe Evaluation System and Reliability of its Fixed Tests. *Methods Inf Med* 2006 45 3: 310-315.

[15] Zvarova J, Zvara K, Hanzlicek P. Dissemination and Evaluation Tools for eHealth Products, Services and Distant Education. In: Jordanova M, Lievens F (Edrs.) *E-Health.* Proceedings of Med-e-tel 2006. Luxexpo, Luxembourg, 2006, 106-109.

[16] Zvarova J, Hasman A (Edrs.) Tempus International Conference on Information, Health and Education. *Int J. Med Inform* 45, 1-2, 1997

[17] Zvarova J, Kulikowski P, Mansmann U (Edrs.) Statistical Methodology in Bioinformatics and Clinical Trials. *Methods Inf Med* 2006

[18] Zvarova J, Van Bemmel JH, Mc Cray A (Edrs.) Biomedical Informatics and Biomedical Statistics Education. *Methods Inf Med* 45, 3, 2006

[19] Zvarova J, Blobel B (Edrs.) Electronic Health Record, Healthcare Registers and Telemedicine. *Int J Med Inform* 75, 3, 2006

[20] Zvarova J, Paralic J (Edrs.) European Potential for Building Information Society in Healthcare. *Int J Med Inform* 75, 4, 2006

[21] Kaiser K, Miksch S and Tu SW (eds.): Computer-based Support for Clinical Guidelines and Protocols. Studies in Health Technology and Informatics, Vol 101, IOS Press 2004

eHealth for Personalized Care

eHealth: Combining Health Telematics, Telemedicine, Biomedical Engineering and Bioinformatics to the Edge. Edited by B. Blobel, P. Pharow and M. Nerlich.
IOS Press, 2008

The Personal Health Record: Consumers Banking on their Health

Marion J. BALL [a,1], Melinda Y. COSTIN [b] and Christoph LEHMANN [c]

[a] *IBM Center for Healthcare Management, IBM Research, Baltimore, Maryland, USA*
[b] *Baylor Information Services, Baylor Health Care System, Dallas, Texas, USA*
[c] *Johns Hopkins University School of Medicine, Baltimore, Maryland, USA*

Abstract. With personal health records (PHRs) acting much like ATM cards, increasingly wired consumers can "bank on health", accessing their own personal health information and a wide array of services. Consumer-owned, the PHR is dependent upon the existence of the legal electronic medical record (EMR) and interoperability. Working PHRs are in place in Veterans Health Administration, private health care institutions, and in the commercial sector. By allowing consumers to become involved in their own care, the PHR creates new roles and relationships. New tools change the clinician's workflow and thought flow, and pose new challenges for consumers. Key components of the PHR include the EMR and regional health information organizations (RHIOs); key strategies focus on human factors in successful project management. Online resources provided by the National Library of Medicine and Health On the Net help address consumer needs for information that is reliable and understandable. The growth of self-management tools adds to the challenge and the promise of PHRs for clinicians and consumers alike.[2]

Keywords. Personal Health Record, eHealth, human factors

1. The Personal Health Record: Consumers Banking on their Health

In 2000, Ramsaroop and Ball described the concept of individuals "banking on health", using their personal health records (PHRs) in the same way they use their personal bank or credit cards to withdraw and deposit information at automatic teller machines (ATMs) [1-2]. Under their concept, PHRs would function like ATMs, giving consumers a secure vault for storage, monthly updates of their accounts, worldwide accessibility, and optional personal services.

The single most important strategic innovation in retail banking, the ATM radically changed the way consumers bank and interact with banks. This did not come cheap. According to Retail Banking Research, it cost over US $40 billion just to buy the machines, and many times that amount in running them [3]. To build upon this investment, the banking industry is creating new services that allow consumers to pay

---

[1] Corresponding Author: Marion J. Ball, PhD, IBM Center for Healthcare Management, IBM Research, 5706 Coley Court, Baltimore, MD 21210, U.S.A.; Professor Emerita, Johns Hopkins University School of Nursing, Baltimore, Maryland, USA; Email: marionball@us.ibm.com
[2] This information was first presented at the 2006 Annual HIMSS Conference and Exhibition in San Diego, Calif. Reprinted with permission from the Healthcare Information and Management Systems Society (HIMSS).

traffic tickets or child support via ATM, and employers to issue "plastic paychecks" [4].

In health care, consumers are demanding new services. In 2004, one in three U.S. residents, or eight in ten internet users, went online to find information on a medical problem [5]. In 2005, nine out of ten so-called "cyberchondriacs"—those who search for health information online—reported having successful searches and finding reliable information [6]. These same cyberchondriacs looked online for other health-related information, including answers to their diet and fitness questions (51 percent and 42 percent) [7]. In addition, the California HealthCare Foundation reported growing demand for "patient self-management tools". These tools, "used by consumers to manage their health issues outside formal medical institutions", range from home surveillance systems to decision support aids and more [8]. Revenues for home and portable peripherals are expected to total $2.65 billion 2005, with annual sales growth projected at 8.5 percent [9].

These trends suggest that health care consumers "want their experiences to mirror their expectations as consumers in other areas of their life" and they want "more involvement in deciding what health care they want to receive and how they want it delivered" [10]. They also support the conclusion of U.S. business leaders, including chief executive officers from FedEx, General Motors, Target, and six other major employers: Consumers "are ready for change, as they increasingly seek more health care information and choices….and would be the ultimate beneficiaries of HIT and the resultant transformation of America's health care system, as they have been for previous technological revolutions" [11]. It is within this context that the PHR is emerging as "an Internet-based set of tools that allows people to access and coordinate their lifelong health information and to make appropriate parts of it available to those who need it" [12]. PHRs are becoming the ATMs of health care as consumers become increasingly "wired" and the concept of "banking on health" evolves. Progress to date has been made possible by the adoption of standards and security protections. Though a few health care organizations which are advanced in their healthcare technology do support PHR's, more progress will depend upon interoperability of the scope envisioned as the National Health Information Network (NHIN). Experts estimate that establishing an NHIN will require $156 billion in capital investment over five years and $48 billion in annual operating costs. Although these costs seem (and are) high, $156 billion is equivalent to only 2 percent of annual health care spending for five years [13].

2. Personal Health Records

2.1. Defining the PHR

Efforts in both the public and private sectors have given new life to the concept of using the PHR to "bank on health". Since its publication in 2003, the final report of the Personal Health Working Group has served as a base document for defining and operationalizing PHRs. This report, generated as part of the Markle Foundation's public-private initiative known as Connecting for Health, acknowledged that, although the PHR can take many forms, all forms share six attributes:

1. "Each person controls his or her own PHR.
2. PHRs contain information from one's entire lifetime and all health care providers.
3. PHRs are accessible from any place at any time.
4. PHRs are private and secure.
5. PHRs are transparent. Individuals can see who entered each piece of data, where it transferred from and who has viewed it.
6. PHRs permit easy exchange of information across the health care system" [12].

As described in the report, the PHR "connects each of us to the incredible potential of modern health care" at the same time it "gives us control over our own information". This requires that the PHR give an integrated and comprehensive view of information, "self-generated as well as from doctors, pharmacies and insurance companies". It assigns the PHR the role of a communications hub, for emailing physicians, transferring information to specialists, receiving test results, and accessing educational and decision support tools [12].

In 2005, the American College of Medical Informatics (ACMI) symposium on Personal Health Records made the Connecting for Health report the launching pad for its deliberations. Breakout groups addressed three distinct areas: (1) definition of PHR, policy, and requirements standards; (2) technical architecture supporting interoperable PHRs; and (3) business model and strategies for PHR adoption and use. Although the group on interoperability considered responsibilities and roles in the implementation process, the issues it focused on were predominantly technical.

In contrast, the other two breakout groups listed human factors as topics for consideration. The group on the definition of PHR explored "Who owns the data? What level of control should the patient have over access to their records (and how)? How is information updated (or corrected) by the patient? ….How does patient-entered data get incorporated into the provider's record? What is the legal liability of providers to review patient-entered data?" In examining the "value proposition" for key stakeholders, the business model group emphasized consumers/patients.

A recent HIMSS Analytics white paper distinguishes the patient's electronic health record (EHR) from the electronic medical record (EMR): "The EMR is the legal record created in hospitals and ambulatory environments that is the source of data for the EHR. The EHR represents the ability to easily share medical information among stakeholders and to have a patient's information follow him or her through the various modalities of care engaged by that individual." Authors Garets and Davis state that "EHRs are reliant on EMRs being in place, and EMRs will never reach their full potential without interoperable EHRs in place" [14] The PHR is dependent upon them both - and upon the consumer.

2.2. Public Sector Exemplars

Federal initiatives offer models of working PHRs. One of the earliest was PCASSO (Patient Centered Access to Secure Systems Online). Funded by the National Library of Medicine for a six month evaluation in 1996, PCASSO offered proof of concept, with high patient satisfaction ratings of its safeguards, ease of use, and value [15].

In an ongoing initiative, the Veterans Health Administration has rolled out its PHR on its web portal, My HealtheVet, www.myhealthevet.va.gov. Users are offered an audio introduction to the PHR or closed captioning if they need it. On Veterans Day

2003, the PHR gave veterans access to details on benefits and services, health information, and a health assessment tool. On November 11, 2004, new functionalities were added. Veterans who registered had access to a Personal Health Journal (demographics, contact information, providers, etc.), Health eLogs (blood sugar, blood pressure, pain levels, etc.), and room to enter information such as military history and drug records (prescriptions, over the counter medications, herbal preparations). This new version included improved security and enhanced online help features throughout. Added features allow PHR users to arrange for prescription refills online and print out wallet sized identification cards. On Veterans Day 2005, patients were given access to their electronic medical records over the Internet through My HealtheVet. According to Jonathan Perlin, MD, the then acting undersecretary for health at the VA, "The patient is often the forgotten partner in health care." Sharing those records "recognizes a person has interests in how his care is managed" [16].

2.3. Private Sector Exemplars

2.3.1. In Health Care Institutions

In 2000, CareGroup information systems and Beth Israel Deaconess Medical Center implemented PatientSite to provide patients with services, education, and their own PHR. By February 2003, there were 11,000 patients enrolled and 120 physician users in 40 practices [17]. Available at http://www.patientsite.org, the PHR offers Services (email, prescriptions, appointments, referrals, links, and account statements), About Me (records, personal profile), Support (help features). As a registered user signs on, she sees a list of her appointments, providers, and email. PatientSite is today considered a success; at the same time, it has introduced "controversial and interesting issues". According to Sands and Halamka, these include, "Should patients have full electronic access to their record? Should certain types of data be restricted? Is it necessary for physicians to review results before patients can view them? Should patients be permitted to use PatientSite to view their record if their physician does not use PatientSite? What should happen to patient-entered information in the personal health record? Should physicians be able to view the patient's personal health record? Should they be required to do so?" [17]

Adult patients of primary care physicians at the Cleveland Clinic can register for the eCleveland Clinic MyChart® at https://mychart.clevelandclinic.org and use it to review past appointments, manage prescription renewals, make or cancel appointments, and access reliable health information about the topics of concern to them. Winona Health Online provides the registered "consumer patient" with a personal health profile, health assessment, online prescription refills, drug information, and the ability to receive lab and test results through secure messaging. According to the homepage to be found at www.winonahealth.org, "This free service allows you to actively manage your own health and the health of your loved ones", and it is "a secure site…safer than on-line banking or as safe as using your ATM card".

In September 2005, the University of Texas Southwestern Medical Center healthcare system in Dallas began rolling out a web-based system giving patients access to their medical information and a connection to their doctors. Also named MyChart, the system comes from Epic Systems and is used by over 300,000 people throughout the United States at a number of large healthcare institutions. The first phase of implementation allows patients to go online to review their records, order prescriptions, get messages from their physicians, and check upcoming appointments [18]. Other organizations using this same technology include Sutter Health in California, Geisinger Health System in Pennsylvania, and Fairview Health Services in Minneapolis. Healthcare consumers in Seattle can go to http://www.ghc.org/ the web site for Group Health Cooperative in Washington to receive preventative health reminders, refill prescriptions, understand their Medicare Prescription Drug Benefit, join a Smoking Cessation Plan, access their children's medical records, as well as requesting appointments, reviewing their test results, and e-mailing their physician.

2.3.2. In the Commercial Sector

WebMD is a major force in this sector. Approximately 15 million people have access to WebMD's PHR through their employers' or health plans' websites. More than 20 million unique visitors to webmed.com each month provide an opportunity to offer even greater PHR access [19]. In its present version, WebMD's PHR offers valuable services, including personalized health and benefit information, benefit and treatment decision support, and targeted clinical messages. It integrates self-reported and professional data, including medical and medication claims, to create a complete profile of health history and health status. These capabilities will grow. As of June 2005, six professional data feeds were enabled, and many more planned.

In September 2005, IBM offered its employees their own PHRs, customized for IBM by WebMD and Fidelity. The PHR allows individuals to tailor content to their personal needs and manage all of their health information in one Web-based place.

3. New Roles and Relationships

The PHR allows consumers to become directly involved in their own health care, creating new roles and relationships. According to Goldsmith and Safran, "The actively engaged patient brings high expectations into healthcare relationships. These expectations can improve the way the system interacts with the patient and the way care is delivered." [20]. It is in these interactions that the potential for better quality and improved outcomes lies. As tools enabling these interactions, PHRs must be accepted by patients and clinicians alike. Neither innovation nor consumer autonomy is "more important than a relationship with a trusted physician" or, more accurately and inclusively, with a trusted clinician [21].

This relationship was defined by more than 200 patient and physician participants at a national consensus conference [22] focused on "an increasingly central role for patients" emerging as a result of changes "within and outside the health care sector - such as the growing preponderance of chronic illnesses, new medical technologies, shifting reimbursement practices, the Internet, government regulations, rising costs and changing social norms" The ideal patient-physician relationship they envisioned includes seven principal elements, shown in Table 1.

Table 1. Seven Principal Elements Essential to the Patient-Physician Relationship [3]

<table>
<tr><td>1.</td><td>"**COMMUNICATION:** including means of communicating; information gathering; the role of patient self-assessments and feedback; delivery of information; and adequacy of information.</td></tr>
<tr><td>2.</td><td>**OFFICE EXPERIENCE:** including access to care; office-patient communication; processes for obtaining prescriptions and refills; information forms; and the care environment.</td></tr>
<tr><td>3.</td><td>**HOSPITAL EXPERIENCE:** including expectations for personalizing care; the physician in charge; communication among members of the health care team, patients, family and patient advocates; discharge planning and the emergency room experience.</td></tr>
<tr><td>4.</td><td>**EDUCATION:** including information provided by physicians to patients; addressing patients' individual situations; non-physician sources of information; and the role of self-care.</td></tr>
<tr><td>5.</td><td>**INTEGRATION:** including the sharing of information among all members of the health care team; navigation of the health care system; medical records; and health plan information.</td></tr>
<tr><td>6.</td><td>**DECISION-MAKING:** including the patient's role; the patient advocate's role; the right of patients to know all evidence-based options; and non-clinical factors that impact medical decisions.</td></tr>
<tr><td>7.</td><td>**OUTCOMES:** including clinical outcomes; patient-centered outcomes; and physician-centered outcomes" [22].</td></tr>
</table>

Significantly, each of these elements maps all or in part to capabilities, services, and outcomes targeted by health information technology (HIT), including the PHR. Equally significantly, none of these elements functions without human interaction. What Levinson noted in 1987 still holds true: "No computer will ever detect the subtleties of interaction between clinician and patient that occur in the examining room or at the bedside. The computer can liberate the patient to exercise these uniquely human skills while, at the same time, placing complex diagnostic and therapeutic decisions on a far more accurate, dependable, and scientific basis than is now the case." [23].

4. Human Factors

Optimal health care and the optimal value of the consumer's PHR can be realized only within the patient-physician relationship, within the human context. The importance of human factors here is intensified by the fact that PHRs are predicated upon the existence of the EHR environment and of the national health information network (NHIN) advocated by President Bush and originally coordinated by David Brailer, the first National Health IT Coordinator, and now coordinated by Dr. Robert Kolodner, Director of the Office of the National Coordinator (ONC). As a standalone accounting of personal health information, the PHR has little value; as an interactive account with

---

[3] Source: Defining the Patient-Physician Relationship for the 21st Century, pp. v-vi, ©2004 American Healthways

the health care system as a whole, it offers a wide array of benefits. Ultimately, it promises to complete the transformation to the patient-centered model of care envisioned by the Institute of Medicine.

Over a decade ago, Postman made a series of three observations:

- "First, technology is not a neutral element in the practice of medicine: doctors do not merely use technologies but are used by them.
- Second, technology creates its own imperatives and, at the same time, creates a wide-ranging social system to reinforce its imperatives.
- And third, technology changes the practice of medicine by redefining what doctors are, redirecting where they focus their attention, and reconceptualizing how they view their patients and illness" [24].

This concept has been expanded upon by Ball and Bierstock in their paper, "Clinician Use of Enabling Technology: The Missing Link", where the concept of "thought flow" is introduced. Postman's first two points are why, as Stead and Lorenzi conclude, "It is natural to resist information technology, because it changes roles and the social order" [25]. They are also the reasons why attention to human factors is so important. His third point underscores the role of information technology as enabler in creating a new health system for the 21st century and of the PHR in making it patient-centered.

The bottom line for banking on health is clear: For PHRs to become the ATMs of health care, they must become part of the routine practice and conduct of health care, for clinicians and consumers alike.

4.1. For Clinicians

Even a "simple" tool like electronic prescribing fundamentally changes "what docs do" [26]. It involves more than a digitized prescription pad; it requires the physician to enter the patient's recent history, note recalls, complete interactions and allergy checks, and specify other indications such as patient weight and co-morbid conditions [27]. Not surprisingly, physician resistance to change is a primary challenge.

Bierstock's model illuminates why a tool like electronic prescribing has the impact it does and why physicians resist technology adoption [27]. In a mature electronic environment, data arrive as quickly as they are generated, for the clinician to process, prioritize, and act upon. However, the immature environments in which most clinicians now practice often disrupt thought flow and force workflow. New tools require relearning, which can be both time-consuming and frustrating. However, while there is initially an additional time commitment required, as physicians gain experience with the PHR, they have found that it is a time-saver.

4.2. For Consumers

The counterpart to clinician resistance is consumer demand. They are seeking this technology and organizations that provide it will build loyalty to their delivery system. PHRs and internet-enabled self management tools allow consumers to do what they have not been able to do before. Unlike most health care professionals, they do not have to unlearn old skills and old tools. That said, however, consumers must learn much more that is new.

As a recent California HealthCare Foundation issue brief acknowledges, "Consumers who go online to choose or manage their own care often encounter clinical information and technical jargon that they are unable to decipher because it is presented in a format that reflects the provider's point of view (diagnosis, treatment, option)" [28]. The average consumer needs content that is qualitative and descriptive, not raw lab data or diagnostic codes. When consumers access information online, they need assurances that it is trustworthy and that they can use it to help in making decisions about their own health care.

Increasingly, consumers can find this type of assurance on the web. Recognizing the need for information that is comprehensible to persons who are not healthcare professionals, the National Library of Medicine went beyond Medline, its database for medical professionals, to develop PubMed and MedlinePlus. PubMed includes citations to more journals, links to other sites and to citations for related articles, and a clinical queries search filter. MedlinePlus offers information on more than 700 topics, about prescriptions and over-the-counter drugs, and local resources, even locations for flu shots. The Library (NLM) collaborated with the National Institute on Aging to develop NIH SeniorHealth, including options to enlarge text size or have it read aloud, or view videoclips. Topics range from Alzheimer's and other common diagnoses to issues of daily living, including Dry Mouth, Exercise, and Problems with Smell and Taste.

5. Key Components and Strategies

5.1. Components

As already mentioned in Section 2.1., the white paper for HIMSS Analytics differentiates clearly between electronic medical records (EMRs) and electronic health records (EHRs) [14]. As a subset of information from various care delivery organizations (CDOs), the EHR relies upon two key components: electronic medical records at those CDOs and connections via regional health information organizations (RHIOs), which form the base for what will eventually be the National Health Information Network (NHIN).

5.1.1. Electronic Medical Records

Bierstock observes that health record technologies require "full integration of physician workflows with…the workflows of every other discipline in a healthcare enterprise" [27]. This level of integration is critical. Yet, according to HIMSS Analytics 2005 data, most US hospitals (68 percent) are still in the early stages of clinical transformation, and almost a third (29 percent) do not have all three ancillary systems (laboratory, radiology, and pharmacy) installed, much less components of EMRs. This renders them incapable of participating in EHR initiatives, because "The EHR environment relies on functional EMRs that allow care delivery organizations to exchange data/information with other CDOs or stakeholders within the community, regionally, or nationally." The CDO, not the patient, owns the EMR [14].

5.1.2. Regional Health Information Organizations

Currently 20 plus RHIOs were swapping data, more than 100 have been created, and the Department of Health and Human Services had pledged $139 million over five years "to provide direct assistance to several pilot RHIOs and support other RHIO activities" [29]. The Robert Wood Johnson Foundation has awarded 20 information-exchange grants between $75,000 and $100,000 each [30]. The state of Arizona announced it would build a statewide health information network [31] and Blue Shield of California Foundation announced it would donate $1 million to the California RHIO launched in April 2005, rising its funding to a total of $4.82 million [32]. For physicians in practice, however, the concept may still be "in relative obscurity" [33]. This grassroots movement is moving rapidly and in places faster than the federal government could move. For success, we believe federal leadership is crucial [34].

5.2. Strategies

Reed Gardner's 80/20 rule states that success in IT implementations is only 20 percent dependent on technology and 80 percent dependent on social and political interaction skills. Implicit in this rule is the recognition of the importance of human factors - a basic tenet for healthcare informatics for over two decades that finally began to gain widespread acceptance in the 1990s.

In implementing EHRs, the primary focus has been on human factors involving physicians. Costin described one approach to achieving physician involvement in successful EHR adoption in a presentation at HIMSS 2005 [35]. Used at multiple sites and refined based on lessons learned, the approach begins by developing a strategy and road map based on the right people making the right decisions at the right time and by establishing a physician-focused body for governance and decision-making during and after implementation. It recognizes the complexity of the physician culture, including the differences between, for example, hospitalists and community physicians as well as hierarchy and decision-making dynamics. The methodology and processes throughout are designed to foster physician involvement and address the challenges physicians and other leaders, including nursing, face in planning for and adopting the new technology. The approach acknowledges that clinical systems affect workflow and require involvement of the total organization. Hence, the approach makes use of intensive and highly visible programs for communication, and for training and support. Project champions are a must, as are highly engaged end users.

As PHR technology is included in the implementation of EHR's, the patients themselves should be involved in the implementation approach. A community communication plan is recommended as well as establishing patient advocates. As processes are designed, patients should be included in the decision-making. Successful organizations have focused on a pilot implementation and obtained patient and physician testimonials before moving forward.

As was the case in the well-known failure of computerized physician order entry at Cedars-Sinai Medical Center in Los Angeles, physician resistance can bring down an IT implementation [36]. Despite the fact that the PHR is owned by the consumer, physician resistance can severely limit its effectiveness and curtail its usefulness within the patient-physician relationship.

6. Consumer Needs and Resources

The report *Lost in Translation* [28] acknowledges the many challenges posed by a consumer-oriented approach to health information sharing: "Patients who undergo medical tests, for example, need information organized around three moments in care", namely, decision support, test preparation, and the presentation of test results. "To be relevant and useful, the information patients retrieve must take into account their demographics (such as age and gender), health risks, and other medical conditions. Consumers also need to know how a decision at any one moment of care, such as choosing a treatment, might affect other aspects of care, such as paying for it."

According to *Lost in Translation*, a chief advantage of consumer-owned PHRs is that they allow consumers who have switched providers or insurers to access their full history and compare old test results with new results. But the report concludes that consumers do not yet have the electronic tools and information they need to manage their own care: "Much of the information is arcane, scattered, inaccessible, or unusable, partly because it doesn't address the unique circumstance of each patient at any moment of care. Tools to retrieve and manage the information -if they even exist- often are designed for medical and technical professionals rather than lay people. Nor do the tools provide a consistent way for consumers to link to information across the continuum of care from any delivery point." The report concludes with a call to integrate consumer health information standards into the NHIN framework.

If consumers are to be responsible for managing their own care, they too must be able to interpret health information and even raw data in some instances, as *Lost in Translation* makes clear. Accessing information is preliminary to the critical task of assessing it. With the growth of online information, consumers need to be able to determine what is valid and what is relevant to them. The National Library of Medicine provides such help at its site, www.healthfinder.gov, with its health library, online checks ups, provider information, and selected topics organized by gender, age, race, and ethnicity. Other valuable resources are provided by Health On the Net (HON). Based in Geneva, HON provides access to trustworthy health information through its HONcode toolbar at www.hon.ch/HONcode/Plugin/Plugins.html and through WRAPIN (Worldwide online Reliable Advice to Patients and Individuals) at www.wrapin.org, a new facility that allows consumers to compare health information in any format or length with established benchmarks and what is available in the published literature.

The discussion of consumer needs in *Lost in Translation* does not take note of the trend indicated in *Patient Self-Management Tools: An Overview* [8] or the impact these tools have on patient-physician relationships. These tools "straddle the health care and consumer sectors" and are clearly designed to be used and owned by the consumer in their roles as patients. With revenues of $2.65 billion for home and portable peripherals (e.g., blood pressure/pulse cuffs, blood glucose monitors, coagulation meters, pulse oximeters, fetal/pediatric monitors, etc.) in 2005 and annual sales growth predicted at 8.5 percent, these tools are a force to be reckoned with. Interfacing them to the PHR is only a first step. Unless information entered by the patient using a given tool (e.g., a glucometer or pressure cuff), is interpreted and acted upon, it adds no value. The physician must be ready to accommodate and to use data entered by the patient, and to do so outside the traditional face-to-face encounter. In Goethe's words, quoted by the Institute of Medicine in *Crossing the Quality Chasm*, "Knowing is not enough; we must apply."

References

[1]   Ramsaroop P, Ball MJ. A model for more useful patient health records. MD Computing, July/August 17(4) (2000) 45-48.

[2]   Ramsaroop P, Ball MJ. Banking on good healthcare. *Healthcare Informatics* July 2000, 143-148.

[3]   Retail Banking Research. www.rblondon.com/report/atmstrategy. Accessed 8/20/05.

[4]   www.atmmarketplace. Accessed 07/13/05

[5]   Pew Internet and American Life Project. Health Information Online. 2005. www.pewinternet.org

[6]   Harris Interactive. Number of cyberchondriacs—US adults who go online for health information— increases to estimated 117 million. www.harrisinteractive.com, July 15, 2005.

[7]   Harris Interactive. July 15, 2005.

[8]   Barrett MJ. Patient Self Management Tools: An Overview. Report prepared by Critical Mass Consulting for the California HealthCare Foundation, June 2005.

[9]   Patient Monitoring Devices: U.S. Forecasts to 2008 and 2013. www.freedoniagroup.com.

[10] Darkins AW, Cary MA. *Telemedicine and Telehealth: Principles, Policies, Performance, and Pitfalls.* Springer Publishing Company, 2000.

[11] Health Information Technology Leadership Panel. Final Report. Prepared by the Lewin Group, Inc., for the Department of Health and Human Services, March 2005.

[12] Connecting for Health. The Personal Health Working Group: Final Report. Markle Foundation, July 1, 2003.

[13] Kaushal R, Blumenthal D, Poon EG, Jha AK, Franz C, et al. The costs of a National Health Information Network. *Annals of Internal Medicine* 143(3) 2005 (August 2) 165-173.

[14] Garets D, Davis M. Electronic Medical Records vs. Electronic Health Records: Yes, There is a Difference. A HIMSS Analytics White Paper. Chicago: HIMSS Analytics, August 26, 2005.

[15] Baker DB, Masys D. PCASSO: Vanguard in Patient Empowerment. In: Nelson R, Ball MJ (Edrs.) *Consumer Informatics: Applications and Strategies in Cyber Health Care.* New York: Springer, 2004, 63-74.

[16] Gaul GM. Revamped Veterans' Health Care Now a Model. Washington Post, A1, A7, August 22, 2005.

[17] Sands DZ, Halamka JD. PatientSite: Patient-Centered Communication, Services, and Access to Information. In Nelson R, Ball MJ (Edrs.) *Consumer Informatics.* New York: Springer, 2005, 20-32.

[18] Precker M. Your checkup account. DallasNews.com, September 20, 2002.

[19] Marshall P. Personal Health Records. An Overview. Presented to the NCVHS Hearings, June 6, 2005.

[20] Goldsmith D, Safran C. Collaborative Healthware. In: Nelson R, Ball MJ (Edrs.) *Consumer Informatics.* New York: Springer, 2004, 9-19.

[21] Abramson J. *Overdosed America: The Broken Promise of American Medicine.* HarperCollins Publisher: New York, 2004, p. 10.

[22] Defining the Patient-Physician Relationship for the 21st Century. 2004. 3rd Annual Disease Management Outcomes Summit, October 30-November 2, 2003, Phoenix, Arizona, v.1. ©2004 American Healthways, Inc.

[23] Levinson D. *A Guide to the Clinical Interview.* W.B. Saunders Company, Philadelphia 1987, 279.

[24] Postman N. Technopoly: the surrender of culture to technology. New York: Alfred A. Knopf, 1992.

[25] Stead WW, Lorenzi NM. Health informatics: linking investment to value. *J Am Med Inform Assoc* 6(5) 1999, 341-348.

[26] Hagland M, quoting Peter Basch. Reduced errors ahead. Healthcare Informatics. 2003. www.healthcare-informatics.com.

[27] Bierstock S. Physician Adoption and Acceptance of Tools of Technology: Key Factors for Successful Electronic Health Record Implementation. Presentation at MIE 2005, The XIX International Congress of the European Federation for Medical Informatics, Geneva, Switzerland, August 30, 2005.

[28] J Seidman. 2005 (September). Lost in Translation: Consumer Health Information in an "Interoperable" World. California HealthCare Foundation. www.chcf.org

[29] iHealthBeat. Health officials seek to expand RHIOs. www.ihealthbeat.org, June 10, 2005.

[30] Weier S. Interviews: Robert Wood John foundation announced information exchange grants, iHealth Beat. www.ihealthbeat.org, June 29, 2005.

[31] Arizona embarks on IT Network effort. HealthData Management. 9/6/05, (September 02, 2005). www.healthdatamanagement.com

[32] iHealthBeat. Blue Shield of California Foundation gives $1M grant to help fund RHIO. www.ihealthbeat.org, September 8, 2005.

[33] T Lee. Commentary: The evolution of RHIO economics. iHealth Beat. 08/23/2005.
      www.ihealthbeat.org
[34] Health officials seek to expand RHIOs, op cit.
[35] Costin M. Physicians and the EHR: Achieving successful adoption. Presentation at HIMSS 2005,
      Dallas, TX.
[36] Connolly C. Cedars-Sinai doctors cling to pen and paper. Washington Post, A01, March 21, 2005.

eHealth: Combining Health Telematics, Telemedicine, Biomedical Engineering and Bioinformatics to the Edge. Edited by B. Blobel, P. Pharow and M. Nerlich.
IOS Press, 2008

Bioinformatics and Genomics for Opening New Perspective for Personalized Care

Hiroshi TANAKA [1]
School of Biomedical Sciences, Tokyo Medical and Dental University, Tokyo, Japan

Abstract. A new perspective for personalized care which genomics and bioinformatics cooperatively open was described, with emphasis on promising possibilities which "genome/omics-based personalized care" is thought to bring about. In doing so, we took it into consideration that, along the rapid progress of the genome/omics and bioinformatics, the contents of "genome/omics-based personalized care" have evolved, mainly through three generations. The first generation is personalized care based on (1) the polymorphism of the "germline" genome sequences, such as personalized medication depending on the individual genetic differences concerning the pharmacodynamics/phamarcokinetics or estimation of genotype relative risk for individual's disease occurrence, the second generation is that based on (2) the information pattern of vast amount of omics data of diseased "somatic" cell, which brings about detailed classification, early diagnosis and prognosis of the disease, and the third generation is that based on (3) the system level understanding of complex diseases which enables wholistic comprehension of the mechanism of diseases, with special reference to disease pathway.

Keywords. eHealth, bioinformatics, genomics, personal health

Introduction

Recent advances in genomics and the subsequent comprehensive molecular information collectively called "omics" [1], such as transcriptomics, proteomics, metabolomics and so forth, are giving rise to a new possibility of medicine, especially in cooperation with rapidly progressing bioinformatics, which processes these omics data to produce the medically meaningful information. This new medicine is now called various names, for example, genomic medicine, genome-based medicine or omics-based medicine. We consider the cooperation between genome/omics and bioinformatics would open a new perspective for personalized care, which we would properly call "genetically-based" or "genome/omics-based personalized care". But what is the content of genome/omics-based medicine in concrete, and what kind of possibilities does genome/omics-based personalized care bring about to the present medical and health care?

In this article, we will describe a new perspective for personalized care; especially focusing on the various promising possibilities which genome/omics-based

---

[1] Corresponding Author: Hiroshi Tanaka, MD, PhD, Director General and Professor, University Center for Information Medicine, Tokyo Medical and Dental University, Koyasu Building, 1-5-45 Yushima Bunkyo-ku, Tokyo 113-8510, Japan; Email: tanaka@cim.tmd.ac.jp

personalized care is thought to bring about. In doing so, we took into consideration that the genome/omics study and their computational counterpart, bioinformatics, have progressed rapidly and, along this progress, the contents of "genome/omics-based personalized care" have evolved through the various generations and now a plenty of new possibilities is expected for medical and health care.

Thus, in the following, we will first describe the progression of generations in genomics and bioinformatics, by investigating the leading concepts viewing life with respect to its biological information. Second, we will describe the contents of genome/omics-based medicine corresponding to each generation along their progress.

1. Generations in Viewing the Biological Information

In regard to the general concept viewing the life with respect to biological information, it is considered that there have been three generations. The first is the generation of biological sequence information, the second is that of the whole information pattern of omics, and the last is the systems biology or system level understanding of biological pathway/network. We will describe the features of each generation (Figure 1).

The first generation is the dawn of the genetics and bioinformatics. In the beginning of molecular genetics, we consider genetic information exists in the biological sequences such as those of amino acids and nucleotides. The homology, mutational differences and polymorphism of these biological sequences, genes or proteins, with respect to their differences of biological functions have been mostly concerned and bioinformatics studies were directed to provide the means to realize these kinds of sequence analyses. This leading concept was continued to be central until the end of the human genome project. Hence we call this generation that of bio-sequential information.

In the second generation, many kinds of "post-genomic" comprehensive molecular information, "omics", become available such as transcriptomics, proteomics, metabolomics and so forth. These kinds of post-genomic information are not usually presented by sequential data, but they are given rather by whole information patterns, such as "heat map" of genetic expression, or "spectrogram" of mass spectrometry and so on. The interests were directed to the difference of whole information pattern of the omics causing the difference of biological meanings. Hence we call this generation that of whole bio-information pattern.

Now that we have entered upon the omics era where a plenty of comprehensive molecular information have been available, the challenge in the third (present) generation is how this plenty of omics information should be utilized to understand the whole spectrum of the life. It becomes widely recognized that a framework to

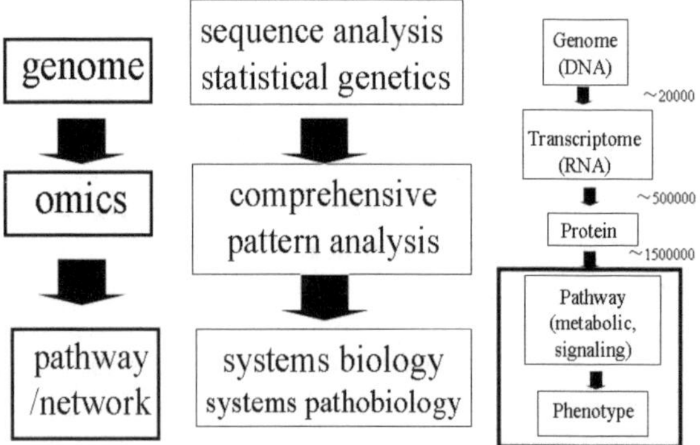

Figure 1. Three generations in genomics and bioinformatics

understand such a vast amount of omics data is critically needed. The systems biology which understands life as a unified system is the key concept in the third generation. Systems biology aims to grasp the structure which explains the underlying mechanism behind the various pattern of omics information and tried to obtain the system level understanding of biological function. Hence we call third (present) generation that of systems-level understanding of bio-function.

2. Personalized Care Based on Genetic Polymorphism – Genome/Omics-Based Medicine of the First Generation

2.1. Genetic Polymorphisms

Along the advances of the concept viewing biological information, the content of genome/omics-based medicine has rapidly expanded. Genetically-based personalized care starts based on the polymorphism of the genomic sequences. We call the difference of the nucleotide "polymorphism" if it occurs more than 1% of the population and if it is less than 1% we call it "mutation".

Accompanied with human genome project, it became widely known that human genome has individual congenital (germ-line) difference. Other than mutation, there are various kinds of polymorphism in human genome. The first polymorphism of genome noted was the difference of the length of fragmented genome sequences after the restriction enzyme is applied. This fragmentation polymorphism is called RFLP (Restriction Fragment Length Polymorphism), and occurs due to the single genomic nucleotide difference which we will explain later.

The next polymorphism is the variable number of tandem repeat of several nucleotides (VNTR). VNTR is the number of tandem repeated nucleotides which is more than 10 bp but, ordinarily, several tens bp. A well-known example is type I diabetes where VNTR of 14 bp in 600 bp upstream of insulin gene affects the efficiency of its transcription, thus increasing the susceptibility. The third polymorphism is the micro-satellite, which is also the repeat of short nucleotide sequences but shorter than VNTR (less than 7 bp). Famous example is CA repeats which are used as marker to detect the disease causative gene.

The fourth polymorphism is single nucleotide polymorphism (SNP), as in Figure 2. In human genome, on average, one nucleotide for about 1000 nucleotides is different from the major type of the genome (3B bp). The relative frequency is 0.1% of genome and totally 3M~10M SNPs exist for an individual. There is many database of SNP in the world. The most widely-known database is dbSNP at NCBI (National Center for Biotechnology Information) which contains the 6M data of SNPs [2]. We tabularized the advantage and disadvantage of these

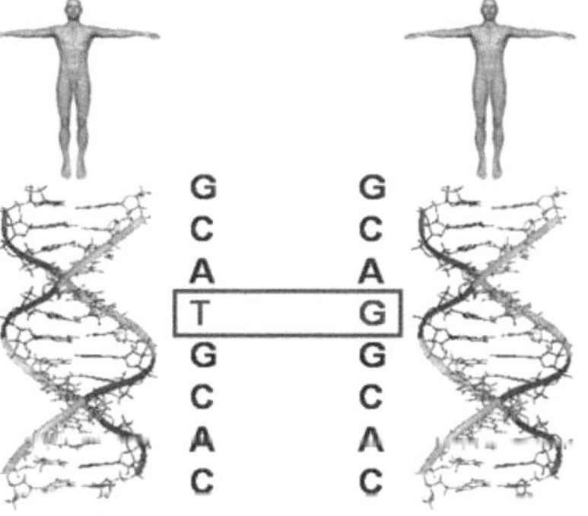

Figure 2. Concept of SNP

polymorphisms (Table 1). It is now widely recognized that most important and well-used polymorphic information is SNPs. We hereafter focus mainly on the genetic polymorphism known by SNPs.

The SNP polymorphism could be used for genetic typing to predict the following individual differences;

    1.   Drug responsiveness
    2.   Disease susceptibility

The former drug responsiveness shows the personalized difference in response to drugs. The certain SNPs might have effects on functions of genes related to the drug effects, which make the individual differences in

Table 1. Various genetic polymorphism

	RFLP	VNTR	MS	SNP
Number	~10000	~1000	~10000	3M~10M
Diversity	△	◎	◎	△
Linkage Analysis	△	△	◎	○
Disease Susceptibilty	△	○	△	◎

the drug response, ranging between responder and non-responder. The branch of pharmacology studying such influence of genetic or genomic variation on drug response in patients by correlating gene expression or SNPs with a drug efficacy or toxicity is now called pharmacogenomics or pharmacogenetics (PGx, abbreviation for both).

The latter, disease susceptibility shows the personalized difference in risk of disease occurrence. The certain SNPs might be linked to the disease related genes, or in some cases, more directly to the disease-causative genes, through the mechanism of linkage disequilibrium, which increases genotype relative risk (GRR) of that disease.

In both cases single SNP might be sometime sufficient for genetic typing of drug responsiveness and disease susceptibility, but, for multifactorial diseases, especially for disease susceptibility, single SNP is not sufficient to obtain the efficient estimation of disease risk. Hence, in order to strengthen genomic polymorphic information, the combination of multiple SNPs is observed to estimate the haplotype of patients.

2.2. Personalized Medication Based on the Genetic Polymorphism

As mentioned previously, pharmacogenomics or pharmacogenetics (PGx) are now revealing the personalized difference in drug responsiveness due to the genomic polymorphism or variation. JAMA (The Journal of the American Medical Association) described in 1998 that 2 million patients per year suffered from drug side-effect and among them about 100 thousand patients died, which amount to the 4th or 5th major cause of death in the United States [3]. Prediagonistic DNA test to examine the drug responsiveness has started to be imposed by FDA (Food and Drug Administration, US) to avoid useless side-effect.

Individual differences of drug response might be ascribed to two categories of gene polymorphisms. One is linked to genes coding the proteins at the site of drug action such as drug receptor and is called pharmacodynamics (PD) polymorphism. The other is linked to genes coding the proteins responsible to absorption, distribution, metabolism and excretion (ADME) of the drug, such as drug metabolizing enzymes or transporters and is called pharmacokinetics (PK) polymorphism. We will describe each type of the personalized medication in the followings.

2.2.1. PD (Pharmacodynamics) Pharmacogenomics: PD-PGx

The PD polymorphism is mainly related to molecular target chemotherapy of cancer. PD-PGx shows individualized difference of drug response due to polymorphism or variation of receptor gene or drug-targeted molecules. The well known example is Gefitinib (Irressa), which is the anticancer agent to lung cancer, especially for advanced non-small cell carcinoma. This drug has very remarkable effect for " super responder" who would recover even if he has cancer of, for example, 5cm diameter. The rate of effect is 25 to 30% for Japanese, and especially effective for Asian female, but about 3%for US people but for US female 17%. But it might cause "serious side effect" of affecting interstitial lung disorder for 2% of Japanese, and one among three dies from chronic interstitial lung disorder. Hence, to avert risk for medication to non-responder, genetic screening is absolutely necessary. Now the polymorphism in responsiveness of this drug is ascribed to the specific mutation of EGF (Epidermal Growth Factor) receptor and it is reported that drug effect becomes 10 times bigger for the patient who has this mutation.

Other well-known example is Herceptin (Trastuzumab) which is anticancer drug of breast cancer using a monoclonal antibody. This drug is effective for the patients who suffer from breast cancer and express HER2 (human epidermal growth factor type 2) receptor [4]. FDA determined that prediagnostic DNA test using immunohistochemistry (IHC) and fluorescence in situ hybridization (FISH) test is compulsory for administration of this drug.

2.2.2. PK (Pharmacokinetics) Pharmacogenomics: PK-PGx

This kind of personalized medication is, as described previously, based on the patient genetic polymorphism or variation in drug metabolizing enzyme and transporter gene during ADME process of the drug. Individualized drug response among the patients range from "extensive metabolizer" who has highly efficient metabolizing enzyme so that the drug is less effective, to "poor metabolizer" who metabolize the drug poorly so that the drug remains longer within the patient body and becomes too effective. The most well-known polymorphism of drug metabolizing enzyme is the family of cytochrome P450 (CYP). This enzyme has more than 80 isoenzymes known up to now. The classification of this enzyme is based on the homology of the genetic sequences; drug is classified by numeral figure of 1 to 4 into groups within 40% homology, and by alphabetical character of A,B,C,D…. into more detailed subtype within 55% homology. It is already known that many types of CYP are very important because their polymorphism is remarkably related to the drug effects. Especially the effect of anticancer drug frequently depends on the polymorphism of CYP. Some of the well-known isoenzymes are tabulated in table 2.

Personalized medication is now partially realizing. As the example of g-POC (genetically-based Point of Care), FDA guidance recommended pre-diagnostic DNA test to examine the drug responsiveness, which is ranged between compulsory, recommended, and arbitrary. We might predict that 30% of drug will be g-POC in about less than 10 years. It is anticipated that drug market and pharmaceutical industry will drastically change by the spread of personalized medication; market will shrink but some drug comes back because, in the conventional random clinical trial without taking the genetic type related to drug effect, drug effect might be reduced on average by including the non-responders as the test population. If we eliminate them, the response rate (RR) might increase to exceed the criterion.

Table 2. Various types of cytochrome P450 (CYP)

Types of CYP	Description
CYP2D6	First identified polymorphic drug metabolizing enzyme, many variants; metabolizing many clinically important drugs, completely deficit type, 5-6% Caucasian, for homozygote of half-deficit type, drug effect is 6 times effective
CYP2A6	Metabolizing well-known anticancer drug 5-FU, completely-deficit type, 4-5%, for Japanese, variable effect (breast anticancer drug retrosol) , completely deficit type, low risk of lung, colon cancer occurrence
CYP2C19	2C19*2 type slow but effective (Helocobacter pylori eradication)
CYP3A4	Related to the drug effect of many anticancer agents (irinotecan, paclitaxel, docetaxel, gefitinib)
CYP3A5	Similar to CYP3A4 but sometime different drug effects, increase the dose for CYP3A5 patient
NAT2(N-acetyl-transferase 2) slow type	10% for Japanese, 60~70% for Caucasian (isoniazid; antituberculous)
TPMT	Thiopurine S-methyltransferase, metabolizing leukemia drug

2.3. Estimation of Disease Susceptibility

Another important utilization of genetic polymorphism for the personalized care other than genetically-based medication is to relate SNPs with the occurrence of disease. Since SNPs are genome-widely distributed, they have been used as a linkage disequilibrium maker of disease related genes or, in some cases, disease-causative genes. A lot of methods in statistical genetics such as Mendelian linkage analysis and association analysis has been invented to identify the loci of the disease related genes. But for the personalized care, these SNPs information can be utilized as estimation of relative risk of occurrence of disease, that is, index for disease susceptibility. For the monofactorial disease, the observation of certain mutation of specific gene means occurrence of future disease. But, almost 95% multi-factorial diseases is mutifactorial and is "common disease" like hypertension, cancer, diabetes. So we only know relative increase of the risk of disease occurrence (GRR; genotype relative risk) by the observation of SNPs. For example, the mutation of Met235Thr of angiotensionogen, and linked mutation of A6G in its promotor increase the susceptibility of hypertention.

Other than genotype relative risk, clinical and environmental, and life-style factors affect the risk of disease occurrence. Their composite effects are not straightforward. For example, in the relative risk estimation of colon cancer of Japanese Hawaiians who have American lifestyle but Japanese genetic background but the lifestyle risk factors such as "smoking" and "likes well-done meat" together with genetic factors of NAT2(slow and rapid type) and CYP1A2 (slow and rapid type) cooperate to make the composite disease occurrence risk. The relative risk of disease occurrence are ranged from 0.6 to 1.5, but when they are mixed, nonlinear effects is active among these risk factors and, for specific combination of risk factors, composite risk becomes 8.6 by far more than just multiplication of each factors risk.

3. Personalized Care Based on the Disease Omics – Genomics/Omics-Based Medicine of the Second Generation

3.1. Omics for Personalized Care

Various high-throughput equipments have been developed in the post-genomic era such as DNA microarray or TOF-MS, etc to provide a vast amount of omics data. These rapid advances in omics such as transcriptomics, proteomics, metabolomics and so forth in the post-genomic era have revolutionized genomic medicine to open a new stage of personalized care, which we call "genomics/omics-based medicine of the second generation" or more simply "omics-based medicine". The concept of omics collectively call the various kinds of comprehensive molecular information, which are originally derived from the common genomic information, though, by the modification of post-genomic mechanism, each omics also has its own original information to contribute to the personalized care.

But, then, what kind of new possibility does this omics information bring about to personalized care in addition to the first generation of genome-based medicine?

Omics information is genome-wide comprehensive molecular information. Unlike the first generation of genome-based medicine which utilizes congenital polymorphism of the "germline" genome sequences, most of the omics data is related to comprehensive molecular information of "somatic cell", that is, "diseased cell". Hence, unlike the first generation which suggest, for example, "only" the possibility of future occurrence of the disease, the second generation genome/omics-based medicine utilizes more direct disease-related molecular information so that it could predict "when disease will occur "and "how disease will develop" more directly.

The main reason that disease omics could be used to predict the disease is that the omics information has sufficiently direct and comprehensive information about the distortion of molecular activity of the diseased cell. Omics information provides detailed and comprehensive molecular information about current disease state. That is, omics provides the following information to medicine:

1. Detailed information to identify the subtype or fine structure of disease type,
2. Comprehensive information to enable wholistic understanding of disease.

In the following sections we will describe contribution of these advantages to personalized care. Of course, by omics we also include genomic information so that the second generation genome/omics-based medicine includes the advantages of the first generation. It might be better to say that the second generation has been expanded from the first generation.

3.2. Omics Provides Detailed Information for Subtyping of Disease

Omics provides detailed information to reveal the fine structure of molecular activity of the cell. For example, omics data provides clinically and pathologically unobservable information which could be used to distinguish the difference of prognosis or disease course. We would take transcriptomics, the genome-wide gene expression pattern observed by microarray. There are many studies about the predictability of the disease transcriptome. The gene expression pattern does not just give the molecular activities of diseased cell, but microscopic information in the most bottom molecular layer contains most macroscpic information about the prognosis of disease, rather intermediate level information such as clinical and pathological layer the information can not be observed [5]. The conventional routine pathological test of diseased tissue and clinical observation can not give the exact prediction of the prognosis.

We show the example of the gene expression pattern called heatmap where gene expression activities of thousands of genes are depicted for each of the patients observed (Figure 3) [6]. The example is the DNA microarray (Affinmetrix, GeneChip HU) of the hepatocellular carcinoma where gene expression pattern (totally 33 patients) of the recurrent (20 patients) or non-recurrent patients (18 patients) is illustrated.

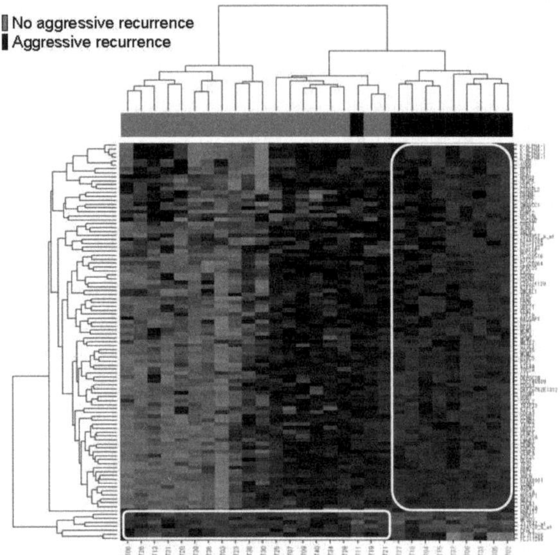

Figure 3. Gene expression pattern of hepatocellular carcinoma

3.3. Diagnostic Ability of Proteome and Conventional Tumor Marker

As we described earlier, the omics data contains the comprehensive and molecular information of the diseased cell more directly, so that it can predict not only the prognosis after the disease has definitely appeared, but also can detect the onset of disease in very early period when conventional clinical and pathological observation can not discover. Especially as for the cancer, we have many well-established tumor makers but when these huge proteins, tumor makers, are appeared, it is already too late; the cancer is definitely established.

On the contrary to the tumor maker, the observation of disease proteome by new type of mass spectrograph provides the spectral pattern of the proteins. Many studies report that the allover pattern of peaks of the mass spectrometry not just specific peak of single protein contains the information which could be used to detect the cancer in very early stage, although we still can not observe very heavy protein by this method.

Statistical and data-mining methods have been applied and detection sensitivity is very high. For example, it is reported that ovarian tumors can be discovered in very early stage, by proteome examination of patients' serum using Seldi-TOF-MS at the rate of 99 and machine learning approach [7].

The example is shown where we compared the detection sensitivity between the proteomic information and conventional tumor markers with respect to the hepatocellular carcinoma (HCC). It is well known that the patients suffering from the liver cirrhosis will contract HCC. We collected the patients of liver cirrhosis (LC: 20 subjects) early HCC (E-HCC: 20 subjects) and advanced HCC (A-HCC: 20 subjects) We investigate the presision of early cancer detection. For proteome measurement, SELDI-TOF-MS was used to analyze the patients' serum, and for tumor marker, AFP PIVKA-II was investigated. For serum protein spectral profile, three components were extracted from MS spectral pattern by using partial least square method. The classification is used (Table 3). Classification results showed that the early HCC could be detected with high sensitivity by proteome examination whereas the conventional tumor marker had poor performance in detecting early HCC but they can be used to confirm the well developed cancer.

Table 3. Classification of proteome and tumor marker

SELDI-TOF-MS Components estimation	True class		
	LC	E-HCC	A-HCC
LC	11	3	3
E-HCC	8	12	10
A-HCC	1	5	7

proteome only

AFP + PIVKA estimation	True class		
	LC	E-HCC	A-HCC
LC	16	8	0
E-HCC	4	8	2
A-HCC	0	4	18

tumor maker only

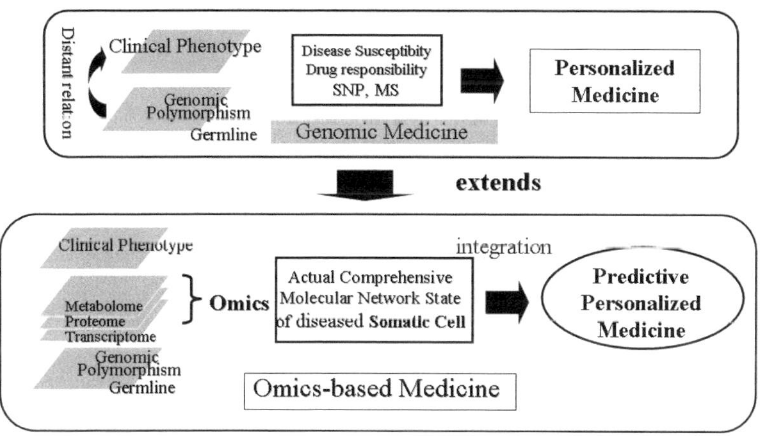

Figure 4. Concepts of omics-based medicine

4. Personalized Care Based on the Systems Pathobiology – Genome/Omics-Based Medicine of the Third Generation

As with the background to need the emergence of systems biology in the third generation of life science, also in the personalized care, the same situation have come up where systems approach is urgently needed to fully utilize the genome/omics data

for clinical diagnosis/therapy. We propose "systems pathobiology" which is the counterpart in genome/omics-based medicine to the systems biology in life science. Comprehensiveness of omics data makes possible to understand a disease as an integrated whole. Try to find underlying mechanism of disease behind the omics data.
In developing the systems pathobiology, we established the basic principles in the systems approach to the disease. The following principles are mostly directed to the common complex diseases like cancer, hypertension and diabetes. We will exclude the rare genetic disease.

1. The principle of hierarchically integrated systemness of disease

Disease is hierarchically organized integrated system, which might be composed of molecular network level, intercellular/tissue level and individual level. Bottom-up causality and top-down causality are acting together to make disease as an integrated whole system of disease

2. The principle of existence of self-sustaining mechanism of disease

Disease is not just ad hoc failure of biosystems but disease organize itself as sustainable system according to the own systems logic. There should be some mechanism such as looping one to sustain the disease

3. The principle of systems evolution of disease within the patient

Disease develops and changes itself in the course of time. Some disease like cancer, disease system evolves itself to reach the complex state or chaos. Some disease follow the developmental process; from stem cell, progenitor to matured cell. Cell lineage-based understanding of disease makes it possible to understand the disease from morphological organization process of tissue-organ level structure

4. The principle of take-over of host's self-organization ability by the disease

The self-organizing ability of the disease comes from take-over of patient's normal systems organizing ability. The disease does not have original system organizing ability.

With the above mentioned system principles in mind, we can comprehend the disease in the whole spectrum. Disease is distorted bio-systems where normal pathway is modified to form "sustained disease pathway".

As the example of the fact that disease is hierarchically organized integrated system, we suggest that other than the bottom up causality from genetic cause to tissue level and individual level of the abnormality, systemic (in large) environment causes gene abnormal (disease-adaptive) function. In hypertension, blood pressure raises by some abnormal supporting mechanism like genetic one at early stage, but after several months, if hypertensive condition is sustained, the genetic activity begins to start remodeling of capillary vascular to have more stiff vessels in order to sustain high blood pressure (adaptation by gene expression). This shows the organization of disease system is done by integration of bottom-up and top-down causality.

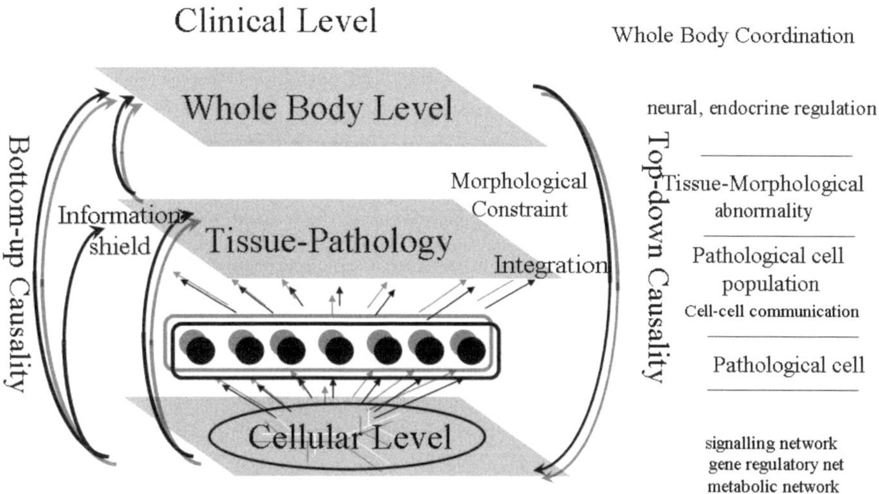

Figure 5. Organization of disease system

From the systems pathobiology approach, system-theoretical methods such as systems analysis modeling, and simulation, is accommodated to use for disease pathway to determine which pathway is out of order based on the collective observation of differentially expressed genes (Figure 6).

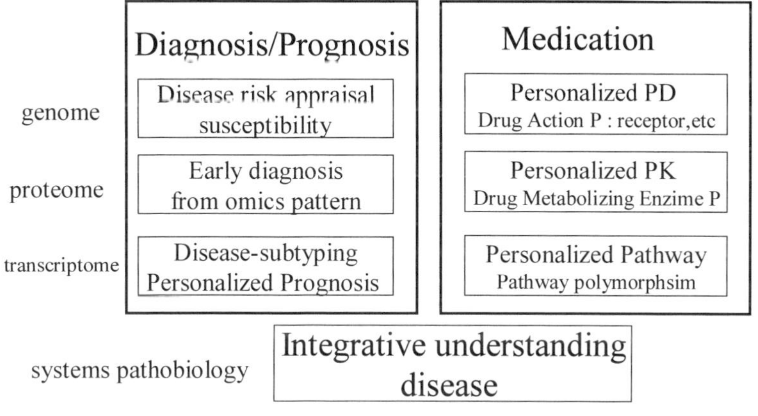

Figure 6. Summary of genome/omics-based personalized care

5. Conclusion

A new perspective for personalized care which genomics and bioinformatics cooperatively open was described, focusing on future possibilities which "genome/omics-based personalized care" is thought to bring about.

At last we should ask what about the genetically-based healthcare? We think EHR (Electronic Health Record) and PHR (Personal Healthcare Record) should contain genomic information. With longitudinal evaluation of disease risk, life-long management of own health joined with ubiquitous healthcare IT, the era of longitudinal health attainment will come.

References

[1]　Weinstein JN, Myers TG, O'Connor PM, Friend SH. Fornace AJ Jr., et.al. An information-intensive approach to the molecular pharmacology of cancer. *Science* 275(5298):343-9, 1997

[2]　Sherry ST et al. dbSNP- databasse for single nucletiode polymorphisms and other classes of minor genetic variation. *Genome Res* 9, 677-679, 1999

[3]　Lazarou J, Pomeranz B, Corey P. Incidence of Adverse Drug Reactions in Hospitalized Patients: A Meta-analysis of Prospective Studies. *JAMA* 279:1200-1205, 1998

[4]　Slamon DJ, Leyland-Jones B, Shak S, Fuchs H, Paton V, et al. Use of chemotherapy plus a monoclonal antibody against HER2 for metastatic breast cancer that overexpresses HER2. *N Engl J Med.* 344: 783-92, 2001

[5]　Alzdeh AA, Michael BE, et al. Distinct types of diffuse large B-cell lymphoma identified by gene expression profiling. *Nature* 403:503-537, 2000

[6]　Tanaka S, Arii S, Yasen M, Mogushi K, Su N, Cho C, Imoto I, Eishi Y, Inazawa J, Miki Y, Tanaka H. Aurora kinase B is a predictive factor for the aggressive recurrence of hepatocellular carcinoma after curative hepatectomy. *British Journal of Surgery* 2007 in press

[7]　Petricoin III EF, Ardekani AM, Hitt BA, Levine PJ, Fusaro VA, Steinberg SM, Mills GB, et al. Use of proteomic patterns in serum to identify ovarian cancer. *Lancet* 359: 572-577, 2002

[8]　Ohta T, Iijima K, Miyamoto M, Nakahara I, Odagawa R, Naitoh1 S, Mimaki S, Sakiyama T, Tanaka H, Ohtsuji M, Kobayashi A, Shibata T, Yamamoto M, Hirohashi S. Activation of Nrf2 by Loss of Keap1 Function Provides Advantages in Growth of Lung Cancer. *Cancer Research*, in press

eHealth: Combining Health Telematics, Telemedicine, Biomedical Engineering and Bioinformatics to the Edge. Edited by B. Blobel, P. Pharow and M. Nerlich.
IOS Press, 2008

EHR Architectures – Comparison and Trends

Bernd BLOBEL [1]
eHealth Competence Center, University of Regensburg Medical Center, Regensburg, Germany

Abstract. For meeting the requirements for high quality and safe of care as well as efficiency and productivity of health systems, latter have to move towards job sharing, communicating and cooperating structures. This paradigm change must be supported through sustainable and semantically interoperable architectures for health information systems, especially for Electronic Health Record (EHR) systems as the core application in any eHealth environment. Advanced system architectures are characterized as being highly distributed, component-oriented, model-based, service-oriented, knowledge-based, user-friendly, lawful and trustworthy, based on a unified development process, a harmonized ontology and reference terminologies. Existing and emerging approaches for EHR systems are to be compared using the Generic Component Model (GCM) as architectural reference. Any system can be assessed according to GCM dimensions: transparent domain representation, composition/decomposition behavior and reflection of the systems' viewpoints as well as their components' interoperability level. All those aspects have to be interrelated for real systems analysis, design, implementation, and deployment by that way enabling the migration of different EHR approaches on the basis of GCM.

Keywords. Electronic Health Record, EHR architectures, standards, semantic interoperability, Generic Component Model

Introduction

The realization of requirements for high quality and safe care as well as efficiency and productivity of health systems under the well-known constraining conditions is seen in increasingly distributed and specialized healthcare that becomes strongly oriented on actual personal health status and the needs of the subject of care. Through the transition from standardized organization-centered care to a disease-specifically optimized and process-controlled care (also named disease management or managed care), health systems are moving on to meet the aforementioned challenges. Standardized process-controlled solutions based on best practice clinical guidelines enable a more regular care quality with minor dependencies from resources, e.g., the experience of the care team. However, the paradigm has to further be enhanced towards personalized care for responding to the individual status and conditions of the patient, called Personal Healthcare. When such process includes prevention and home care addressing citizens

<hr>

[1] Corresponding Author: Bernd Blobel, PhD, Associate Professor, eHealth Competence Center, University of Regensburg Medical Center, Franz-Josef-Strauss-Allee 11, D-93053 Regensburg, Germany; Email: bernd.blobel@klinik.uni-regensburg.de; URL: http://www.ehealth-cc.de

before becoming patients, the Personal Health paradigm has been met. A highly distributed, specialized, integrated, and individualized care necessarily requires sharing all information including the actual contexts and underlying concepts.

If communication and cooperation is provided independent of constraints in time, locality, or resources for optimally caring a patient even in rural areas at night, health telematics has to be combined with telemedicine, permanently miniaturized biomedical devices, and genomics for individualizing diagnostics and therapeutics. This altogether is called eHealth. Personal Health is finally the personalization of eHealth.

1. eHealth Core Application Electronic Health Record

Common interests, common information, its common understanding and common actions derived are essential for any cooperation. Common availability of data, information and services is the most important prerequisite for an eHealth environment. In clinical and nursing documentation, all data and information (meaning the interpretation of data on the basis of pre-existing domain knowledge) about patients or -in the Personal Health paradigm's context- about citizen, and related processes are summarized. The medical documentation's electronic counterpart forms the Electronic Healthcare Record (EHCR) or the Electronic Patient Record (EPR). Extended by social, prevention or lifestyle information, the Electronic Health Record (EHR) is becoming established. The EHR enhances to become the core application of any eHealth platform and service [1].

2. Characteristics for Information Systems Evaluation

For evaluating information systems, many parameters have to be considered. Not only the offered functionality but also user friendliness is of interest for the end-user. Both aspects are defined by exploited paradigms and architectures on the one hand, and by implementation details on the other. Because implementations have -contrary to architectures- a shorter lifecycle and the same architecture can be implemented on different platforms, only implementation-independent aspects will be considered here. Aspects to be further investigated include, but are not limited to, the information cycle and the interoperability level. Reality is typically described by simplified and simplifying models reflecting intentions and interests of the person creating and using the information. In the information cycle, the observed data is being interpreted according to intended objectives to perform the right actions for achieving those objectives. Both steps require knowledge of experts operating in the domain of interest. The information cycle is represented in the different information definitions provided by C. E. Shannon, L.-M. Brillouin, and N. Wiener. Regarding the interoperability level, technical interoperability, structural interoperability, syntactic interoperability, semantic interoperability, and service-oriented interoperability can be distinguished. While technical interoperability establishes harmonization at the plug&play, signal, and protocol level, structural interoperability is based on exchange of agreed data, syntactic interoperability provides harmonized messaging and document exchange, Semantic interoperability requires harmonized information model based on common references and agreed, ontology-based terminology. The higher level of semantic interoperability –service-oriented interoperability- is realized through invocation of services accessed via standardized interfaces. Here, common business models are needed. Interoperability levels reflect information cycle aspects. While communication focuses on exchange of meaningful and correctly interpreted messages, cooperation depends on the applications' behavior and functionalities, defined by their structural components, their functions and the components' interrelationships. Therefore, applications' behavior and functionalities is defined by the application architecture. The assessment of systems regarding their interoperability has to be provided by analyzing their architecture and the completeness of the information cycle [2]. In the next sections, the aforementioned general principles and statements for information systems will be constrained to EHR systems.

3. Characteristics of Semantically Interoperable EHR Architectures

Before discussing the characteristics of semantically interoperable EHR architectures, some basic terms have to be introduced. An EHR is considered a repository of information about a person's health status and all processes directly or indirectly related to this person's care, provided .in a computer-readable format. An EHR system is therefore a set of components for realizing the mechanisms for creating, using, storing, and retrieving an EHR. An EHR architecture defines a model of generic properties required for every EHR to be communicable, comprehensive, useful, effective, ethically-legally binding, bewaring its integrity independent of platforms and systems as well as national specialties over the time.

For providing advanced and sustainable communication and cooperation, architectures for sustainable health information systems such as EHR systems have to be open, scalable, flexible, portable, distributed, standard-conform, semantically interoperable, service-oriented, user-accepted, and lawful. Therefore, the following architectural paradigms have to be met: Distribution; component-orientation; model-driven and service-oriented design, considering concepts, context and knowledge; comprehensive business modeling; separation of platform-independent and platform-specific modeling (separation of logical and technological view); agreed reference terminologies and ontologies, unified development process, advanced security and privacy services embedded in the architecture. The aforementioned architectural paradigms arc rcflected in the Generic Component Model (GCM) which provides a multi-model approach to any system architecture [3]. It can be used for analyzing, designing and implementing EHR architectures, but also for developing migration strategies [3], [4].

EHR systems as well as standards and projects defining them have to be assessed in reference to the GCM. So, usability of the approach, gaps and the capability for migration can be evaluated, and migration paths can be derived.

4. EHR-Related Standards

Currently, three different streams for specification and implementation of advanced EHR architectures exist that have their roots in legacy systems, traditional imaginations and methodologies: Data approach (data representation), concept approach (concept and knowledge representation), and process/services approach (business process and service representation).

Because of their rational roots, all approaches have their at least temporary right to exist. All three approaches undergo a further development, offering a convergence. As the GCM considers all aforementioned aspects, the distance of evaluated approaches to the GCM as well as the reflection of the presented principles allows for evaluation of developed or emerging solutions as well as for description of missing characteristics.

4.1. HL7 Version 3

Following the tradition of structured messaging, the HL7 Reference Information Model as well as step by step improved modeling methodologies and tools are established for faster and more consistent message development. The RIM design followed existing developments and traditions, some basic paradigms and the objectives behind the information model, not fulfilling the requirements for an ontology, however. Through separation of message definition and message exchange format and introduction of a unified process (Message Development Framework – MDF), a quite open standard has been developed. However, this standard is suffering from claiming that it does not define any requirement to the communicating information systems, but compensates existing structures with optional attributes. Basis of specifications are data or information of common interest. For overcoming obvious inconsistencies as well as for assuring step by step semantic interoperability (without guarantee), a comprehensive vocabulary has been introduced and permanently developed further while going back to existing terminologies. With

- the further development of MDF towards a comprehensive HL7 Development Framework (HDF),
- the transition from proprietary to open development environments and tools, and
- the definition of meta-models at different aggregation levels from a domain (here: not the OMG definition, but medical specialties or aspects) up to single communication scenarios and the definition of generic domain-crossing concepts (Common Message Element Types – CMETs),

prerequisites for semantic interoperability have been established which are able to support future architecture developments. Thereby, HL7 supports -step by step- the GCM dimensions composition/decomposition as well as the separation of platform-independent and platform-specific information models. It does not reflect at all the separation of system views, business modeling, the representation of technical concepts (GCM domain concepts), and the separation of GCM domains.

With the introduction of Clinical Document Architecture (CDA) and Clinical Templates, a move towards the description of business processes was enabled. This move is now being perfected towards EHR functionalities and services with the EHR-S Functional Model Draft Standard for Trial Use, the EHR-S Interoperability Model, and even more with the CORBA-related Service Object Architecture. So, the transfer from the message paradigm to the architecture paradigm enabling real semantic interoperability is being carried out [5].

4.2. HL7 CDA

CDA is an XML-based standard for exchanging and storing clinical documents such as discharge or transfer letters, care documentations, and surgical reports. CDA defines clinical documents as structured, persistent, human-readable and machine-processable objects for a specific purpose. The CDA interoperability level enhances with more structured CDA Releases from R1 up to R3. Thereby, only the structural representation of concepts in R3 providing real semantic interoperability at the level of knowledge representation (semantic information) is supported, but not at the level of services (pragmatic information). Therefore, the term Clinical Document Structure (CDS) would fit much better.

A CDA document consists of the CDA Header and the CDA Body. The latter contains information about CDA Structure, CDA Entries and CDA External References. A care record consists of a series of CDA documents which have to be appropriately aggregated according to the context. CDA only enables the GCM dimensions structural composition/decomposition and partially that of separation of domains [6].

4.3. CDA Clinical Templates

The generic HL7 Version 3 specification allows developers either internal or external to HL7 for generating, maintaining and distributing Template Packages to describe certain use cases. Thus, intentions as well as knowledge about concepts and workflows can be communicated between domain experts and users on the one hand. Cooperative workflows can be improved on the other hand. HL7 Templates are constraint models based on HL7 Version 3 message specifications or CDA documents including needed guidelines for implementation and use. They can be used, e.g., for control of data and information entry, validation of messages and documents, or qualification of processes (e.g., the representation of rules, decision support, alert generation). Clinical Templates describe clinical concepts and workflows. In relation to the GCM, Clinical Templates partially supply the missing business process descriptions of CDA documents [6].

4.4. HL7 EHR-S Functional Model and EHR Interoperability Model

As described, the HL7 EHR-S Functional Model DSTU offers a service-orientation considering business processes and supporting the qualification of HL7 Version 3 towards an architecture paradigm. It describes functional requirements for an EHR system and thereby its behavior using a user-oriented language. It classifies those requirements in Direct Care, Supportive Functions, and Information Infrastructure with all of them being specialized in a hierarchical way. So, stakeholders get a systematic description of parameters and criteria for quality assurance and possible certification. For GCM conformance, the EHR-S Functional Model needs a corresponding formalization. While the EHR-S Functional Model describes requirements from the user perspective, the EHR-S Interoperability Model specifies technical requirements in relation to the Functional Model [6].

4.5. HL7 CCD

The HL7 Continuity of Care Document (CCD) specification demonstrates the application of the Template paradigm using constraints and mapping to translate the ASTM Continuity of Care Record (CCR) specification. Beside common constraints on data types, sources, identifiers, roles, and terminology conformance, Document ID, language, creation date, patient, communication partner, and purpose as well as the CCD Footer are specified in the CCD Header. The CCD Body contains information about actors, functional status, problem, social and family history, allergies, medications, immunizations, vital signs, results, procedures, accounts and care plans. CDA characteristics in extending and restricting CCR remain unchanged [6].

4.6. Continuity of Care Record

The ASTM Standard E 2369 "Standard Specification for Continuity of Care Record (CCR)" describes a basic data set containing administrative, demographic, and clinical information that are most important for patient's medical care. For improving the communication of that information, the data set is coded in XML. It has been developed by the American Society for Testing and Materials (ASTM) with contributions from numerous American medical association and corporations. The CCR provides an effective, simply implementable, practicable means to providers and their supporting information systems for summarizing and communicating selected relevant data about the patient, thereby supporting continuity of care. For this purpose, the CCR contains a summary of the patient's health status (e.g. problems, medications, allergies) as well as basic information about insurance, advance directives, care documentation, and the patient's care plan. It also includes identifying information of all principals involved (e.g. systems, applications, devices, documents) and the purpose of the CCR. The CCR is a non-persistent and itself permanently actualizing ad-hoc snapshot of the basic documentation about the patient and his/her care process. Thereby, it provides a means for a single healthcare practitioner, system, or setting to aggregate all of the pertinent data about a patient, and to forward it to another practitioner, system, or setting for supporting the continuity of care. It does not replace either special documents such as discharge letters nor comprehensive EHRs. Because of the sensitivity of personal health information as well as ethical and legal requirements, advanced data security and privacy mechanisms shall be supported. Therefore, the CCR also contains information relevant for privilege management, authorization and access control. Communication security has to be guaranteed through the deployment of corresponding standards and protocols (e.g. W3C specifications for digital signature and encryption of XML documents). The user-specific and purpose-related recording and presentation of information is assured using XML Schema definitions. Those XML Schemes are specified in annexes recently amended to the standard. Professional societies can define further XML Schemes appropriate for their specific needs. As with HL7 conformance statements and implementation guides, standard-conform implementation of the CCR specifications for assuring interoperability of solutions and products is supported by normative implementation guides.

A CCR consists of its core components CCR Header, CCR Body, and CCR Footer which are specialized in sections with detailed data fields. The CCR Header defines all information relevant for the document such as unique identifier, language, version, time stamp (data/time), information about the patient, the principal generating the CCR (doctor, nurse, patient, system, and application), target/recipient, and purpose of the CCR. The CCR Body contains patient-specific basic data such as medical problem, health insurance, medication, procedures, etc.), while the CCR Footer describes the actors in the care context, comments, and references to external documents and information.

The CCR covers neither the semantic richness of GEHR or CDA specifications nor the structural depth of EN/ISO 13606 EHR Reference Architecture, not talking about behavioral aspects. Here, it is pointless that CCR only provides a document structure, but not an architectural approach. It does not support context-related re-use of elements on the basis of knowledge representation. Contrary to the still forthcoming long-term process of developing concept specifications (Archetypes) for EN/ISO 13606 or domain-related (D-MIM) and process-related (R-MIM) CDA specifications, CCR is immediately applicable, however. The CCD specification jointly developed by HL7 and ASTM diminishes the differences a little, without wiping off the basic advantages or disadvantages of the approaches. The persistency of objects as basis for service-oriented interoperability is such a difference [7].

4.7. EN/ISO 13606 Health Informatics – Electronic Health Record Communication

Four parts CEN ENV 13606 "Health informatics – EHCR communication" -approved in 1999 and restricted to medical care- defines a component-based Electronic Health Record (EHR) Reference Architecture without describing the domain concepts to be filled in the containers. Its revision -EN/ISO 13606 "Health informatics – Electronic Health Record communication"- extends the further developed and HL7 RIM conformant Reference Architecture (Part 1: Reference Model) by Archetypes. Archetypes have first been developed in the context of the GEHR/openEHR project (EN Part 2: Archetype Interchange Specification). Terminology important for semantic interoperability and presented in the former Part 2 (ENV Part 2: Domain Term List) as list of terms will be extended in the new Part 3 by a set of Archetypes reflecting the diversity of clinical requirements and basic conditions. In its revision, the privacy-relevant Part 3 (ENV Part 3: Distribution Rule) will be completed towards a comprehensive view on data security and privacy as new Part 4 (Part 4: Security Features), unfortunately insufficiently bridging to the corresponding ISO TS 22600 "Health informatics – Privilege management and access control". The last part of both the old and the new version of the standard (EN Part 5: Exchange Models) provides examples for implementing the standard. In the context of cooperation of Standards Developing Organizations (SDOs), a harmonization takes place between EN/ISO 13606, HL7 Version 3 in general and HL7 CDA in particular. Thereby, the mapping of sets of data type definitions, the development of the EHR Domain Information Model as well as a series of Refined Message Information for certain structures and functionalities occur.

Following the architecture paradigm, the revision of CEN ENV 13606 provides a specification for semantically interoperable EHR systems supporting communication and cooperation of EHR extracts, but also of comprehensive EHRs. The EN/ISO 13606 Reference Architecture enables the structural composition/decompositions as well as the representation of concepts of the related component models through platform-independent information models. The GCM architecture is not completely covered, however. Especially the consideration of component views and their separation is as missing as a sufficient modeling of processes and domain management. Contrary to the strict system theoretical GCM approach and the approach of related established standards, the definition of Archetypes does offer neither strict paradigms for defining components nor rules for their composition/decomposition, semantic composition/decomposition cannot be addressed at all. Behavioral aspects are currently completely ignored [8].

5. Programs and Projects for Advanced EHR Systems

5.1. GEHR Project and openEHR Foundation

Based on the "Good European Health Record – GEHR" project funded by the European Commission within the Third Framework Programme but also considering other research and development initiatives (e.g. SYNAPSE, PICNIC) as well as existing standards, the Australian Government started the "Good Electronic Health Record – GEHR" project back in 2000. The fundamental challenge of the GEHR project is interoperability at knowledge level requiring adequate methods for knowledge representation. Already in the past, so-called Constraint Languages have been developed for knowledge representation, allowing for deriving a disciplinary domain concept from a general concept by deploying domain-specific knowledge. As an example, the Object Constraint Language (OCL) as part of the Unified Modeling Language (UML) is used for knowledge and concept representation in an object-oriented world. For the Web Services world, e.g., the Web Ontology Language (OWL) has been developed; but there are also other recent developments. Also the GCM follows this approach by further evolution of syntax and semantics, i.e., underlying rules and expression means combining meta-languages and logics representation.

The GEHR model consists of two parts: the concrete GEHR Object Model (GOM) providing the EHR information containers, and the GEHR Meta-Models for clinical concept representation. GEHR Meta-Models describe medical knowledge using domain-specific, organization-specific, or even individual views and constraints. Those (user-defined) meta-models are called Archetypes, thereby referring to the term for user-defined database tables. The separation of structures and concepts in a two model approach allows for separating the IT world from the domain world (medical world) with its special requirements, domain languages, and communication problems. The concepts can be developed step by step and flexibly combined like LEGO® bricks, following construction plan laid down in the Archetypes [9].

As any other knowledge representation language (e.g. Medical Knowledge Modules of the HL7 Arden Syntax for communication of knowledge concepts), Archetypes consists of the Header Part (Archetype ID and meta-data), the Body Part (Archetype definition, generic concept representation) and the Terminology Part (definition of terms and their bindings to existing terminologies such as SNOMED-CT™). For describing Archetypes, the Archetype Definition Language (ADL) has been developed [10]. Contrary to GCM, the GEHR approach only allows for describing structural aspects of the concept components (knowledge) in question, not their behavior, however. Because of missing rules, Archetypes are not being aggregated, but replaced by Archetypes of higher complexity. In general, the GEHR approach still demonstrates essential mathematical, system-theoretical, and informatics weaknesses thereby remaining behind the GCM methodology. In the future, the aforementioned weaknesses have to be overcome.

It should be mentioned that the term constraint model -introduced long time ago-still covers all aspects essential in the given context without any need for introducing a new term. Therefore, the Archetype term is first of all a marketing term which itself enhances the danger of isolation for the medical domain. This could be contra-productive in an environment looking for integration of all fields characterizing the open approach of Personal Health up to an eSociety.

5.2. IHE XDS

Starting in the USA and meanwhile adopted at many countries and regions, the healthcare user community has launched the IHE initiative, which aims at standard-based semantic interoperability. IHE stands for "Integrating the Healthcare Enterprise", defining the objectives for that initiative. Inaugurating standards used by IHE have been DICOM (Digital Image Communication) and HL7. Meanwhile, other SDO's work products have been included as well. These and other standards, however, are necessary but not sufficient for the successful integration of heterogeneous information systems. This is caused by different requirements established at different sites as well as the optionality offered by many standards to fit in any environment [11]. This problem can only be managed by an advanced architectural approach sharing any concepts, contextual information and knowledge in a formalized way. Intermediately, the variety of possible solutions must be reduced by profiling or constraining use cases and approaches according to common agreements, implementing, testing, and certifying the results. Such an approach is known in specifications not only communicating information but also sharing services such as DICOM with its conformance statements [12].

The IHE Cross-Enterprise Document Sharing (XDS) Integration Profile for exchanging structured documents supports navigation through distributed EHR systems, while IHE XDS-MS Content Profile and XPHR Content Profile provides the medical summary or the patient created summary information to be shared, both being based on constrained HL7 CDA R2 specifications [13]. There are many other IHE profiles dealing with further services for enabling health information systems and especially EHR systems interoperability, dedicated to certain aspects such as the dedication to specific media (e.g. images), document availability notification (NAV), Cross-Enterprise Document Media Interchange (XDM), Cross-Enterprise Document Reliable point-to-point Interchange (XDR), etc.

6. Security Requirements and Solutions for Advanced EHR Systems

Advanced and sustainable EHR systems following the GCM architectural paradigm are based on the following computational principles: mobile computing, pervasive computing, and autonomous computing [14]. Being completely distributed intelligent, adaptive, and flexible, security and privacy services cannot be predefined or separately managed by system administrators anymore. As a special domain (legal, regulatory, policy-related), they have to be an integrative part of the system's architecture. Therefore, all principles established for advanced and sustainable systems architectures must be comprehensively applied to security and privacy issues as well. Following, security and privacy services have to be analyzed, designed, implemented and deployed according to the GCM approach [15].

EN/ISO 13606 is the only approach slightly tackling this view in reference to ISO TS 22600 "Health informatics – Privilege management and access control" [15]. The preliminary instance established in EN/ISO 13606-4 only meets some of the principles, however, nevertheless allowing for further migration.

7. National Initiatives

7.1. EHR Blueprint

The Canadian EHRS Blueprint establishes an extensible, flexible EHR Enterprise Architecture, which provides the necessary framework for distribution of right information to the right people at the right time based on pan-regional EHR-systems and a set of infrastructural services. It supports all decisions leading to better health in a better health system for Canadian citizen [16].

Based on a distributed system approach allowing for both centralized and decentralized implementations, the EHR architecture comprises the EHR solution consisting of point of service applications and viewers, the EHR infostructure containing the components ancillary data and services, a health information data warehouse, EHR data and services, registries data and services, and longitudinal record services, as well as an EHR solution locator service. All components and services mentioned are connected through the health information access layer. This layer established a set of common services for integration, interoperability, context handling, privacy and security, subscription, system management and general services (e.g. auditing, logging, exception and error handling).

7.2. National Programme for IT

The National Programme for IT of the English National Health Service is a revised edition of establishing IT in the English healthcare system [17]. After defining and implementing an infrastructure –the SPINE, following partial programs are currently running:

*   NHS Care Record Service
*   Choose & Book
*   Electronic Transmission of Prescriptions
*   N3, the National Network

IT projects at NHS have a long tradition consuming covered by incredibly high expenditures. Being well observed by the other countries as success and failure experiment, from different perspectives this work provides a basis for many development.

7.3. Shareable EHR in Finland

Finland pursues a concept of distributed EHR systems. In that context, inter-organizational and inter-domain communication is supported by regional EHR systems, offering legally binding EHR extracts within advanced security architecture. EHR architecture and communication are based on HL7 using HL7 CDA and HL7 V3 Messages. Additionally, service-oriented architectures (SOA) are under consideration [18].

7.4. Australian HealthConnect Project and Nehta Architectural Map

Aiming first at an integration-driven approach for connecting loosely-coupled systems with shared semantics, a single control point deploying standards, Australia moves strategically towards an interoperability-driven and standard-driven eHealth platform based on multiple semantics and multiple control points. The Australian HealthConnect Project is focused on the first approach, while the National E-Health Transition Authority (NETHA) Architectural Map follows the advanced methodology and strategy based on a service-oriented architecture [19].

7.5. Electronic Health Record Vendors Association (USA)

After having a long tradition of tackling the EHR challenge and offering regional projects and domain-specific solutions (e.g. in the VHA domain), the USA started recently an industry-driven initiative for establishing a national EHR solution to met the 2004 President's Order challenge for offering an EHR to every American citizen by 2014.

The HIMSS Electronic Health Record Vendors Association (EHRVA) was formed in 2004 to provide a collective voice with which to respond to governmental and other external initiatives affecting electronic health records (EHRs) and the creation of a nationwide health information network (NHIN). EHRVA's mission is [20]:

- to improve healthcare by advancing the EHR industry as a whole and promoting the rapid adoption of electronic health records;
- to deliver immediate and future value to healthcare providers and patients by providing a unified voice and a forum for cooperation for the EHR vendor community; and
- to serve as leaders in standards development, EHR certification, interoperability, advancing performance and quality measures, and other EHR issues subject to an increasing number of initiatives and requests by government, payers, patients and physician associations.

EHRVA developed a four phase approach towards EHR standardization, specification, implementation, and deployment from exchanging medical summaries between healthcare providers up to collaborative and intelligent care. It which provides a four granularity level framework from high level business use cascs through communication services and integration profile down to basic standards and technical protocols. The work is part of the formation of a nationwide health information network (NHIN) for transforming healthcare delivery.

Regarding the NHIN infrastructure, five services have to be established: identification services, security and access control services, persistent information management, dynamic information access, and workflow/quality services.

7.6 National Health Information Infrastructure Programs in Asia

Following the aforementioned and long-term examples, many other countries are facing the challenge of changing their health systems towards the personal health paradigm. In that context, especially Asian countries (Japan, Korea, Taiwan, China, Malaysia, etc.) are setting up ambitious, partially well financed programs and projects finally focusing on advanced eHealth infrastructures and EHR or Personal Health

Record (see, e.g., the next section). All solutions are considering international standards and especially HL7 specifications such as the HL7 v3 methodology, HDF and CDA as foundation. The solutions tend towards the component paradigm and its implementation through Web Services, thereby emphasizing the need for privacy and security services.

7.7. Electronic Health Record and Personal Health Records

Future advanced and sustainable eHealth architectures for individualized care with regional or European dimensions are described in the eHealth Action Plan of the European Commission and the EU Member States. This challenging program defines the Electronic Health Record as the core application for every eHealth platform. There are different approaches towards EHR system implementations in the various countries, however. The variant established are ranging from Medication Files in The Netherlands as well as in England over Sharable EHR as the Finnish solution up to the comprehensive EHR in Denmark. In the long term, all countries will approach a comprehensive EHR. Because of the individualized focus putting the person in the centre of the business and empowering him/her to play an important role in his/her health, the person will also contribute to the documentation of his/her status and processes applied. Therefore, EHR systems in Personal Health setting are also called Personal Health Records (PHR).

Beside the Electronic Health Record, the improvement of quality and safety of care through evidence-based medicine und decision support plays an extraordinary role. In this context, ePrescribing using decision support systems has been prioritized in Europe and in other eHealth regions as well.

8. Discussion and Conclusions

The core application EHR is in the center of considerations for all regional (e.g. EC eHealth Action Plan) and national (UK, Denmark, USA, Finland, Australia, Canada) eHealth Programs. With the move from organization-centered to process-controlled care and even more by the paradigm change towards personalized healthcare, comprehensive communication and cooperation between all participants in the process including semantic interoperability between supporting information systems is inevitable.

Different advanced approaches for future-proof architectures, EHR specifications, and the implementation of semantically interoperable EHR systems (e.g. HL7 Version 3 Standard Set with CDA, CCD, EHR-S Functional Model, EHR Interoperability Model, GEHR/openEHR, EN/ISO 13606, CCR) have been demonstrated, discussed and evaluated using the Generic Component Model (GCM) as reference architecture for sustainable and semantically interoperable health information systems.

Currently, no one of the specifications investigated from an insider's perspective meets the requirements for semantic interoperability at service level – but this is what almost all of them claiming to do. The maturity of the approaches is very different, whereby history of specifications and originating organizations, the chosen paradigm as well as scope and objectives are of importance.

The HL7 Version 3 methodology in connection with the definition of system requirements by the EHR-S Functional Model and the EHR-S Interoperability Model (it remains a question to the author, why both models have not been brought together) provides the best approach so far to the GCM without solving domain-crossing aspects and the connection of non-IT views to ICT views. Furthermore, the formal business process specification and the dynamic behavioral/functional aspects of the components are still missing. The service-orientation missing could be overcome by current efforts of the SOA SIG in liaison. Additionally, present concept representations have not been adequately integrated, probably due to a missing HL7 ontology. Surmounting the many solution islands, the complex HL7 Standards family could -in collaboration with CEN, openEHR and CORBA- demonstrate some progress.

The second rather comprehensive approach to semantic interoperability is EN/ISO 13606, even if many deficiencies and inconsistencies have yet to be removed. Contrary to the HL7 Version 3 approach, the problem of semantic composition/decomposition is insufficiently solved. The same counts for business processes. On the other hand, the project orientates from the beginning to the architecture paradigm despite of the irritating title of the standard, and it goes beyond the HL7 approach in this perspective. GEHR/openEHR has to be evaluated partly analogue to EN/ISO 13606 due to the close connections and the common knowledge representation based on Archetypes. It constraints itself in essence to parts 2 and 3, however.

The two promising approaches suffer from the complexity of the healthcare domain. So, it will take some time until a critical mass of model-based services (meta-models at different levels or Archetypes respectively, as well as tools for instantiation) will be available for revolutionizing health. Since 2001, different pathways are followed. While EN/ISO 13606 still focuses on its architectural approach, the openEHR Foundation project focuses to concepts, leading to different structural components. At the same time, commonalities with HL7 CDA and HL7 Clinical Templates are growing

Contrary to the HL7 Version 3 Standard Set and to EN/ISO 13606, CCR provides an immediately applicable record solution without claiming semantic interoperability, however. All ways offered allow for migration using the GCM. A closer cooperation between standards bodies is absolutely helpful. During the evolution, the user community has to decide which interim solutions are needed.

The necessity of meeting all paradigms of the GCM has been emphasized through experience from national project in different countries the author is involved in. For a long time being the internationally leading program for introducing a national EHR, the Danish approach started with the underlying business processes in an exemplary way. The problem of structural and functional composition/decomposition has been ignored, however. This deficiency braked down the project, now resulting in a comprehensive restart. Other projects and standards including the ones discussed here ignore the business processes, at the same time providing reasonable solutions for the other aspects. This has adverse effects as well, if the gaps have not been single-mindedly closed [21].

An important requirement for achieving semantic interoperability has been, and still is, the establishment of a unified process including the definition of conformance statements as well as the quality assurance for specifications and implementations. Here, projects such as the European Q-REC project led by the EuroRec Institute or the work of the US Certification Commission for Health Information Technology (CCHIT), pushing testing, quality labeling or certification, respectively, of EHR specifications and EHR systems [??], [23].

The eHealth Competence Center at the University of Regensburg Medical Center is involved in most of the international standards activities and national programs related to the EHR. While the work in many regions is ongoing and more or less evolved, the German EHR development started with the bIT4health (better IT ore better health care) launched some years ago by the German Federal Ministry for Health is comparably immature. Recently, the eHCC has been appointed to specify the German EHR architecture.

Acknowledgement

The author is indebted to the colleagues from standards bodies and institutions such as ISO, CEN, HL7, the EuroRec Institute as well as related projects like GEHR/openEHR and Q-REC for kind cooperation and support.

References

[1]   Blobel B. Advanced EHR architectures – promises or reality. *Methods Inf Med* 2006; 45: pp 95-101.
[2]   Blobel B. *Analysis, Design and Implementation of Secure and Interoperable Distributed Health Information Systems*. Series "Studies in Health Technology and Informatics" Vol. 89. IOS Press, Amsterdam, 2002.
[3]   Blobel B: Educational Challenge of Health Information Systems' Interoperability. *Methods Inf Med* 2007; 46: pp. 52-56.
[4]   Blobel B: eHCC Conference Introductory Address. (in this volume)
[5]   Blobel B, Engel K, Pharow P: Semantic Interoperability – HL7 Version 3 Compared to Advanced Architecture Standards. *Methods Inf Med* 2006; 45: pp 343-353.
[6]   Health Level Seven Inc.: http://www.hl7.org
[7]   American Society for Testing and Materials: http://www.astm.org
[8]   EN/ISO 13606 "Health informatics – EHR communications": http://www.centc251.org
[9]   Australian Ministry for Health and Aging: The GEHR Project: http://www.gehr.org
[10]   Beale   T.   A   Model   Universe   for   Health   Information   Standards   (2003): http://www.deepthought.com.au
[11]   Oemig F, Blobel B. HL7 Conformance: How to do Proper Messaging. In: Bos L and Blobel B (Edrs.) *Medical and Care Compunetics 4*, pp. 298-307. Series Studies in Health Technology and Informatics, Vol. 127. IOS Press, Amsterdam, 2007.
[12]   National Electrical Manufacturers Association, Inc.: Digital Imaging and Communication (DICOM): http://www.nema.org
[13]   Integrating the Healthcare Enterprise: www.ihe.net, see also www.rsna.org
[14]   Blobel B, Pharow P, Norgall T. How to Enhance Integrated Care towards the Personal Health Paradigm? In: Kuhn KA, Warren JR, Leong T-Z (Edrs.) *MEDINFO 2007*, pp. 172-176. IOS Press Amsterdam, Berlin, Oxford, Tokyo, Washington, DC, 2007.
[15]   Blobel B, Nordberg R, Davis JM, Pharow P. Modelling privilege management and access control. *Int J Med Inf* 75, 8 (2006) pp. 597-623.
[16]   Canada Health Infoway Inc.: EHRS Blueprint, Version 2, March 2006. http://www.Infoway-Inforoute.ca
[17]   National Health Service: National Programme for IT, 2002. http://www.connectingforhealth.nhs.uk/
[18]   Harno K and Ruotsalainen P. Shareable EHR Systems in Finland. In: Bos L, Roa L, Yogesan K, O'Connell B, Marsh A, Blobel B (Edrs.) *Medical and Care Compunetics 3*, pp.327-336. Series Studies in Health Technology and Informatics, Vol. 121. IOS Press, Amsterdam, 2006
[19]   HealthConnect and NEHTA Road Map: http://www.nehta.gov.au
[20]   EHRVA. EHRVA Interoperability Roadmap. HIMSS EHRVA, Version 2.0, October 2006 http://www.himssehrva.org

[21]　Bernstein K, Bruun-Rasmussen M, Vingtoft S, Andersen SK, Nøhr C. Modelling and implementing Electronic Health Records in Denmark. International Journal of Medical Informatics, 2004
[22]　The Eurorec Institute: http://www.eurorec.org
[23]　Certification Commission for Healthcare Information Technology: http://www.cchit.org

Legal, Ethical, Political and Social
Challenges for the Advancement of
eHealth Systems

*eHealth: Combining Health Telematics, Telemedicine, Biomedical Engineering and
Bioinformatics to the Edge. Edited by B. Blobel, P. Pharow and M. Nerlich.
IOS Press, 2008*

Ethical Aspects of Future Health Care: Globalisation of Markets and Differentiation of Societies – Ethical Challenges

Eike-Henner W. KLUGE [1]
Department of Philosophy, University of Victoria, Canada

Abstract. The shift in health care to an aggregate corporate and distributed model dominated by electronic methods of diagnosis, record-keeping and communication spanning jurisdictional boundaries raises technical, social and paradigmatic issues. The technical issues concern the material natures of the tools, devices, procedures and protocols; the social issues gravitate around abstract matters like individual rights and models of responsibility within a corporate setting and accountability in inter-jurisdictional contexts; the paradigmatic issues centre in the question of how the rights and duties of traditional and direct health care translate into the mediated context of the globally expanded corporate model of eHealth and telemedicine. The present discussion presents a brief overview of the issues and sketches some of their implications for the evolution of contemporary health care.

Keywords. eHealth, ethics, health care globalization, privacy, telemedicine

Introduction

Health care, both in the private and the public sector, is rapidly moving into eHealth and telemedicine and, in the course of rationalizing administrative and delivery structures, is increasingly outsourcing diagnosis, consultation (both informatic and medical), data storage and manipulation etc.. In that sense — and to that extent — it is rapidly becoming an international affair. This globalization is especially pronounced in the private sector as health care providers, taking advantage of market niches, move beyond their original national boundaries with a concomitant distribution of administrative and delivery structures. This development, which is still in its infancy, presents a series of ethical and legal problems that touch not only health care associated professionals but also institutions, policy makers and societies at large.

More specifically, the scale of health care delivery is shifting from the traditional, more-or-less immediate setting that involved direct inter-personal contact and accountability, to an aggregate corporate model that is dominated by electronic methods of diagnosis and communication where contact is frequently mediated rather than direct, is spread out among a changing variety of individuals, and responsibility is

---

[1] Corresponding Author: Eike Henner W. Kluge, PhD, Professor, Department of Philosophy, University of Victoria, Canada; Email: ekluge@uvic.ca

distributed among a whole host of players whose roles are intricately choreographed into a complicated service-delivery ballet whose every facet is necessary for the process to function, but where accountability tends to be seen in institutional terms instead of personally and direct. The situation is further complicated by the fact that the delivery model itself is in the process of moving from a jurisdictionally localized approach to one that transcends national boundaries.

The process and the attendant issues have three distinct sets of parameters. One set is technical; the other, for want of a better term, could be called social and the third is paradigmatic. The technical parameters centre in issues that focus in the material natures of the tools, devices, procedures and protocols that are involved in the delivery of this expanded and distributed kind of health care; the social parameters gravitate around issues that involve more abstract matters such as individual rights and models of responsibility within a corporate setting, accountability in inter-jurisdictional contexts and ownership of (or control over) data. The third, paradigmatic, set of issues is perhaps the most difficult of all. It gravitates around the question of how the rights and duties that were more or less clearly understood in the immediate context of traditional and direct inter-personal health care delivery translate into the mediated and expanded context of the globally expanded corporate model of eHealth.

Health informatics in the larger sense of the term — which is to say, health informatics in the sense of the discipline that deals with the development and deployment of the tools that are necessary for providing health care in an electronically assisted mode — is of course only one player in this scheme of things. However, not to put too fine a point on it, it is a central player. It is the glue that facilitates eHealth, telemedicine and its associated developments and that holds the whole process together. This imposes special responsibilities on the discipline. These responsibilities were recognized from the very beginning, and have been addressed by various individuals and at various levels. Thus, on the technical level, issues such as reliability, quality control and usability of the electronic tools involved in the implementation of eHealth [1], the interoperability of data-processing, handling and communication devices and protocols [1], [2], [3], [4], the standardization of electronic health record (EHR) structures and of nomenclatures, syntax and semantics for EHRs [5], [6], [7], etc. all have been seriously considered and continue to receive close attention. Similarly, the social parameters have become a matter of some concern, and issues such as consent to data collection and usage [8], [9], [10], [11], [12], [13[, [14], legality of record exchange [8], [9], [10], [11], [12], [15], [16] and the question of record ownership and right of disposition have been closely scrutinized [8], [9], [10], [11], [12], [13], [15], [17]. Finally, right from the very start it was realized that the ethics of professional behaviour would be integral to the deployment of telemedicine and eHealth, and a move was initiated to develop relevant of codes of ethics for health information professionals (HIPs) as well as for health care professionals [18], [19], [20], [21]. However, treatment of the social issues has been piecemeal at best and various issues remain to be resolved — or at least resolved in a consistent fashion.

The paradigmatic issues have received even less attention, and indeed do not even seem to be on the intellectual horizon of many players. They are issues that are as abstract as they are profound and yet, because of their very nature, they condition any systematic deployment of telemedicine and eHealth and affect every aspect of the move to globalize health care delivery. They are the central issues that were mentioned in the beginning, and they can be captured in the following general question: How should the informatic rights and duties that were more or less clearly understood in direct inter-personal health and profoundly material health care delivery be translated into the mediated and expanded context of the globally expanded corporate model? The remarks that follow are intended as a brief overview of some of their manifestations.

1. The Logic of the Issues

With but a few exceptions, traditional health care delivery involved immediate and direct interpersonal contact between health care professionals and patients. It used material records for gathering, storing, using, manipulation and transmitting patient-relative data, and recognized a distinct line of physician-centred responsibility. While ethical and legal difficulties arose on occasion, by and large the overall framework was clear because it was conditioned by the Hippocratic model of the physician-patient relationship whose ethics set relatively clear boundaries on privacy, security, ownership and disposition of patient-relative information. Even administrative and epidemiological uses of patient-relative data were conditioned by this Hippocratic model, and relative clarity existed as to who had what responsibility. The relative clarity of this situation was also functionally related to the limited (and limiting) nature of paper-based records.

The development of EHRs fundamentally changed this. Personal health records, rather than being essentially nothing more than aides-memoir developed by physicians to assist in their treatment of individual patients, evolved into (more-or-less complete) patient analogues [22] where access to these records could take the place of direct contact with the patients themselves for diagnostic and treatment purposes. This not merely facilitated increased expert consultation among physicians but also allowed the development of eHealth as a real-time method of health care delivery, thereby changing the logic of health care delivery from that of a localized field of personal interaction to a distributed field of data-centred relationships that are not inherently confined to a particular juridical or cultural setting. It also facilitated the systematic expansion of patient-relative data for administrative and epidemiological purposes.

On the one hand, of course, this immediately increased the ability to provide appropriate, economical, efficient and timely patient care; on the other, however, it also complicated the ethical and legal landscape — and that on two levels: intra-jurisdictionally and inter-jurisdictionally. In particular, complications gravitating around questions of privacy, ownership, control and responsibility came to assume increased importance.

1.1. Intra-jurisdictional Issues

That is to say, the shift to EHRs and to a distributed mode of health car delivery separated the direct line that previously linked individual physicians and health care providers to their specific patients and put in its place a logically distributed complex. With this development, just as the therapeutic model became a mosaic with distinct parties, each contributing directly but distributedly to the therapeutic whole, so the record itself has become a multifactorial composite where multiple originators and contributors are the rule and lines of responsibility for content have become shared and thereby tend to become blurred.

Likewise, the electronic nature of the record itself and its increasingly distributed nature raise the question of who has responsibility for maintaining the records and for safeguarding their accessibility, integrity, usability and privacy. Where previously records were the responsibility of the health care provider and record-keeping personnel and professionals served in an essentially ancillary capacity, the very nature of the EHR, and the very nature of eHealth and telemedicine, injected the health information professional (HIP) as an important player into the mix and introduced a line of responsibility that was not inherently therapeutic in nature. This line of responsibility, therefore, cannot be evaluated in Hippocratic terms but requires a completely new approach. The situation is complicated still further by the increasing use of, and reliance on, computerization and diagnostic algorithms.

Moreover, as EHRs become increasingly more complete, expanding to include genetic and other data, and as the domain of who is affected or implicated by these data increases, jurisdictions can no longer afford to ignore questions of ownership and of control of the records themselves, and of the data that are contained in them. The issue becomes more and more pressing because of the potentially significant economic implications of some of these data. Rights of access and usage therefore become critical.

Finally, as health care delivery migrates from purely private or purely public delivery models to mixed public-private partnerships, and as outsourcing of different services, even within the same jurisdiction, becomes more common, the problematic assumes an even greater degree of complexity. The danger that obtains in this connection is that the rules, regulations and guidelines that are devised to deal with the problems and the issues that arise are formulated on an *ad hoc* basis in response to specific problems rather than in a principled fashion. This raises the real possibility of internal conflict, and sets the potential for litigation.

1.2. Inter-jurisdictional Issues

The situation becomes even more complicated as health care is increasingly seen as a commodity, rather than a right, as health care delivery on the international level is increasingly dominated by multi-national corporations either providing health care directly or on a mixed private-public partnership basis, and as telemedicine and eHealth start to move to the global plain. Information- and data-exchange are instrumental to, and integrally involved in, this development. By that very token, however, they present potentially serious problems.

Thus, in some jurisdictions, any information that is contained in a patient record belongs to the patient and, except for a few carefully delimited circumstances, may not be accessed, manipulated or communicated without the patients explicit or implied consent. In these jurisdictions, therefore, the overarching presumption that governs all informatic actions is that data access and disclosure will be governed by the values and standards of the patient.

On the other hand, there are jurisdictions in which this is not the case, and where control of patient-relative information either lies entirely in the hands of the health care provider or is controlled by the provider/professional to some significant degree. Examples here include the selective "blacklisting" of patient-information by health care providers so that patients will have access to this information only at the discretion (and under the supervision of) relevant professionals or institutional structures.[2]

It therefore follows that if the assumption of a single and consistent model of access control and determination no longer holds true — and this is increasingly the case in the distributed delivery context of global markets — the stage is set for serious complications. Lines of responsibility and matters of rights and duties become opaque. Consequently the move to globally situated health care providers and to inter-jurisdictionally based telemedicine and eHealth raises the problem of how to reconcile these conflicting approaches. Some jurisdictions — the European Union is here the most obvious example — have recognized the problem and have attempted to deal with it through regulatory provisions and by quasi-legislative means. However, these cannot be considered an unqualified success because the provisions still allow national laws and rules to predominate in critical and troublesome cases [23]. To put it bluntly, they leave unsolved precisely the central question of which laws and standards apply.

Nor is the situation resolved by issue-specific and overarching international treaties. Unless the treaties capture all players in the field of health care, they leave unresolved the question of what rules apply when health care delivery is truly global but some members of a health care team or corporate structure operate in jurisdictions that are not part of the treaty process. Nor is this an idle and merely academic speculation. Outsourcing of consultation to India by USA health care providers is a fact, and raises precisely this issue [24]. Consequently, prudent corporate management would suggest that in the absence of global treaties that regulate informatic issues, the development of multi-national corporate models of health care delivery, of globally-based mixed private public health care partnerships, of global outsourcing and of the use of eHealth on an international scale should confine itself to jurisdictions that share the same ethical and juridical perspective.

1.3. Collectivities and Consent

An especially difficult wrinkle is added to this problematic by the emergence of collectivities as ethically and juridically identifiable players. The issue already surfaced in the context of medical research, when investigators from one jurisdiction and from one cultural setting had access to tissues and genetic data from subjects in another setting. However, the globalization of markets and the use of eHealth has moved the issue squarely into the overall context of health care delivery; yet so far, with but a few exceptions, it has remained below the horizon of most health care- and informatics services providers. Specifically, then, it is the question of how to structure consent to health care and how to structure the collection, use, storage, manipulation etc. of the data that are acquired in the course of treating the collectivities themselves epidemiologically and as a group, on the one hand, and the individuals who are members of such groups on the other.

That is to say, collectivities may be defined as indigenous or ethnically distinctive groups that have no formal status as nation states but that are identifiable as the inheritors and practitioners of socio-culturally distinct customs and ways of life [25].

They may or may not be geographically defined [26], [27]. The first and best-known example of a collectivity that was not geographically based but received international recognition was that of Jews. This recognition was initially enunciated in the Balfour Declaration of 1917, was reasserted in several later international statements, and ultimately led to the establishment and recognition of Israel as an independent and sovereign nation state. Further expansion of the notion and recognition of the concept of a collectivity itself came with Article 27 of the International Covenant on Civil and Political Rights. This recognition of collectivities as ethically and juridically distinct entities that are similar in their rights to nation states was made still more explicit in 1982 when the United Nations passed ECOSOC Resolution 1982/34,7 which established an International Working Group to consider the rights of collectivities and indigenous peoples [28, 29]. Still more blatant recognition occurred in 1990 when the UN General Assembly passed Resolution 45/164 recognising 1993 as the International Year for the World's Indigenous People [30].

The reason that collectivities require special attention in the informatic context is that at least some collectivities — in particular those that are geographically localized — tend to hold the position that the genetic data of their members (and indeed any medical data that may yield information about members of the collectivity as such) are not entirely under the control of the subjects from whom the data are derived but, to a significant degree, are communal property. A good example of the issues that can arise in this connection is the case of patent No. 5,397,696 for PNG-1. The patent is for a genetic sequence found among the Hagahai of Papua-New Guinea. The sequence appears to confer resistance to the human T-lymphotropic Virus-1 (HTLV-1). The US researchers who were involved in its discovery apparently obtained permission to isolate and use the gene from the individual subjects whom they studied, but failed to obtain permission from the collectivity. The US, as funder of the researcher, patented the gene under United States Patent No. 5,397,696 but ultimately, in the face of international pressure and objections from UN agencies, had to abandon its claim and reassign it to the collectivity itself [31]. Clearly, this constitutes *de facto* recognition of collectivity-rights at the international level.

The example just cited deals only with genetic data. However, the underlying logic of the case — and there are others [25] — strongly suggests that in the case of collectivities, consent to the use, disclosure etc. of any data by any individual of a collectivity will be insufficient. A similar problematic, although in the opposite direction — whether a collectivity has control over the data of individual members of the collectivity — emerged in the case of Icelandic [32], [33] and Estonian [34] data banks. Unless eHealth in all of its aspects includes a consent process that honours these distinct perspectives, it will violate what are perceived to be fundamental ethical tenets. It may also encounter legal hurdles that are better addressed and solved at the outset rather than waiting for the problems to materialize. It will be a particular challenge for the HIP to design software templates that recognise these considerations.

2. Ethics, Commerce and Security Directives

Another difficulty that is beginning to emerge derives from a difference in philosophies about the relationship between individual rights and society as a whole. Strictly speaking, it is an issue that existed prior to the advent of EHRs, eHealth and telemedicine but that has started to become acute with the advent of searchable records and globally distributed health care and health information providers.

Some jurisdictions have distinct views on the circumstances under which health care related informatic privacy may be breached for non-medical reasons. That is to say, as has been pointed out on another occasion [35], EU Directive 2002/58 [36] and related Directives, as well as the *USA Patriot Act* [37], allow the non-consensual disclosure of personal health information for the sake of national/global security when this is deemed to be necessary in the eyes of relevant security agencies. Whatever one may think about the ethics of such provisions — and one is here reminded of the quote attributed to Benjamin Franklin: "They that can give up essential liberty to purchase a little temporary safety deserve neither liberty nor safety"— it presents problems for the global market.

At a very general level, it requires some international resolution of the question whether security concerns constitute a legitimate basis for abrogating, without the usual safeguards of openness, due process and reasonable doubt, the privacy rights that are integral to the health care tradition, and whether it is ethically appropriate to address problems that have nothing to do with health care by violating the standards and traditions of health care itself. More specifically, however, and in particular reference to globalization, socio-cultural differentiation and conflict of laws, it calls for an international harmonization of privacy and communication legislation so that provisions that are enacted in one jurisdiction do not undermine the laws of another.

More specifically still, and with respect to health care providers and developers of health care related IT and software providers that are US-based or that are subsidiaries under the control of US-based parent corporations, it raises the question whether they have a duty inform their clients of the potential for privacy violations by US intelligence services and intelligence agencies that share information with the latter. Must they disclose the security- and privacy-compromising potential inherent in the rules that govern their operations as US-based corporations or their inherent inability to guarantee the security of the technology and software that they develop, use or provide? The international development of certification standards that clearly spell out these various issues would obviously facilitate the resolution of this problematic. However, whether such certification will be developed will depend not only on the power of nation states to advance their own interests but also corporate considerations about how such certification will impact on competitiveness and the ability to survive as corporations. It is here that we shall see whether self-interest and economics triumphs over ethics.

Analogous questions arise for HIPs who are employed by such corporations and who are involved in the development, deployment and operation of EHR- and health-related software, of telemedicine and of eHealth. Should they ignore the factors that have been outlined, not inform their employers of these dangers and thereby become complicit through their inaction in any privacy violations that might occur, or should they alert their employers to these considerations and advocate that they distance themselves from US products, corporations and affiliates, thereby potentially undermining administrative efficiency and stultifying globally situated health care delivery? Likewise, do they owe it to the subjects of EHRs and to the recipients of telemedicine and eHealth — i.e., do they owe it to patients either individually or collectively as a group — to alert them of such possibilities? In the eventuality that the answer is in the affirmative, is this a duty that falls to the profession as a whole, or does it fall to the individual professional?

The US connection is merely an example — albeit a flagrant one. EU Directive 2002/58/EC Article 4:2 (as well as Article 1:3) may be presumed to give some guidance on this matter, since it states that

> *In case of a particular risk of a breach of the security of the network, the provider of a publicly available electronic communications service must inform the subscribers concerning such risk and, where the risk lies outside the scope of the measures to be taken by the service provider, of any possible remedies, including an indication of the likely costs involved.*

It might therefore be assumed that the issue has already been resolved because other jurisdictions have followed the US example. However, this is not really the case. As a closer consideration of the EU Directive shows, its provision only addresses the duties of service providers and not HIPs, and it only applies to public providers of communication services, not health care institutions or organizations. It therefore provides no guidance for the health care sector or for HIPs. Is it appropriate to assume that the underlying logic of this provision — which clearly goes to informed consent — extends into the health care sector and that it applies both to providers and HIPs? Is there a line of responsibility that connects HIPs to patients as well as institutions in this regard? The situation becomes even more confusing on other continents. With the possible exception of the IMIA Code of Ethics, no institutional or professional codes, rules or guidelines have currently addressed the issue.

3. Standards, Certification and Enforcement

The successful penetration of global markets by health care providers assumes not merely a secure and interoperable technical infrastructure but also an integrated and comparable set of professional standards for the informatics professionals who are responsible for its development and operation. This, in turn, necessitates some means not merely for assessing and certifying these qualifications but also of enforcing the standards and, if necessary, for administering disciplinary actions. As yet, only limited steps have been taken in this direction. In an ideal world, standards, certification and discipline would ultimately be referable to an independent body. It remains to be seen whether the real world will approximate this ideal for HIPs or whether it will leave it to the market place to provide a solution.

It may be worthwhile in this connection to reflect that globalized health care delivery also cannot function without the participation of informatically proficient health care professionals (HCPs). Consequently there arises the question whether it would be appropriate to require informatic qualifications from health care professionals engaged in eHealth and telemedicine. Given that there is currently no mechanism for ensuring internationally comparable standards in medical qualification, this may pose an immense challenge.

4. Identifiers

Finally, there is the question of personal identifiers. Personal identifiers of course are nothing new. For obvious reasons, and in one form or another, they have existed as long as there has been health care that made use of records. The advent of EHRs, eHealth and the globalization of health care delivery therefore changed nothing in this respect. What did change was that distributed health care delivery necessitates *unique* personal identifiers (UPIs) so that patient-relative data in distinct data bases can be linked.

At the same time, the very suggestion that UPIs might be necessary if electronically assisted health care delivery is to achieve its full potential raises two concerns. One focuses on the use to which such UPIs might be put by a nation state, the other on how they might be used by multi-national health care organizations. The first is the fear that by establishing UPIs, societies would make it easy for governments to link different data-bases and thereby facilitate the rise of surveillance societies that would fulfil our worst Orwellian nightmares. The second concern centres in the fear that with UPIs in the hands of commercial and international health care providers (who of course require distributed data lines and data bases for their operation), information privacy would no longer be governed by the rules of the patient's jurisdiction, and that the rights and responsibilities that had previously been demarcated in a relatively straightforward manner could no longer be clearly defined and could no longer be enforced effectively.

In one sense, this issue is technical in nature. Is it technically possible to guarantee that only duly qualified individuals (or agencies) using appropriate means can have access to personal data for medically justified reasons in a world of electronic records and globally distributed health care? If current developments are any indication, the answer is in the affirmative.

However, in another sense the issue is not technical at all. It is an issue of paradigms and perception. Specifically, it involves the paradigm of health care and the perception of how the individual is situated in the evolving social framework of health care delivery. That is to say, traditional health care delivery was localized and direct, and the individual's identity was materially grounded in the body of the individual her/himself. Moreover, the individuals' place in that framework was not defined in terms of data about that individual in a particular record or set of records but in terms of personal interactions between the individual as patient and the individual health care professional. Records merely functioned as professional and administrative aids.

By contrast, distributed health care delivery depends on records, uses a changing variety of diverse professionals who may not even be in contact with the patients. The record, therefore, becomes central in no merely accidental sense — and this threatens the individual patient's perception of himself as a person. It raises the paradigmatic fear of becoming re-defined as a mere set of data distributed among a variety of players and data banks [38]. This, in turn, prompts the inchoate fear that the ethical lines that governed the treatment of the patients in the old-style system will be replaced by a diffuse web of purely administrative considerations, where rights are trumped by efficiency and where responsibilities are shrugged off for the sake of for the sake of administrative ease and profit.

5. Conclusion

In other words, when all is said an done, the hurdles that eHealth, telemedicine and the globalization of health care face are not merely technical in nature — although these should not be underestimated. In a much deeper sense, they are paradigmatic. The paradigm of how health care is delivered is shifting because the new technology and the administrative structures which the latter has facilitated invalidate it.

Paradigms are anchored in cultures and in perceptual frameworks; that is why paradigm shifts are resisted. A paradigm shift can only be successful if there is a bridge that allows a transition from the old to the new. In this case, what is required is some means for translating the rights and duties that were more or less clearly understood in the context of direct inter-personal health and profoundly material health care delivery into the mediated and expanded context of the globally expanded health care delivery corporate model that relies on EHRs and electronic communication.

The most difficult task that faces the evolution of health care in this electronically assisted and globally distributed world, therefore, may not be that of finding technical solutions but of identifying the underlying ethical bridge that ties old and new together, and of clarifying the ethical framework that allows the paradigm shift to occur and that validates it.

References

[1]　SEISMED Consortium. *Data Security for Health Care vol. II, Technical Guidelines.* IOS Press, Amsterdam, 1996.

[2]　Blobel B, Pharow P (Edrs.) *Advanced Health Telematics and Telemedicine: The Magdeburg Expert Summit Textbook.* IOS Press, Amsterdam, 2003.

[3]　Marsh A, Grandinetti L, Kaurame T (Edrs.) *Advanced Infrastructures for Future Healthcare.* IOS Press, Amsterdam, 2000.

[4]　ISHTAR Consortium. *Implementing Secure Health Telematics Application in Europe.* IOS Press, Amsterdam, 2001.

[5]　Rooksby J and Kay S. Clinical Narrative and Clinical Organization: Properties of Radiology Reports. Proceedings of MedInfo 2001, 680-684.

[6]　Peleg M, Boxwala A, Tu S, Greenes RA, Shortliffe EH, and Patel VL. Handling Expressiveness and Comprehensibility Requirements in GLIF3. In: Patel VL, Rogers R and Haux R (Edrs.) *Proceedings of the 10th World Congress on Medical Informatics.* IOS Press, Amsterdam, 2001, pp.241-245.

[7]　Kushniruk AW and Patel VL. Cognitive approaches to the evaluation of healthcare information systems. In: Anderson JG and Aydin C (Edrs.) *Evaluating the organizational impact of healthcare information systems, 2nd ed.* Springer-Verlag, New York, 2005, pp. 144-173.

[8]　EU Directive 95/46 EC. Data Protection (Amendment) Act, 2003.

[9]　Canada. Privacy Act, R.S., 1985 c. P-21 and Personal Information Protection and Electronic Documents Act. R.S.C. 2000, c. 5.

[10]　New Zealand, Privacy Act, 1993.

[11]　Taiwan, Computer-Processed Personal Data Protection Law, August 11, 1995.

[12]　Germany, Bundesdatenschutzgesetz, 2003.

[13]　e-Health Ethics Initiative, "e-Health Code" (2000) accessed June 28, 2005 at http://www.ihealthcoalition.org/ethics.

[14]　Hi-Ethics, "Ethical Principles For Offering Internet Health Services to Consumers" (2000) accessed June 28, 2005 at http://www.hi-ethics.org/Principles/index.asp.

[15]　van Eecke P, Rienhoff O, Laske C, Wenzlaff P and Piccolo U (Edrs.) *A Legal Framework for Security in European Health Care Telematics.* Studies in Health Technology and Informatics, Vol. 74. IOS Press, Amsterdam, 2000.

[16]　Allaert F Blobel B and Barber B (Edrs.). *Security Standards for Health Information Systems.* IOS Press, Amsterdam, 2002.

[17]　Kluge E-H. *The Ethics of Electronic Patient Records.* Peter Lang, Bern and New York, 2001.

[18] IMIA Code of Ethics for Health Informatics Professionals .http://www.imia.org/code_of_ethics.html
[19] American Psychological Association, Ethics Committee issues statement on services by telephone, teleconferencing and internet, APA Monitor, 29:1 (January, 1998), p.38.
[20] Iverson KV. E-Health: A Proposal for an Ethical Code. *Camb. Q. Healthc. Ethics*, 9:3 (Summer 2000) 404-6.
[21] Rippen H and Risk A. E-Health ethics initiative, e-Health Code of Ethics. *Journal of Medical Internet Research* 2:2 (2000) e9 URL: http://www.jmir.org/2000/2/e9/
[22] Kluge, E-H. .Medical Narratives and Patient Analogues: The Ethical Implications of Electronic Patient Records. *Meth Inform Med* 38 (1999) pp 1-7.
[23] EU Directive 94/56 EC Article 4, Article 8.4, Article 13:1, etc. updated in EU Directive 2002/58.
[24] Vijaya K. Teleradiology Solutions: Taking expertise to hospitals in US. Express Health Care Management, Issue dtd. 16th to 29th February 2004, accessed September 25, 2006 at http://www.expresshealthcaremgmt.com/20040229/innews07.shtml.
[25] Wasserloos A. Die genetische Diversität des Menschen als Herausforderung für Bioethik und Humanwissenschaften. Berlin Weißensee, 2005
[26] Morgan. Advancing Indigenous Rights at the United Nations: Strategic Framing and its Impact on the Normative Development of International Law. Social and Legal Studies 13 (2004) 481–500.
[27] Xanthaki A. *Indigenous Rights and United Nations Standards.* Cambridge University Press, 2007.
[28] E/CN.4/Sub.2/1991/39.
[29] UN General Assembly Resolution 45/164.
[30] UN Doc E/CN 4/Sub 2/AC 4/1996/2, Working paper on the concept of Indigenous peoples.
[31] 1993 Mataatua Declaration on the Cultural and Intellectual Property Rights of Indigenous Peoples, and the 1995 Treaty for a Lifeforms Patent-Free Pacific and Related Protocols.
[32] Knoppers BM.. Of Populations, Genetics and Banks. Genetics Law Monitor, January/February 2001, 3-6.
[33] Hauksson P. Consent in Genetic Research in Iceland. accessed at http://www.insurancetranslation.com/Language_Perils/current.htm.
[34] Estonian Gene bank. accessed at http://www.geenivaramu.ee/mp3/Biotech%20in%20Estonia%202004%20sh%20Kalev%20Kask.pdf.
[35] Kluge E-H. Secure e-Health: managing risks to patient health data. Int J Med Inform 76(5-6): (2007) 402-6.
[36] Directive 2002/58/EC
[37] Uniting and Strengthening America by Providing Appropriate Tools Required to Intercept and Obstruct Terrorism Act (HR 3162) §215.
[38] van der Ploeg I. Biometrics and the Body as Information. Normative Issues of the Socio-Technical Coding of the Body. In: Lyon D (Edr.). *Surveillance as Social Sorting: Privacy, Risk and Digital Discrimination.* Routledge, New York, 2003, pp. 57-73.

Ubiquitous Care in Aging Societies - A Social Challenge

Sabine KOCH [1]
Centre for eHealth, Uppsala University, Sweden, and
Department of Learning, Informatics, Management and Ethics, Karolinska Institute,
Stockholm, Sweden

Abstract. The phenomenon of an aging society is frequently raised in scientific, public and political discussions in the developed world. It is well known that a number of challenges related to the demographic, economic and societal development will lead to increasing demands for health and social care. To cope with these challenges, effective delivery of health and social care will be more dependent on different technological solutions. The objective of this paper is to identify emerging technological solutions and to relate them to the expected changes occurring in an aging society. Results from an analysis of existing literature show that ubiquitous care in aging societies is merely a social than a technical challenge as it will require a redesign of today's healthcare processes. Supportive technologies have to be adapted to older people's needs, self-care processes and coping strategies, and to support new ways of healthcare delivery under close surveillance of patient safety, legal and ethical issues.

Keywords. Aging society, health information systems, smart homes, telecare, ubiquitous technologies

Introduction

In most developed countries, healthcare systems face a number of challenges leading to an increased demand for health and social care. These challenges are mainly related to;

1. The demographic development – a decreasing number of younger people will have to support increasing numbers of older, retired people. The old age dependency ratio in Europe is expected to double by the middle of this century[2] and the number of persons aged 80 and over (oldest-old) is expected to nearly triple, rising from 18 million in 2004 to 50 million in 2051 [1].

2. The economic development – higher standards of living will lead to greater expectations of the quality of healthcare systems. At the same time, public health services have to cope with financial resource constraints and shortage of skilled labor [2].

---

1 Corresponding Author: Sabine Koch, PhD, Associate Professor, Centre for eHealth, Uppsala University, Sweden, and Department of Learning, Informatics, Management and Ethics, Karolinska Institute, Stockholm, Sweden; Email: sabine.koch@ehealth.uu.se

[2] This means that whereas in 2004 there was one elderly inactive person (>65 years-old) for every four persons of working age (15-64 years-old), in 2050 there would be about one inactive person for every two of working age.

3. Societal factors – an increasing number of elderly people live alone, and increased mobility in society results in families/relatives distributed over large geographical areas. The challenge facing all western societies is twofold: ensuring that present and future elderly can look forward to improvements in their function and care, and countering the decreasing societal commitment to the elderly, who are often perceived as a "burden" [3].

Effective delivery of healthcare will be more dependent on different technological solutions supporting the decentralization of healthcare, higher patient involvement and increased societal demands.

The goal of this article is therefore to identify healthcare trends and new technological developments that appear due to an ageing society and to reflect upon the kind of upcoming technologies that should be introduced to meet the needs of a changing society.

1. Who Forms the Aging Society?

Population aging is characterized by changes in the proportion of different age groups and usually based on a three age group population model – young people (<20), those of working age (20-64), and elderly people (>64). According to Robine and Michel [4] this model does not reflect current population changes where we will see a decrease in the proportion of young people, followed by an increase in the working age group, leading to an immense increase in the oldest age group. Due to a higher life expectancy, this oldest age group will consist of younger retired people, the so called "sandwich generation", and very elderly people [5]. As these oldest old are expected to make up an increasing proportion of the number of retired people, the sandwich generation will play a pivotal role as informal caregivers [6]. Robine et al therefore propose to move to a four age group population model comprising young people, those of working age, younger retired people, and the oldest people (>84) [5]. Accordingly, Robine et al. also propose to use the oldest old support ratio[3] for monitoring changes in the age structure as a rough indicator of informal care resources for very elderly people, complementing the demographic ratio [5].

1.1. The Oldest People

The oldest people will be the pre-dominant patient group requiring health and medical care and/or social care. However, not all oldest people require help with their everyday needs. According to the US national long term care survey, for instance, only about half of Americans aged 85 or older are dependent on others to perform personal care or instrumental activities of daily living [6]. Moreover, the future oldest people, having benefited from higher education and better working and living conditions and being more wealthy, may prefer to pay for formal care rather than rely on family support [5].

1.2. Younger Retired People

The younger retired people are the active retired generation and will be the main contributors to long term care of the oldest people by providing informal care to their

---

[3] The number of people aged 50-74 divided by the number of aged >84.

parents. However, oldest old support ratios are expected to decrease. This will lead to a decrease of informal carers and may lead to an increase in formal care services [5]. This may also imply a greater need for different technical solutions to support informal carers and other relatives.

1.3. People of Working Age

In the light of an aging society, this age group will be represented by care professionals, informal family carers and patients. All three user categories will, depending on their current roles, need different kinds of technology in order to stay informed and play an active role in the care process.

1.4. Living Environments for the Elderly

Many communities market themselves as "Elder-friendly communities", that is places that actively involve, value, and support older adults, both active and frail, with infrastructure and services that effectively accommodate their changing needs. Alley et al identified the following as the most important characteristics of an elder-friendly community: accessible and affordable transportation, housing, healthcare, safety, and community involvement opportunities [7].

2. Emerging Ubiquitous Technologies

Computing applications in healthcare have become ubiquitous in the non-technical sense of being present everywhere [8]. They are, however, not yet ubiquitous in the true sense of the word, but rather are 'novel', being at the research, pilot, and selective use stage [9]. They present a major contribution to new models of care allowing for patient monitoring and telecare as well as information access and documentation at the point of need.

2.1. Smart Homes and Telecare

A more recent development in home based applications is the design of "Smart homes". A "smart home" is a residence setting equipped with a set of advanced electronics and automated devices specifically designed for care delivery, remote monitoring, early detection of problems or emergency cases and maximization of residents' safety and quality of life. The origins of the concept are to be found in the late 1970s and the1980s, when "intelligent buildings" were designed with the aim to improve energy efficiency and ventilation [10].

Smart home features nowadays focus among other things on monitoring the health status of the residents and improving their well-being using for example, motion-sensing devices to assess activity levels, temperature control devices, fall detection sensors, gait monitors etc. Such an infrastructure can address the prevalence of neurological and/or cognitive disorders in the elderly, and enhance their ability to function independently within their residence [10].

Current developments strive towards ambient intelligent environments where bio- and environmental sensors are combined with new methods for context-aware computing to allow for ageing in place (e.g. [11]).

One of the main challenges for smart homes is, however, not technological but social. It must be a sanctuary that is secure and private, and provide a harmonious space for relaxation and socialization [12]. Moreover, the increasing introduction of medical devices into the homes of the elderly and their interaction with different kinds of ICT solutions requires close surveillance and analysis of the medical, legal and ethical responsibilities [13].

2.2. Elderly-centric Information Systems

We observe a shift from organization-specific towards patient-centric care models regarding formal care. In medical informatics and related fields considerable research has been conducted to develop suitable technologies that support this shift in formal care [14]. Current research in the field of health information systems (HIS) is for example focused on supporting trans-institutional healthcare processes [15].

Also, health enabling technologies in form of unobtrusive, active, non-invasive technologies are emerging in form of personalized HIS [14]. Further, new approaches for sensor-enhanced regional health information systems (rHIS), integrating personalized HIS and institutional HIS, and their challenges for implementation are discussed in the literature [16].

However, the development of health information systems has often been too technology-centric [17] and the underlying process models are usually care professional driven and do not reflect the patient's point of view.

3. Future Care Models and Elderly Specific Design

Older people are not a homogenous group. They may belong to the oldest old or younger retired people, they may suffer from functional or mental disabilities or not and, in general, their needs and goals of life are not fundamentally different from those of any other adults. They want to remain independent as long as possible and to keep control over their lives once outside help is needed, thereby maintaining the feeling of independence [18].

A common prejudice by care professionals is that older people are unable or not willing to use new technology. 80% of Europe's home care decision makers e.g. believe that the acceptance of ICT-based services amongst older adults is very low [19]. However, the 2005 Eurostat ICT survey in all 25 member states revealed that 24.9% of the private individuals in age group 55-74 used the Internet over the past 12 months [20] and a recently published study shows that two third in the age group 55-64 use the Internet in Sweden [21]. We know that the future generation of elderly is more educated, more demanding and has experienced the fastest technology development ever. More than 80 percent of baby boomers fully expect scientific and technological advances to improve their lives as they age [22].

Future elderly are predicted to be more responsive to technology and technology is able to meet the demands of managing age-related diseases and disabilities. But what kind of technology will the demanding generation of future elderly accept? Products for disabled users are often thought to be used for elderly users, too. Whilst the physical needs may be similar, the elderly person, acquiring a disability slowly over time, often does not show the same level of awareness or acceptance that usually accompanies disabilities at birth or by accident [23]. Instead other family members or informal carers are often the first to realize the need for specific technologies or aids. This accentuates the increasing role of family members, relatives and informal carers not only as future care resources but also as target costumers for new product design.

Ongoing developments in our society towards a more fragmented, multi-cultural society further accentuate the demand for highly individual, personalized solutions. The paradigm shift regarding care models does not only include a shift towards integrated care models from a care professional's point of view. It also includes a shift towards partnership models, involving the family carer as expert [24] or the patient as expert, demanding a redesign of traditional HIS. Elderly people tend to apply self-care strategies that develop from active to passive towards the end of life [25]. Although coping strategies are strongly related to the personality, active coping strategies can be supported by for example access to information, informal networks, web communities and active participation in shared care planning. Often suffering from multiple diseases, the elderly need proactive management from healthcare professionals following agreed protocols, shared care plan and personal life goals [26]. This requires an ICT infrastructure with improved support for coordination of work and cooperation, including decision support, between different healthcare professionals but also between patients and their relatives which are today a fairly unused resource.

The combination of formal and informal care giving and self care, both locally and at a distance, involving a large number of different actors, can be supported technically. However, implementation of these technical solutions requires the redesign of healthcare processes from a patient's perspective and close surveillance of patient safety, ethical and legal issues.

4. Conclusions

An ageing society requires increased accessibility of care outside traditional care settings turning home healthcare into one of the most challenging healthcare areas from a technological point of view with large social implications if the patients can stay in their well-known daily environment. More specifically, the main challenges can be summarized as follows:

- Home healthcare is dependent on patient-centric shared care models that require a more efficient work organization and better communication and cooperation between medical specialists, formal and informal carers, patients and relatives.

- Home healthcare is characterized by highly mobile work situations, different user profiles (care professionals, next-of-kin and different patient groups with different cultural backgrounds) and a need for access to information from a variety of technically and locally distributed databases and medico-technical equipment. This puts high demands on interoperability, usability, safety, security, availability and accessibility as well as on legal and ethical aspects.

- Home healthcare really requires user-friendly, personalized and reliable solutions as there is no technical support nearby as e.g. in a hospital.

- Talents, behaviors and active involvement of residents in a specific household and their next-of-kin complement the work in healthcare institutions. In taking increasing responsibilities for their own health, laypeople face growing health information management challenges. Consequently, what was an optional choice by an individual to engage in becomes an essential responsibility.

In order to fully exploit the emerging new technologies, the debate must move from focusing solely on the technologies, and move to their systematic application and their embedding into the local health system [27]. Indeed, given the future challenges of the ageing population, ubiquitous technologies must not just be bedded into the health system, but by very definition produce a paradigm shift in the design and functioning of that system [28]. This requires a cross-disciplinary research approach to fully understand the social dimension, to consider the clinical pre-requisites, to accommodate the probability of co morbidity but the need for a holistic integrated service, to analyze the individual needs of all stakeholders and to develop appropriate and usable technological solutions under close surveillance of a legal and ethical regulatory framework.

References

[1]   Lanzieri G. Eurostat Statistics in focus "Long-term population projections at national level". Newsletter 3/2006 http://www.europa.eu.int/comm/eurostat/ (last accessed September 23, 2007).

[2]   Cabrera M, Burgelman J-C, Boden M, da Costa O, Rodriguez C. eHealth in 2010: Realising a Knowledge-based Approach to Healthcare in the EU. Challenges for the Ambient Care System – Report on eHealth related activities by IPTS. Technical Report EUR 21486 EN http://forera.jrc.es/documents/eur21486en.pdf (last accessed September 29, 2007).

[3]   Gordon M. Problems of an Aging Population in an Era of Technology. *J Can Dent Assoc* 2000; 66: 320-2

[4]   Robine JM, Michel JP. Looking forward to a general theory on population aging. *J Gerontol A Biol Sci Med Sci* 2004; 59: M590-7.

[5]   Robine JM, Michel JP, Herrmann FR. Who will care for the oldest people? *BMJ* 2007; 334: 570-71.

[6]   Spillman BC, Pezzin LE. Potential and active family caregivers: changing networks and the "sandwich generation". *Milbank Q* 2000; 78: 347-74.

[7]   Alley D, Liebig P, Pynoos J, Banerjee T, Choi IH. Creating elder-friendly communities: preparations for an aging society. *J Gerontol Soc Work.* 2007; 49 (1-2): 1-18

[8]   Roger-France FH. Progress and challenges of ubiquitous informatics in health care. In: Hasman A et al. *Ubiquity: Technologies for Better Health in Aging Societies.* Stud Health Tech Inf, (2006), 124: 32-6

[9]   Rigby M. Applying emergent ubiquitous technologies in health: The need to respond to new challenges of opportunity, expectation, and responsibility. Int J Med Inf 2007; article in press: doi: 10.1016/j.imedinf.2007.03.002

[10] Demiris G. Home based e-health applications. In: Demiris G (Edr.) *E-Health: Current Status and Future Trends.* IOS Press, Studies in Health Technology and Informatics, Vol 106 (2004), 15-24.

[11] http://www-static.cc.gatech.edu/fce/ahri/index.html (last accessed September 30, 2007)

[12] Punie Y. A social and technological view of Ambient Intelligence in Everyday Life: What bends the trend? EMTEL Report 2003. http://www.lse.ac.uk/collections/EMTEL/reports/punie_2003_emtel.pdf (last accessed September 30, 2007)

[13] Koch S. Facing the challenges – the role of medical informatics in an ageing society. In: Hasman A et al. *Ubiquity: Technologies for Better Health in Aging Societies.* Stud Health Tech Inf, (2006), 124: 25-31

[14] Haux R. Individualization, globalization and health – about sustainable information technologies and the aim of medical informatics. Int J Med Inform 75, 2006; 795-808

[15] Bott OJ. Health Information Systems: Between Shared Care and Body Area Networks. Findings from the Section on Health Information Systems. *IMIA Yearbook of Medical Informatics 2006*: 53-6

[16] Bott OJ, Marschollek M, Wolff K-H, Haux R. Towards New Scopes: Sensor-enhanced Regonal Health Information Systems – Part 1: Architectural Challenges. *Methods Inf Med* 2007; 46 (4): 476-83

[17] Stefanelli M. Knowledge Management in Health Care Organizations. In: *Yearbook of Medical Informatics 2004.* Towards Clinical Bioinformatics. IMIA and Schattauer GmbH, 2004; 144-55.

[18] Aronsson J. Elderly people's accounts of home care rationing: missing voices in long-term policy debates. Aging and Society 2002; 22: 399-418.

[19] SeniorWatch Report "Older People and Information Society Technology". http://www.seniorwatch.de (last accessed September 27, 2007).

[20] Ottens M. Eurostat Statistics in focus "Use of the Internet among individuals and enterprises". Newsletter 12/2006 http://www.europa.eu.int/comm/eurostat/ (last accessed September 23, 2007).

[21] Sverige i Europa, Rapport 0704220, World Internet Institute, http://www.wii.se/content/view/55/32/lang,se/ (last accessed October 11, 2007)

[22] Rehabilitation Institute of Chicago http://www.ric.org/aboutus/mediacenter/press/2003/1210a.aspx (last accessed September 29, 2007)

[23] Coughlin JF. New Expectations From Older Users: Five Lessons for Product Design & Innovation in an Aging Marketplace. AgeLab 2007-01. Cambridge, Massachusetts: Massachusetts Institute of Technology. http://web.mit.edu/agelab/ (last accessed September 24, 2007)

[24] Nolan M, Grant G, Keady J. Understanding family care. Open University Press, Buckingham, 1996

[25] Dunér A, Nordström M. Intentions and strategies among elderly people: Coping in everyday life. Journal of Aging Studies 2005; 19: 437-51.

[26] Augusto JC, Black ND, McAllister HG, McCullagh PJ, Nugent CD. Pervasive Health Management: New Challenges for Health Informatics. Journal of Universal Computer Science, 2006; 12 (1): 1-5.

[27] Rigby M. Ubiquitous Technologies in Health: New Challenges of Opportunity, Expectation, and Responsibility; in Hasman A, Haux R, van der Lei J, De Clercq E, Roger France FH. Ubiquity: Technologies for Better Health in Aging Societies – Proceedings of MIE2006; IOS Press, Amsterdam, 65-70.

[28] Decentralization of Healthcare via Distributed Diagnosis and Home Healthcare (D2H2): MA, AMIA, and IEEE Conference, Washington, DC, April 2006. http://icsl.ee.washington.edu/d2h2/program.html (last accessed October 1, 2007).

eHealth: Combining Health Telematics, Telemedicine, Biomedical Engineering and Bioinformatics to the Edge. Edited by B. Blobel, P. Pharow and M. Nerlich.
IOS Press, 2008

eHealth for Service Delivery – Special Considerations for Resource-Challenged Health Systems

S. Yunkap KWANKAM [1]
Department of Knowledge Management and Sharing, World Health Organization, Geneva, Switzerland

1. Background Information on eHealth in WHO

Developments in information and communication technologies (ICT) have ushered in an era of profound opportunity and potential for world-wide advancement in public health and clinical care, and eHealth systems today constitute a third major industrial pillar on which the health sector is built. There is a tendency to think that eHealth is a tool exclusively for the industrialized world. This is not true, as evidenced by the number of telehealth projects in developing countries [1]. However, in resource-constrained health systems special considerations need to be made in order to best take advantage of these developments.

The World Health Organization has carried out a number of key actions at policy level, aimed at bringing the power of ICT to bear positively on health challenges at national, regional and global levels. These include: the development of an Organization-wide eHealth strategy, the passage by the World Health Assembly (the highest organ of WHO), of a resolution on eHealth in May 2005; the endorsement by the WHO Executive Board, in January 2006, of a set of priority action areas, and the establishment of a Unit on eHealth to coordinate activities in this area.

eHealth is also one of five strategic directions of WHO's knowledge management strategy. The others are: a) access to health information; b) translating knowledge into policy and practice; c) sharing and reapplying experiential knowledge; d) creating an enabling environment for knowledge management (through culture change, and other mechanisms).

1.1. Resolution on eHealth

World Health Assembly resolution WHA58_28 calls on Member States to carry out a number of activities in the area of eHealth, including: drawing up long-term strategic plans for developing and implementing eHealth services; development of infrastructure for ICT; closer collaboration with the private and non-profit sectors in ICT; reaching communities, including vulnerable groups, with eHealth services appropriate to their needs; mobilizing multisectoral collaboration for determining evidence-based eHealth

---

[1] Corresponding Author: S. Yunkap Kwankam, PhD, Professor, e-Health Coordinator, World Health Organization, Department of Knowledge Management and Sharing, 20, Avenue Appia, Geneva 27, Switzerland; Email: kwankamy@who.int, URL: http://www.who.int/kms

standards and norms; evaluating eHealth activities, and sharing the knowledge of cost-effective models; establishing national centers and networks of excellence for eHealth best practice, policy coordination, and technical support; establishing and implementing national electronic public-health information systems. The resolution further requests the WHO Director-General, inter alia: to provide technical support to Member States in relation to eHealth products and services by disseminating widely experiences and best practices, devising assessment methodologies, promoting research and development, and furthering the development and use of eHealth norms and standards.

1.2. Priority areas

Following the resolution, the 117th session of the Executive Board of WHO approved the following priority areas for eHealth work: i) Legal and ethical aspects of eHealth, ii) a Global Observatory for eHealth, iii) public-private partnerships for ICT R&D and application in health, iv) ICT in support of human resources for health, v) ICT for health education and promotion, vi) eHealth for health care services. These new areas are in addition to the ongoing priorities of a) access to health information; and b) promoting the development and use of norms and standards to enable the exchange of information and knowledge as well as facilitate interoperability among systems.

2. Articulation of eHealth Vision around Four Key Areas

eHealth disconnect? We talk about e"Health", but our discussions are mostly about disease and and curative interventions. Yet we know that a production function for health would necessarily include: a) water and sanitation; b) food and nutrition; c) housing and shelter; d) education; as well as e) health care. Current eHealth efforts have focused heavily on contributing to improved health through supporting health care interventions. There is a need to examine other pathways to health and how ICT can improve their effectiveness At the very least we need to invest more effort to examine how ICT can help reduce health inequalities.

As to an emphasis on wellness, the ecology of medical care shows that in a given month, as many as 20% of those served by the health care system show no signs of illness [2]. Investments in prevention would reap significant benefit in heading off greater expenses in providing care to the sick. Recent evidence points to preventive health as the primary domain of improvement from the use of information technology in health, and decreased utilization of care as the major efficiency benefit realized.

A few examples: Nano-filters in are being used in Bangladesh for removing pollutants and ensuring that water is safe to drink. Similarly, nano-sensors are for monitoring water quality at reduced cost, as well as nano-membranes in the treatment of wastewater.

Sensor technologies for monitor vulnerable environments and prevent or limit natural disasters. In general sensors exist today for water quality, air quality, weather, soil moisture, leaf wetness, biotelemetry, video (web cam), and others. Extensive and effective systems can be deployed to ensure early warning and evacuation, thereby reducing loss of life due to natural disasters. Special robots are now available for mine detection to save lives and limbs in conflict and post-conflict zones [3].

3. Strengthening Health Systems through eHealth

The health system framework proposed by WHO shows not only health status, but also responsiveness and financial fairness as goals of the system. Consider financial protection in that context. In developing countries, out-of-pocket payment is the largest share of the health care dollar - as much as 75c on average. These expenditures are sometimes catastrophic to the economies of the families involved, leading to impoverishment and a cycle of ill-health and poverty. What can eHealth do to mitigate the high cost of health care, especially for the vulnerable and poor?

In general, eHealth can strengthen health systems by focusing on the interactions between ICT and health systems – the development, deployment and use of these technologies to support health system goals and functions. eHealth should provide eHealth policy and implementation options and tools to maximize the capacity of countries to effectively and efficiently deploy ICT to strengthen health systems and improve service delivery. In fact, ICT is seen in the Millennium Declaration as an enabler of for the attainment of all the MDGs. Hence Target 18, which states, "In cooperation with the private sector, make available the benefits of new technologies, especially information and communications."

4. Bridging the Know-do Gap

Knowledge has been a key driver of the health gains recorded in the 20th century. We have indicated earlier that ICT is the third major industrial pillar of the health sector. It supports not only health, but also other sectors of the new knowledge economy. A knowledge economy (including health sector) is "one in which the generation and exploitation of knowledge has come to play a predominant part in the creation of wealth. It is not simply about pushing back the frontiers of knowledge; it is also about the more effective use and exploitation of all types of knowledge." [4] It is also characterized by: "an economic and institutional regime that provides incentives for the efficient use of existing and new knowledge and the flourishing of entrepreneurship; an educated and skilled population that can create, share, and use knowledge well; a dynamic information infrastructure that can facilitate the effective communication, dissemination, and processing of information."

4.1. Knowledge and the Know-do Gap

There is no disputing the importance of new discoveries. So, we should promote cutting edge research, to pushing further affield the frontiers of knowledge. However, we also need balance between investments in new scientific discovery and investments in the application of these discoveries - to improve health in our case. This emphasizes the importance of purpose in knowledge management. There is a growing know-do gap in health: the gap between what is known and what gets done. Most of today's premature death, especially among poor children and women, are due to problems for which are either preventable of for which there are known solutions [5].

This chasm between innovative research and effective practice, often referred to as the contributes to missed opportunities in public health [1, 6]. The knowledge accrued during the 20th century is now ripe for strategic development (i.e. 'translation') and application [7, 8]. New global funds for health, unimaginable a mere decade ago, are reducing financial hurdles [9]. Effective translation would justify increased social investment in strategic research.

4.2. Drowning in Data

A visit at many health facilities or district health offices in remote areas will readily show that health data, when collected and archived on paper, can be overwhelming. One could almost see health workers drowning in data. It is reported that in 2003, 40% of knowledge workers' time was spent managing documents. There are two metaphors inherent in such scenarios of health staff surrounded by stack and stacks of paper records. One is that as more and more data are collected, the average value of an item of data will decrease dramatically, and the real value will be in tools which enable one to sift through the masses of data to get at the nuggets of knowledge that are relevant to one's purpose.

The increasing volume, speed and access to information will require meta-systems to triage and personalize information. It is also reported that in 2004, 60% of IT budgets were spent on managing interfaces to integrate applications and data.

Secondly, such scenarios emphasize the value of tacit or experiential knowledge - that knowledge which comes from experience, insights and relations, and which cannot be easily digitalized - and the challenges inherent in attempting to capture and share this type of knowledge. Paradoxically, IT will also underscore the limits of explicit knowledge and create a premium on tacit knowledge [10].

5. Increasing Productivity of the Health Workforce

The World health Report 2006 highlighted the dearth of health workers world wide. It reported a shortage of over 4 million health workers. In some areas, the needs are staggering. In Africa, for example, the need in the 36 worst hit countries is to train 2.8 million new health workers. Assuming a 20-year time frame to achieve this scale up of the workforce, this need translates to training 140 thousand new workers trained every year. On average then, each country must train 77 thousand over the twenty-year period, or 3,800 workers per year for 20 years. This means producing on average 10 additional health workers per day. Unfortunately, current estimates of training output for Africa range from 10% to 30% of what is needed. In addition, it is estimated that the costs of scale-up, in terms of both training and salaries, will increase the annual health budget by around $10/capita minimum by the year 2025.

Fortunately, there are encouraging signs from a number of successful examples which illustrate the breadth of approaches on how this challenge may be met using eLearning and other ICT-mediated forms of educational delivery.

The PROFAE project in Brazil was able to train 324,000 nurse auxiliaries in 4 years, while in Kenya the skills of 22,000 nurses will be upgraded in 5 years at fraction of cost required using traditional methods. Even more impressive is the time for such training to be completed, which will be cut to less than 10%.

Another example is from The Seychelles, a country made of over one hundred islands. The country recently graduated its first cohort of nurses, without benefit of a brick-and-mortar nursing school, through distance learning supported by ICT.

There are also many content repositories freely available from which courseware could be obtained for adaptation and use locally.

What is clear is that different aspects of ICT support to the development of the health workforce complement one another. Telehealth practice does not only support service delivery, it also facilitates the transfer of knowledge and skills. South Africa has a Health Channel which is not only used for providing health education for the public in waiting rooms, but the infrastructure is also used for updating health professionals with on-demand continuing medical education (CME) courses in 250 sites. And so, even when we focus on scaling up, we should not forget that various ICT interventions need to be considered together.

6. Health Promotion

6.1. Predicting Trends in Health

Health systems, like all systems have natural frequencies – intrinsic response time or built in delays. Today's interventions are in response to yesterday's challenges and will not show effects until tomorrow. We therefore must be able to predict what the challenges will be and design interventions. How can we prepare for the future if we cannot predict it?

WHO has carried out projections on mortality and published these in early 2006. The report shows a shift in the distribution of deaths from younger age groups to older age groups, and from communicable diseases to noncommunicable diseases. It further shows that the four leading causes of death globally in 2030 will be ischaemic heart disease, cerebrovascular disease (stroke), HIV/AIDS and chronic obstructive pulmonary disease. Tobacco attributable deaths are projected to rise from 5.4 million in 2005 to 6.4 million in 2015 and to 8.3 million in 2030. Tobacco is projected to kill 50% more people in 2015 than HIV/AIDS and to be responsible for 10% of all deaths.

The top four causes of mortality in the future are either avoidable or remediable through lifestyle modification. Health promotion using ICT modalities such as eLearning can therefore reap major benefits in prevention. Consider, for example, the impact that electronic information and education campaigns have had in fight against HIV/AIDS.

It is also clear that with people living longer and more deaths occurring from chronic conditions and not episodic illness, there will be a need to manage conditions outside of formal health care institutions. There will not be enough beds to institutionalize the chronically ill and, as we have already seen, there is a shortage of health workers to staff the institutions. Health promotion as well as prevention and telehome care for the sick become important options to consider. Arm the citizen with information and knowledge and the health system will transform itself.

6.2. The Health Academy

WHO has developed the Health Academy, a health promotion program to help create informed citizens, which are key elements in successful prevention and of the therapeutic process when they become patients. The Health Academy aims at investing in people, especially the younger generation, by bringing together technology, health information, and education for the benefit of human development.

The Health Academy transforms learners from passive recipients of information to active participants in knowledge acquisition. Using the concept of eLearning, it provides hands-on practice with automated feedback giving the learner immediate feedback, and offers effective learning and instruction at the learner's own pace. Courses are prepared and validated by WHO technical units and employ text, audio/visual aids, illustrations, photos and animations to convey health information in an attractive and simple language in a multimedia format. Practical activities, instructional games and quizzes are integral components of Health Academy eLearning courses. The courses are distributed to target schools either through the Internet or intranet connection (if available in the country) or on CDROMs, and can be used as part of a school curriculum [11].

A pilot study of the Health Academy eLearning courses was carried out in Egypt and Jordan during 2003/2004 academic year. It involved a total of 6,785 students (4,264 female and 2,491 male) in the age range 12 to 17 years old in 45 schools both government and private. A total of four courses were offered covering the health issues associated with blood safety, road safety, substance use and tobacco use. This experience was very well received in all schools by both students and school teachers (mentors). The students' evaluation of the courses was most positive and many related a positive experience in sharing their new found knowledge with their families.

Course modules cover subject areas such as: water and sanitation, HIV/AIDS, substance abuse, mental health, blood safety, etc. The module on road safety is timely as the WHO projections on mortality indicate a 40% increase in global deaths resulting from injury between 2002 and 2030, predominantly due to the increasing number of deaths from road traffic accidents.

Evaluation conducted by independent entities in both countries demonstrated an overall increase in knowledge and in some aspects a tendency to change attitudes and possibly behavior. This was particularly noticeable with respect to tobacco use.

The initiative collaborates with other organizations, public and private, to fulfill its mission. The new Partnership for African Development (NEPAD) eSchools project, e.g., has connected 120 schools in 20countries to the Internet, with an eventual target 600,000 eSchools. Health Academy content will be shared in the Health Point component of the eSchools.

7. Ensuring Equity

The value of knowledge in health and the economy are increasingly recognized. Gains in life expectancy in the 20th century surpassed those of all of recorded history before the 20th century. But this increase in life expectancy is far from uniform. There are still major disparities between rich and poor countries. Sub-Saharan Africa, for example, has seen setbacks in life expectancy as exemplified by the case of Botswana and South Africa. Health inequalities span the spectrum from life expectancy, to human resources for health, to so-called 10-90 gap in health research, where 90% of health research spending is on 10% of the disease burden. These inequalities exist in technology diffusion, with the term "digital divide" used as the metaphor for disparities in Internet connectivity, availability of servers, the flow of information, etc.

The promotion of equity in health is essential, also including the cutting edge of equity. The health system framework defines as goals to explore health status and to allocate distribution of services properly, including mathematical model for computing health.

Study of trends clearly showed that technology improves averages, but also tends to increase inequalities by increasing the gap between the rich and the poor. The well offs are better able to adopt and otherwise take advantage of technology than the less well offs.

Therefore, there is a requirement to focusing attention on the needs of the less well off through targeted interventions.

8. Examples of Programs that Aim at Reducing Inequalities

8.1. HINARI

Initiated after a study to identify the main constraints to building health research capacity in developing countries, the Health InterNetwork Access to Research Initiative (HINARI) was launched in 2000. It provides free or very low-cost online access to 4,060 major journals in biomedical and related social sciences to local, non-profit institutions in developing countries, and is one of the world's largest collections of biomedical and health literature. There are presently 2,856 participating institutions in 108 countries, and during 2005, users downloaded over 2,000,000 articles. The program is a partnership with 111 of the world's leading biomedical publishers, and other institutions from academia and the UN system. If one estimates the cost of a single subscription to the set of titles at around $2.5million, then the HINARI program represents a value of over $7 billion, annually

8.2. Sharing eHealth Intellectual Property for Development

Despite the potential of eHealth to support health system functions and goals, many resource-challenged health systems are unable to take advantage of these eHealth developments because they do not have access to these proprietary products and services. Inspired by the success of HINARI, a number of organizations are willing to make their products and services available, as appropriate, to all peoples of the world through WHO. Hence the Sharing ehealth Intellectual Property for Development (SHIPD) initiative has been launched.

8.2.1. Vision for the Initiative

Health systems are strengthened and health is improved in low and middle income countries by providing these countries access to eHealth intellectual property rights to appropriate products and services through WHO.

8.2.2. Objectives for the Initiative

The objective of this initiative is to strengthen health systems and improve health in countries through the adaptation and deployment of the donated/shared IP for eHealth products and services. The project will therefore:

- Adapt the eHealth resources to the local context in each country/region:
- Building capacity in countries to use the technology resources

- deploy the resources in countries around the world
- Strengthening WHO capacity to deliver the program
  - WHO staff to manage adaptation and deployment - at Headquarters, Regional Office and Country Office levels
  - Collaborating centers in institutions as needed

8.2.3. Partnership for the Initiative

The vision will be achieved through a partnership. In addition to WHO, all organizations allowing access to their eHealth intellectual property will be members of the partnership on sharing eHealth IP for development. The specific mechanism for such access will be determined on a case-by-case basis.

8.2.4. Initial Partners for the Initiative

Informa – Map of Medicine
Medic-to-Medic (Informa) provides the Map of Medicine for quick access, at the point of care, to the most appropriate clinical information on evidence-based best practices for conditions in all the major areas of medicine. Medic to Medic produces the Map of Medicine, an IT tool that gives an easy-to-use, evidence-based approach to enable healthcare professionals to identify best practices for conditions in all the major areas of medicine [12].

NHS Connecting for Health
NHS Connecting for Health is delivering the National Programme for IT (NPfIT) to bring modern computer systems into the NHS in England which will improve patient care and services. Over the next ten years, the National Programme for IT will connect over 30,000 GPs in England to almost 300 hospitals and give patients access to their personal health and care information, transforming the way the NHS works [13].

NHS National Knowledge Service
Established as part of the Government's response to the Bristol enquiry (Learning from Bristol January 2002), the National Knowledge Service (NKS) is developing a strategic approach to the management of the £150M annual NHS expenditure on knowledge and information services and to obtaining the best value from such investment. The aim of NKS is to ensure that all decisions made in the NHS are informed by best current knowledge.

MEDoctor
MEDoctor Systems is a comprehensive computer-assisted diagnostic decision support system which cross-references symptoms to disease diagnostic categories, providing instantaneous differential diagnoses, and currently operates in five languages.

Other Organizations
Discussion is under way with other organizations with an interest in supporting this initiative, and they will be brought in as appropriate.

8.2.5. Pilot Phase for the Initiative

In November 2007, ten teaching hospitals in six African countries received access to the Map of Medicine in a pilot. The countries are Cameroon, Nigeria, Kenya, Tanzania,

Uganda and Zambia. Other developing regions of other continents are envisaged in the future.

9. Conclusion

There has been rapid growth of ICT in the developing world, as exemplified by average rates of penetration of mobile phones and the Internet which are the highest anywhere today. As expected, the catch-up process for developing countries (which have the most resource-constrained health systems) is occurring much faster with newer technologies than with older ones. Investment in such systems by developing countries represents money well spent, both for immediate benefits and for future gains. It is important to focus attention on the use of available knowledge by underserved communities, such as developing country health systems. Monitoring progress in the assimilation of ICT among the disadvantaged will be important as causal pathways are charted between eHealth technology and health outcomes for both the rich and the poor.

One of the most cited examples of successful application of ICT is the Tanzania essential health improvement project (TEHIP). In this case, basic information systems generated enough evidence to have a more rational allocation of resources, which couple with sound management and a modest investment translated in halving child mortality within 5 years. Similar results have been accomplished in Bangladesh, as well as in Egypt for maternal mortality.

Challenges in health rarely come as well packed problems in one specific discipline, but are often overarching problems that require culling information and knowledge from a number of disciplines to attempt to solve them. It is therefore gratifying to note that the Regensburg conference has focused on combining health telematics, telemedicine, bioengineering and bioinformatics. Through such holistic approaches to ICT in health we can expect to not only increase the benefits for the health sector in all countries from this *great enabler*, but also pay special attention to the specific challenges faced by resource-constrained health systems.

References

[1]   See for example, Telemdedicine and Developing Countries: A report of Study Group 2 of the ITU Development Sector, David Wright, Rapporteur, Study Group 2, Question 6; Journal of Telemedicine and Telecare, vol. 4, supp. 2 1998
[2]   Green LA, Fryer GE, Yawn BP, Lanier D, Dovey SM. NEJ M 344:26 2001
[3]   ITU Internet Report 2005: The Internet of things
[4]   United Kingdom's white paper *Our Competitive Future: Building the Knowledge-Driven Economy (1998)* at (www.dti.gov.uk/comp/competitive/main.htm)
[5]   Ezzati M, Vander Hoorn S, Rodgers A, Lopez AD, Mathers CD, Murray CJL and the Comparative Risk Assessment Collaborating Group. Estimates of global and regional potential health gains from reducing major risk factors. Lancet 2003; 362:271-80.
[6]   Pfeffer J, Sutton RI. The Knowing-Doing Gap: How Smart Companies Turn Knowledge into Action. Harvard Business School Press, Boston, MA, 2004.
[7]   Geiger RI., Research and Relevant Knowledge. American Research Universities since World War II (Oxford University Press, 1993).
[8]   Davis D, Evans M, Jadad A, et al. The case for knowledge translation: shortening the journey from evidence to effect. BMJ 2003: 327:33-35.
[9]   Berwick D. A learning world for the Global Fund. BMJ 2002; 325:55-56.
[10]   Kwankam SY et al. "eHealth" In: Unwin T (Edr.) *ICT for Development.* in press (2008).

[11]   See Health Academy website: www.who.int/healthacademy
[12]   Further information is available at http://www.medic-to-medic.com.
[13]   Further information is available at http://www.connectingforhealth.nhs.uk.

eHealth: Combining Health Telematics, Telemedicine, Biomedical Engineering and Bioinformatics to the Edge. Edited by B. Blobel, P. Pharow and M. Nerlich.
IOS Press, 2008

Legal and Social Responsibility in Health Service Chains

Christian DIERKS [1]
Dierks+Bohle, Attns. Berlin, Germany

Abstract. Personal health settings establishing health service chains lead to new legal challenges. The safe harbor principle of doctor-patient relationships has to be extended for including multilateral relations and other parties by reconciling a broad variety of legal regulations with detailed contractual agreements. Beyond security and privacy, also liability, risk management and reimbursement have to be ruled.

Keywords: Health services chains, safe harbor principle, contract, privacy, safety

Introduction

What are health service chains and what are the legal issues involved? Traditional types of telemedical applications bring about traditional types of legal questions. In telepathology and teleradiology the professional law demands the appropriate standard of care even under remote circumstances. Reimbursement issues are to be discussed if services are not rendered appropriately. Patient/doctor/e-mail also raises national law issues concerning the responsibility in remote therapies. Liability issues need to be added to the legal framework when telemonitoring is involved. Finally data protection needs to be guaranteed throughout all of these services.

1. Scenarios and Relations

Typically the telemedical services mentioned so far are based on bilateral scenarios. It is Dr/patient, Dr/Dr, Dr/service provider or patient/service provider. These bilateral scenarios are typically governed by a traditional legal framework that usually can be applied to the telemedical service in an analogue way. Regularly adjustments are necessary to take into account that the service is rendered at a distance. Special legal or professional duties are part of these bilateral scenarios (see Figure 1).

---

[1] Corresponding Author: Christian Dierks, MD, Ph.D., LL.D., Professor, Dierks+Bohle, Attns. Berlin, Walter-Benjamin-Platz 6, D-10629 Berlin; Email: dierks@db-law.de; URL: www.db-law.de

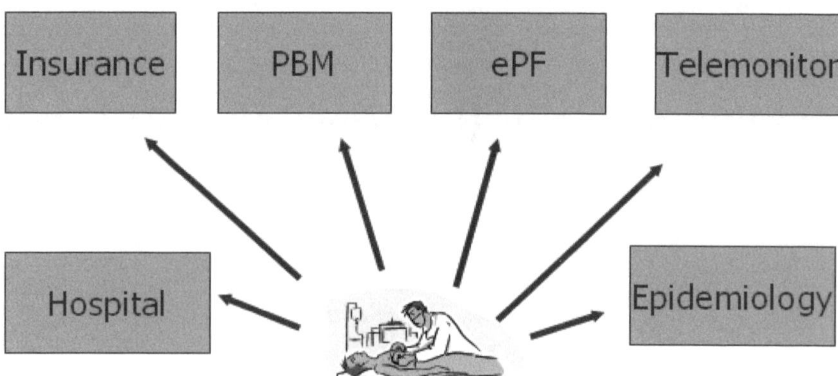

Figure 1. Bilateral relations

Such bilateral services are found between patient and physician, patient and insurance, patient and hospital, doctor and specialist, doctor and pharmaceutical benefit manager, doctor and epidemiology a.s.o. If we understand a chain to be something with more than two links all of these bilateral scenarios are not chains.

2. Legal Framework

In health service chains that have more than two links this bilateral scenario is not applicable and legal issues become far more complicated. One of the common examples is cardiac telemonitoring which on a more extended basis not only involves a patient and a service provider but also the patient's GP, a cardiac clinic, an insurance fund and maybe even a clinical research organization. In such a scenario the patient finds himself and his personal health data embedded in several legal and contractual relations. Whereas the legal framework to the GP is governed by civil law relating to the patient-doctor-relation and the professional duties of the physician, the relation between the physician and the service provider is a contractual one partially governed by the laws of data protection. This contract, however, has not only to ensure the very specific data protection issues involved in dealing with personal health data, but also needs to enable the physician to render his services in accordance with his very own legal duties. Finally the research organization needs to work along the legal framework of clinical research as laid down in the pharmaceutical law. The particular duties of sponsor and investigator need to be integrated into the contractual framework between all the parties of this health service chain.

Another good example of the multitude of legal aspects in health service chains is drug distribution along the work flow of an online pharmacy. Looking at the initial contact between doctor and patient privacy issues and professional duties need to be taken into account. In modern practices an electronic health record (eHR) will be involved. The doctor's therapeutic decision might be supported by a web based expert system and definitely will be carried out with an IT-based decision support system (DSS). In a scenario with electronic prescribing a multitude of legal regulations based on the social security system and data protection issues will be part of the legal framework. We also might expect that health economists will carry out research with the data involved in such an electronic prescribing system. The prescription will be administered by an online pharmacy whose marketing efforts are channeled by specific policy regulations based on European law. The reimbursement issue as a relation between the online pharmacy and the insurance fund is partially governed by social law and partially based on a framework contract between pharmacies and insurance funds. The curious patient will get in touch with the pharmacy's call centre and demand up to date information on the whereabouts of his drug. After delivery he might seek more information than the patient information leaflet can supply and might therefore make use of the Web content as supplied by the online pharmacy or the manufacturer of the drug. These services are governed by European pharmaceutical law.

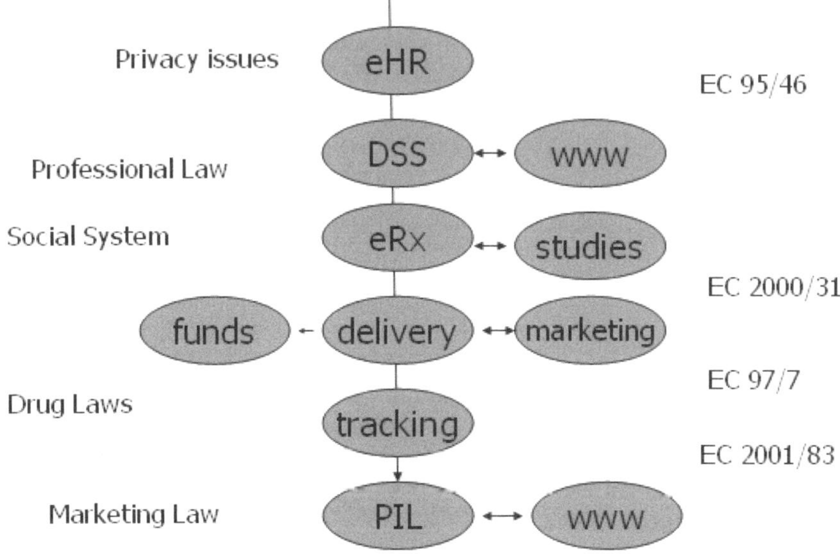

Figure 2. Legal framework for online pharmacies

3. Changing Legal Issues

Most of the legal issues involved in health service chains seem familiar. However, in the far more complicated scenarios of health service chains additional issues arise: A multitude of cooperating parties require clear-cut decisions on responsibilities. There is also a need for a distinct communication management. Provisions have to be made to prevent personal health-related data that have left the safe harbor of the doctor patient relationship from confiscation. Furthermore in a collaborative system of decision-making and patient services mismanagement and mistakes in any organization can yield a shift in the burden of proof in malpractice claims. It is for this reason and the duties of standards of care that risk management systems need to be applied to health service chains.

A decade or longer the focus has been on the medical and technical side of telemedical services. The complexity of health service chains and the legal issues involved to indeed show us that they are still many obstacles along the way before a continuous data flow will enable a competitive market. We are still far from applying the internationally accepted tools of risk management to health service chains, even though this will definitely be necessary.

Contracts require partners, duties and solutions for conflicts. They need to be based on informed consent, which is not particularly easy to achieve when data processing becomes complicated. In the German concept of an eHealth card (see Ficture 3) the patient needs to be informed about content ("Inhalt") management that is either obligatory ("obl") or optional ("fak"), right of access to data ("Zugriffsberechtigt"), requirement of consent ("Einverst") or health professional card requirement for access ("Zugriff mit") as well as a potential claim of deletion ("LöschA"). Evidently these conditions are quite a challenge for anybody who has to explain the details in order to get informed consent.

Inhalt	Stat	Zugriffsberechtigt	Einverst.	Zugriff mit	LöschA
Rezeptdaten	obl	V, A, ZA, Apo, PTA, HE	nein	HPC/Autoris.	ja
EU Berechtigung	obl	?	nein	?	nein
Notfalldaten	fak	V, A, ZA, Apo, HB	ja	HPC/BA	ja
eArztbrief	fak	V, Arzt, ZA, Apo	ja	HPC	ja
AM-Dokumentation	fak	V, Arzt, ZA, Apo	ja	HPC	ja
ePatientenakte	fak '	V, Arzt, ZA, Apo	ja	HPC	ja
eigene Daten	fak	V, Arzt, ZA, Apo	ja	HPC/SMC	ja
Leistungs- und Kostendaten	fak	Versicherter	ja	HPC	ja
Einwilligungserklärung	obl	Arzt	nein	HPC	ja
Protokolldaten	obl	Datenschutz	nein	HPC/Autoris.	nein

Figure 3. The German eHealth Card – as seen from a data protection officer

Finally we need to take into account that health service chains in the future will be a far more complicated than most of the procedures we deal with today. Electronic monitoring will be extended to data derived from an electronic body area network (eBAN – see Figure 4). Monitoring will involve interventions such as defibrillation or injections. Furthermore therapeutic decision making will be based on pharmacogenomic evaluations and made available to epidemiological research. The current concept of the data protection does not supply solutions for such a complex system. Therefore medical researchers, clinicians and technicians alike, need to involve lawyers in a process of developing future concepts that combine legal protection of the human rights especially the right of informational self-determination and contractual safe harbor principles.

Step	Data flow	Content	Participant	Example	Implication	Problems
1	Unidirectional	diagnostic parameter	Patient, MonitoringCenter	Tele-ECG	Diagnosis	
2	Bidirectional	diagnostic parameter feedback to patient	Patient, MonitoringCenter	Telemonitoring	Diagnosis, effecting patient behaviour	dementia
3	Bidirectional	diagnostic parameter control	Patient, MonitoringCenter	Telemonitoring with Teledefibrillation	Diagnosis	
4	Multidirectional	several diagnostic parameter complex control,	Patient, MonitoringCenter, BAN server, elektronische eHR	BAN	Multifunctional data processing and therapeutic control	Unvoluntary diagnosis in public health emergencies
5	Multidirectional und Multilevel	several diagnostic parameter complex control/intervention with web based information e.g. pharmacogenomic	Patient, MonitoringCenter, BAN server, eHR, epidemiology	BAN and Grid	Systematic processing and linking of patient data and control options	

Figure 4. The Future – Step 5

4. Conclusion

Health service chains must be seen as the most relevant prototype of data management in the health system of the future. Their development needs to be undertaken with care and precision in order to avoid the infringement of the patient's right of self-determination. A broad variety of legal regulations will have to be reconciled with detailed contractual agreements in order to extend the safe harbor principle over the full range of data management within a health service chain.

The Challenge for Security and Privacy Services in Distributed Health Settings

Sokratis KATSIKAS [a,1], Javier LOPEZ [b] and Günther PERNUL [c]
[a] University of Piraeus, Greece
[b] University of Malaga, Spain
[c] University of Regensburg, Germany

Abstract. The health care sector is quickly exploiting Information and
Communication Technologies towards the provision of e-health services.
According to recent surveys, one of the most severe restraining factors for the
proliferation of e-health is the (lack of) security measures required to assure both
service providers and patients that their relationship and transactions will be
carried out in privacy, correctly, and timely. A large number of individuals are not
willing to engage in e-health (or are only participating at a reduced level) simply
because they do not trust the e-health service providers' sites and the underlying
information and communication technologies to be secure enough. This paper
considers privacy and security issues and challenges for e-health applications.

Keywords. eHealth services, security, trust, privacy

Introduction

Diffusion, general availability, and potential benefits of Information and
Communication Technologies (ICT) are rapidly changing our society and economy.
They have an important impact on almost any sector in industry, politics and even on
our daily life. Within the health care sector, the use of ICT increases at very fast rates;
health care staff tends to depend all the more on computerized Health Information
Systems (HISs) in order to perform their everyday functions. Moreover, HISs no longer
process only hospital and financial data, as they once did. Nowadays, health care staff
uses HISs to assist themselves in diagnosing, to record information of a purely medical
nature and to assist themselves in patient treatment.

Another fundamental change regarding ICT in health care is the transition from the
traditional model of a stand-alone HIS, that is the HIS operating within the boundaries
of a single Health Care Establishment (HCE), to the networked HIS, that is a HCE's
HIS interconnected to HISs of other HCEs or even of third parties, over national or
international Wide Area Networks (WANs) Moreover, Internet-based e-health services
are already been regularly provided. This increasing use of and dependence on
interconnected Local Area Networks (LANs), WANs, and the Internet, while bringing
important new capabilities, also brings new vulnerabilities and increases the possibility
of security breaches to occur.

---

[1] Corresponding Author: Sokratis Katsikas, PhD, Professor, University of Piraeus, Dept. of Technology
Education & Digital Systems, 150 Androutsou St., 18532 Piraeus, Greece; Email: ska@unipi.gr

This shift to the networked world, a world that provides exciting new possibilities for improving the quality of health care that we are provided with, including the possibility of extending diagnosing, monitoring and treating a patient outside the physical boundaries of a HCE, a shift which has been made possible by the explosive increase in the provision of broadband services not only to organizations but to individuals as well, brings forward the need to open up HISs for access by entities beyond the control domain of the owner of the HIS. Thus, we are now witnessing an inevitable paradigm shift in the security of HISs. We no longer simply need to secure HISs by creating physical or logical barriers to prevent their use by unauthorized entities. Instead, we need to additionally be able to allow their use by all those entities that have a legitimate reason to do so even when these entities do not belong to our immediate security control domain. It is entirely reasonable that, in doing so, as in every paradigm shift, individuals will need increased assurance that their sensitive health information and their privacy is not in the least compromised. Thus, terms like "confidence" and "trust" are coming to complement the traditional concepts of "confidentiality", "integrity" and "availability" of information and of information systems.

The right of humans for keeping their privacy is debated in many fields, including the areas of law, politics, philosophy, sociology, and more recently computer sciences. Privacy is one of the fundamental issues in e-health today and a trade-off between the patient's requirement for privacy and the society's needs for improving efficiency and reducing costs of the health care system is still being sought.

In order for e-health to reach its full potential, the obvious conclusion is that either the organizations involved in the provision of such services need to increase the level of confidence and trust provided by them to their customers or technologies need to be created having strong build-in features to protect the individuals' privacy and the security of the transactions.

In this paper we discuss the major issues involved with securing health information in e-health and with preserving the patients' privacy. We start with a discussion of security issues, including trust issues, followed by a discussion on privacy and privacy enhancing technologies. The discussion follows the one in [1], but is specifically geared towards e-health services.

1. Security

Recognising the fact that, in any given e-health scenario, there are five interconnected and interacting components (people, software, hardware, procedures and data), one comes to the conclusion that e-health systems are (and should be looked upon as) information systems, comprising a technological infrastructure and an organisational framework, rather than pure technological infrastructure. Therefore, addressing the problem of security in e-health must be done in an information system setting.

In such a setting, security can be defined as an organised framework consisting of concepts, beliefs, principles, policies, procedures, techniques, and measures that are required in order to protect the individual system assets as well as the system as a whole against any deliberate or accidental threat [2]. Operationally, in order to compile such a framework, the pertinent requirements must be identified first.

On one hand, the patient needs to be sure that a service s/he is considering is valid, i.e. s/he has to be sure that the integrity of the information that is presented to her/him has not been compromised. On the other hand, the provider must be sure that the service s/he provides is available to the patient. Because of the sensitive nature of the information involved the patient wants her/his information to remain confidential. It is also important to ensure the inability of either party to repudiate their actions. Finally, observe that what is fundamentally different between e-health care and traditional health care is the absence of human face-to-face communication. Machines have no way of knowing who is <u>really</u> on the other end of the line once presented with pre-agreed information that convinces them of her/his identity.

Therefore, e-health security requirements revolve around the need to preserve the confidentiality, the integrity and the availability of information and systems, the authenticity of the communicating parties and the non-repudiation of actions.

1.1. Addressing the Requirements

From a structural point of view, an efficient framework for preserving security in information systems comprises actions that are categorised as legal, technical, organisational and social. Legal actions consist of adopting suitable legislation; these should be and have been undertaken by governments at an international, national, and even local level. Technical and organisational actions need to be undertaken by individual organisations (or by bodies representing organisations of a similar nature and purpose). Last, but by no means least, social actions consist of enhancing the awareness of the public on the need for security and on their rights and obligations stemming from this need.

From a conceptual point of view, the task of technically securing an information system can be broken down into securing its application and communication components. Applications are secured through the combined use of technologies including those for identification and authentication, identity management, access control and authorization, trusted operating systems, secure database systems, malware detection, data integrity preservation, intrusion detection and prevention, audit, and applied cryptology. On the other hand, communications are secured through the combined use of technologies including those for applied cryptology, firewalls, secure transactions, secure messaging, secure executable content, secure network management, network oriented intrusion detection and prevention, web access control, digital rights protection.

It can be seen, therefore, that all of the security requirements of e-health that we identified previously can be addressed by a variety of technical measures, of differing strength and efficiency. Different measures can be and are used for different aspects of these requirements. However, the only measure that can adequately address all but one (the availability) of these requirements is encryption. Indeed, cryptography can be used for ensuring the confidentiality of information, whereas certificates can ensure the authenticity of the communicating parties, and electronic (usually digital) signatures can ensure the integrity of information, and the non-repudiation of transactions. This is why it deserves particular discussion in the current context.

The numbers of entities involved in e-health applications prohibits the use of symmetric encryption, as it is clear that it is impossible to maintain and manage keys and certificates for large numbers of users using small-scale, inter-organization tools, even if these are fully automated. Therefore, a more automated and consolidated approach is required, based on a Public Key Infrastructure (PKI) that consists of five types of components [3]:

1. Certification Authorities (CAs) that issue and revoke certificates;
2. Organizational Registration Authorities (ORAs) that vouch for the binding between public keys and certificate holder identities and other attributes;
3. Certificate holders that are issued certificates and can sign digital documents and encrypt documents;
4. Clients that validate digital signatures and their certification paths from a known public key of a trusted CA;
5. Repositories that store and make available certificates and Certificate Revocation Lists (CRLs).

Additionally, a Time Stamping Authority (TSA) may be thought of as part of the PKI. Entities that collectively operate as CA's, RA's, Repositories, and TSAs have commonly been referred to as Trusted Third Parties (TTPs) or, more recently, as Certification Service Providers (CSPs).

User requirements from a PKI have been recorded in several applications, and are, understandably, quite dissimilar. However, a common ground can be and has been found [4]. A comprehensive list of services that satisfy the above requirements can be found in [5]. The functions required to perform each of these services can subsequently be defined [6].

1.2. Trust

For centuries, people have been provided with health care services on a face-to-face basis. Regardless of the problems and difficulties associated to those different situations, the result of this type of procedures has been reasonably successful. Probably, much of the success of those procedures has been based on the intrinsic trust derived from the face-to-face interactions between persons, a concept that obviously has strong sociological and psychological components.

According to the Webster dictionary, trust can be defined as: (i) An assumed reliance on some person or thing, and a confident dependence on the character, ability, strength, or truth of someone or something; (ii) A charge or duty imposed in faith or confidence or as a condition of a relationship; (iii) To place confidence (in an entity).

When considering a network-based scenario, this issue becomes extremely essential and, as we will see later, its definition is not as trivial as it may have been perceived in the previous paragraph. Moreover, in order for network-based e-health services to achieve similar levels of acceptance as traditional health services, trust needs to become a built-in part of the services themselves. For instance, patients need to trust that physicians or other e-health service providers will not disclose their private information, while service providers need to trust that the patient is eligible for the provision of the service.

This is not easy because people tend to perceive networks, and the Internet in particular, as a more or less anarchic environment, that not only can provide good quality health care services, but is also prone to multiple potential threats. It seems that it does not matter that the number of transactions where dishonest behaviour is detected is negligible in comparison to the number of transactions where the behaviour of the participant is entirely honest. Service providers and service consumers alike are still worried about the threats, and their lack of trust has a negative influence on the wide deployment of the technology.

The problem is accentuated if we consider the increasingly distributed nature of Internet-based e-health applications, where the trust relationships of a specific user with other entities differ depending on many different parameters. Moreover, pervasive aspects of the network itself provide new considerations to bear in mind [2].

1.2.1. The Meaning of Trust

Different definitions of trust have been proposed in the literature during the last years. Some authors have tried to define the concept of trust in a global or general way, while others have defined it attending to the relation with specific types of applications.

One of the first attempts to define the concept of trust in e-commerce can be found in [7], where trust in a system is defined as *"a belief that is influenced by the individual's opinion about certain critical system features"*. As pointed out in [8], that definition *"concentrated on human trust in electronic commerce, but did not address trust between the entities involved in an e-commerce transaction"*.

In fact, the authors in [8] argue that the lack of consensus with regards to trust led them to use the terms trust, authorization, and authentication interchangeably. Further, they define trust as *"the firm belief in the competence of an entity to act dependably, securely, and reliably within a specified context (assuming dependability covers reliability and timeliness)"*. Accordingly, they define distrust as *"the lack of firm belief in the competence of an entity to act dependably, securely, and reliably within a specified context."*

1.2.2. Relation with Authentication and Authorization

We believe that trust, authorization and authentication can not be used interchangeably because authorization and authentication have to be considered as basic security services of applications, while trust can not be considered as a basic security service but as an outcome (a belief, as previous authors mention) resulting of a combination of the appropriate use of basic services. In any case, we agree with [8] on the difficulty and on the lack of consensus of defining the term.

Additionally, we also agree on the importance that [8] gives to authentication and authorization, as both services are essential to get trust from service consumers and providers. In this sense, the concept of the digital certificate has raised as a technical solution that greatly contributes to increase trust on the e-health security technology in general, and on authentication and authorization services in particular.

Identity certificates (or *public-key certificates*) provide the best solution to integrate the authentication service into most applications developed for the Internet that make use of digital signatures [9]. However, new applications, particularly in the area of e-health, need an authorization service to describe what a user is allowed to do. In this case privileges to perform tasks should be considered. *Attribute certificates* provide an appropriate solution, as these data objects have been designed for use in conjunction with identity certificates [10].

It is widely known that the use of a wide-ranging authentication service based on identity certificates is not practical unless it is complemented by an efficient and trustworthy mean to manage and distribute all certificates in the system. This is provided by a *Public-Key Infrastructure* (PKI), which at the same time supports encryption, integrity and non-repudiation services. Without its use, it is impractical and unrealistic to expect that large scale digital signature applications can become a reality.

Similarly, the attribute certificates framework provides a foundation upon which a *Privilege Management Infrastructure* (PMI) can be built. PKI and PMI infrastructures are linked by information contained in the identity and attribute certificates of every user. The link is justified by the fact that authorization relies on authentication to prove who you are, but it is also justified by the fact that the combined use of both types of certificates contribute to increase the trust from users. Although linked, both infrastructures can be autonomous, and managed independently. Creation and maintenance of identities can be separated from PMI, as authorities that issue certificates in each of both infrastructures are not necessarily the same ones. In fact, the entire PKI may be existing and operational prior to the establishment of the PMI.

One of the advantages of an attribute certificate is that it can be used for various purposes. It may contain group membership, role, clearance, or any other form of authorization. Yet another essential feature is that the attribute certificate provides the means to transport authorization information to decentralized applications. This is especially relevant because through attribute certificates, authorization information becomes "mobile", which is highly convenient for digital business applications.

1.2.3. Trust Management

When dealing with trust issues, trust management is probably the most difficult problem to face. Blaze et al. introduced in [11] the notion of trust management. In that original work they proposed the PolicyMaker scheme as a solution for trust management purposes. PolicyMaker is a general and powerful solution that allows the use of any programming language to encode the nature of the authority being granted as well as the entities to which it is being granted.

KeyNote was proposed [12] to improve two main aspects of PolicyMaker: to achieve standardization and to facilitate its integration into applications. Additionally, Keynote uses a specific assertion language that is flexible enough to handle the security policies of different applications.

Later, other similar systems were proposed for trust management purposes. As argued in [8], a common problem is that those solutions are used to identify a static form of trust (usually at the discretion of the application coder). However, trust can change with time, and that is the reason why some authors consider that digital certificates (identity and attribute) can be also considered for trust management purposes. More precisely, the infrastructures used to manage those certificates, PKIs and PMIs, provide procedures and functions that can be seen as an advanced method to manage trust. These are better solutions than the ones mentioned in the previous paragraph in the sense that are less static, but they are too biased towards authentication and authorization services.

In fact, trust management can be tremendously dynamic. This issue has been elaborated upon in [13]. Trust of one entity in another changes due to the following factors: *"(i) After further dealings, the trusting entity has a better idea of the trusted entity's capability and willingness to act the way the trusting entity wants in a given context; (ii) The trusted entity's capability or willingness to act in a given context the way the trusting entity desires might change with time; (iii) The trusting entity, after getting recommendations from other entities, will know more about the trusted entity's capability and willingness to act the way that the trusting entity wants in a given context."* Additionally, [13] defines the dynamic nature of trust as *"the change in the trustworthiness value of an entity, assigned to it by a given trusting entity with the passage of time in different time slots".*

1.2.4. Challenges

As per the discussion above, it can be argued that even the most fundamental issues of trust can be still considered as open issues to be resolved. However, this is only the tip of the iceberg. Additional challenges that can be identified in the area of trust management, include the development of means to initiate and build trust; the creation of formal models of trust; addressing the issues of different types of trust (e.g., trust towards data, or users, or system components); the definition of trust metrics to compare different trust models, the accommodation of trust characteristics (such as context dependency, bi-directionality, and asymmetry) by trust models; the ways in which the trust models handle both direct evidence and second-hand recommendations related to the trusted subjects or objects; the use of trusted parties to initiate and build trust; the investigation of how timeliness, precision, and accuracy affect the process of trust building; the maintenance and evaluation of trust (e.g., credentials, evidence on the behaviour of the trusted objects, recommendations); the discovery of betrayal of trust; the enforcement of accountability for damaging trust; the prevention of trust abuse; the motivation of users to contribute to trust maintenance; the guarantee of scalability, performance, and economic parameters for trust solutions; the engineering of trust-based applications and systems; the experimentation with and implementation of trust-based applications and systems for e-health; the enhancement of system performance, security, economics, etc. with trust-based ideas (e.g., like enhancing role-based access control with trust-based mappings).

Additional research challenges include the social paradigm of trust; the liability of trust; scalable and adaptable trust infrastructures; benchmarks, testbeds, and development of trust-based applications; trust-related interdisciplinary research.

2. Privacy

In this section we will first examine the meaning of privacy in the context of e-health. This is followed by a discussion on what concerns patients may have when using e-health services. Finally we will review some of the currently existing approaches and technologies available that help to preserve or enhance the privacy and discuss their future. The section is concluded with a short discussion of areas in which more research is needed.

2.1. The Meaning of Privacy

In the e-health arena privacy is related to the use of patient information. Altogether, privacy in our context may be defined as the individual right of humans to determine, when, how, and to what extent information is collected about them during the course of the e health service provision; the right to be aware and to control the beginning of any interaction or data gathering process; and the right to choose when, how, and to what extent their personal information is made available to others. Using an e-health service typically makes the transmission of large amounts of sensitive personal data necessary. This may either be necessary for the provision of the e-health service itself (for example: health condition information, insurance data, sex and age, social and financial status, past treatments) or desired by the e-health service provider (for example: collecting patient data that later may be analyzed, shared with other entities). However, because of the high sensitivity of such data, its misuse must be prevented, as, on the one hand, it is a fundamental right of every citizen to demand privacy and, on the other hand, the disclosure of health information may cause serious problems to the patient: a history containing substance abuse or HIV infection might result in discrimination or harassment or an insurance company could use health information to deny health coverage or to increase the insurance premiums for those affected, or an employer might refuse to employ people based on their health records. [14]. The problem is that individual users typically have only little idea about the possible range of uses that the possession of sensitive personal information allows for, and thus have only little idea about the possible violation that might occur to their privacy.

At a first glance the two viewpoints, the first one that supports the service provider's view and favouring their legitimate interests, and the second one that supports the individual's view seem to be mutually exclusive. In practice, however, we face the need to reach a compromise and to arrive at a solution that is mutually beneficial to all.   Such a compromise is called *patient-centric privacy*: for the individual this means to gain the maximum amount of privacy and for the e-health service provider, through the maximisation of privacy for their patients, to gain substantial benefit. The benefit may be resulting from direct effects, like the improvement of the public image of the provider (resulting in additional "customers" and in long lasting trust relationships) or from side effects, like improved brand recognition or more generally, a reduced trust barrier (as discussed in the introduction), leading to an increased e-health level and making many more individuals comfortable with participating in e-health.

2.2. Patients' Concerns

In the digital age distances have been shortened or even diminished. A few years ago, when a patient requested the provision of a health-related service, the service provider and the patient invariably came to direct contact and were, more often than not, located in the same geographical area or country. This is no longer the case. Patients and e-health service providers are now able to transact with almost anyone else in the world.

This new situation has certain characteristics that bring about many concerns regarding trust and privacy. Examples of such characteristics are the indirect contact and the lack of close interaction between all parties involved in the provision of an e-health service, easy and inexpensive collection of information which may happen without notice of the patient at different sites and at different stages of the service provision process, and often an absence of effective regulations or the ineffective enforcement of existing such regulations. The latter is particularly true if different countries are involved, hence different law may apply.

Several concerns to privacy have been identified at times, including *Data gathering*: Once a patient submits personal data there is usually no control how the data may be used; *Lack of regulations*: Privacy laws are different in different countries. Additionally there is no means and effective way to verify that the law is observed; *Privacy statements*: Privacy statements may not be up-to-date, incorrect or may not even be applied at all; *E-mailing*: Unwanted Emails (for example spam mails) may be sent to patients offering services or products; *Site spoofing*: Patients may be linked to other sides where they receive wrong information, or they may be linked to external sites where the published privacy policy does no longer apply.

2.3. Methods to Preserve Privacy

Privacy can be preserved through three classes of methods: through legislation, through organizational means, or through technology. The optimal solution, as usual, involves the efficient combination of solutions from all three classes.

2.3.1. Privacy through Legislation

Because of the high sensitivity of health information, there is increasing social and political pressure to prevent its misuse. This pressure has led a number of countries around the world to establish legislation for the protection of privacy, which usually applies to privacy of all kinds of personal information, but is sometimes complemented by legislation protecting specifically the privacy of health information.

In the UK and Sweden there is a legal restriction on any entity possessing any kind of personal information without the explicit consent of the data owner, and every entity that does store such data has to register this fact with the government. Similar is the situation in Germany. The German privacy law additionally demands the principles of data minimalism and purpose limitation, meaning that only the minimum of data to perform a certain purpose may be collected and that the data may not be used for any other than the specified purpose.

In Japan the Personal Data Protection Act of 2003 regulates the commercial and governmental usage of private data. This act extends an earlier act from 1988, which regulates the storage and use of private data through governmental administration. Additionally the Ministry of International Trade and Industry has published guidelines for businesses how to handle private data and issues a seal for those businesses adhering to the guidelines. In China several relevant laws for data protection exist.

Canada has a very strong privacy law. The Personal Information and Electronic Documents Act (since 2004) determines for businesses how they are allowed to collect, use and disclose private information of their customers as well as their employees.

The United States Department of Health & Human Services Health Insurance Portability and Accountability Act (HIPAA) asks for the protection of any patient data that is shared from its original source of collection.

At the international law level, the processing and movement of personal data is regulated within the EU by the Directive 95/46/EC. A citizen's right to privacy is also recognized in the European Convention for the Protection of Human Rights and Fundamental Freedoms. The Organization for Economic Cooperation and Development, as early as 1998, issued a set of guidelines (the OECD Guidelines on Privacy and Transborder Dataflow of Personal Data, 1980) which sets out the minimum standards for data collection, storage, processing, and dissemination that both the public and private sectors should adhere to. These guidelines are commonly consulted by nations and businesses when drafting privacy laws and policies.

In the age of digital business technology has advanced so far and so fast that the approach of protecting privacy through legal regulations is no longer as effective as it was in the past. Legislators are often far behind the new developments and the legal systems are not fast enough the properly react. Additionally, laws are generally country- specific. This means that a patient, residing in a country whose legislation adequately protects her/his privacy, who receives an e-health service from a provider based in a country without compatible regulations may only enjoy little or no privacy protection at all.

2.3.2 Privacy through Organizational Means

Both the service providers and the patients may have at their disposal simple organizational means that may considerably help in protecting the privacy of individuals during the provision of an e-health service. For example, patient health information can be physically separated into personally identifiable and non-identifiable information. Data collected during a service transaction that refer to the kind of service or the type of information requested is non-personally identifiable as long as it is not combined with personally identifiable information, like name, birth date, address, credit card or banking information. Non-personally identifiable information may be analyzed in any way possible and privacy protection is only applicable to personally identifiable data. It goes without saying that of course it should not be possible to combine the separated data buckets.

Another organizational means is to involve a third party service into the e-health service provision process. Such a service would act as a trusted intermediary that guarantees the outcome of the transaction. Other organizational means to increase trust and privacy are delivering some sort of belief to the patient that a service provider complies to a certain privacy policy. This may be achieved by privacy seals issued by a trusted authority (for example TRUSTe, the "online privacy seal") or through technologies such as the Platform for Privacy Preferences (P3P), that give patients the possibility to evaluate whether the published privacy policy of the provider satisfies their own preferences. However, both approaches mainly show the awareness of a service provider of their patients' privacy concerns but cannot guarantee that the provider will actually behave as expected. Although there is some monitoring involved in the aforementioned privacy seals, we once again have reached a point where the patients have to simply trust the providers to keep their promises.

2.3.3. Privacy through Technology

In order to achieve some level of patient privacy, privacy enhancing technologies (PET) may be used. These technologies attempt to achieve anonymity by providing unlinkability between an individual and any of her/his personal data, i.e. they try to ensure that any information collected cannot link back to an individual's real world identity. Several levels of anonymity have been defined in the literature, ranging from full anonymity (no one can find out who you really are) through pseudo-anonymity (the identity is generally not known but may be disclosed if necessary) to pseudonymity (several virtual identities can be created and used under different situations). Anonymity can be achieved by one of three main methods: anonymising the transport medium, allowing anonymous access, statistical databases.

Technologies for anonymising the transport medium aim at hiding the original identity of the patient in a way that her/his identity cannot be revealed. One of the simplest possible ways to achieve this for a user is to simply set up an account with a free email service provider that the user trusts that they will not log communication details, such as IP addresses. However, this approach is practically not very feasible because many of the free email service providers require personal details to sign up and they have the legal requirement to keep communication details at least for a short period of time. In order to achieve anonymous web browsing another possibility is to use an anonymizing server. When an individual is using such a service all communications are routed through the anonymizing server, thus the recipient has no way to determine the IP address or the identity of the user. However, this technique requires that the anonymizing party is acting as a trusted third-party and that the user can rely on her/his identity not being disclosed by it.

A further step in technical complexity is a setting without a trusted third-party. Reiter and Rubin created a system, called Crowds [15] that groups users into large groups (crowds) and instead of directly connecting requests to a web site the system passes it to the crowd. There the request passes a randomized number of crowd members and finally is submitted to the recipient who is not able to identify who in the crowd is the originator of the request. Another class of privacy enhancing technologies uses encryption. A well known and prominent technology which is using public key cryptography is Chaum Mixes [16]. All messages must be of equal size, they will be cryptographically changed and finally delivered to the recipients in different order. This makes it very difficult to link an incoming message and its sender to an outgoing request and to perform traffic analysis. Chaum Mixes were extended in several ways. For example, onion routing protocols use a network of dynamically changing mixes and the user submits a request in form of a data structure reminding on the layers of an onion. Each point in the communication chain can only decrypt its layer, finding out only where the next point in the route is. For onion routing there are commercial implementations available on the net providing users with anonymity.

Besides anonymizing the transport medium, another privacy enhancing technique is allowing anonymous access to a service. In such systems users are known only by a pseudonym (credential) to the organization they are doing business with. A single user can use different pseudonyms which cannot be linked to each other. Usually credentials are issued by certification authorities and a user can then prove possession of a credential to an organization without revealing his identity. One weakness of such a system is that the legitimate user may transfer credentials on to other users. While this is no risk to privacy it is often not accepted by the service providers or allowed by the law.

Related to anonymous access is the use of an authentication and authorisation infrastructure (AAI). Such infrastructures arose from the fact that it is not always necessary to exactly know who a user is but sufficient to know that the user is authorized to perform a certain action. Often this is outsourced to another organization which is responsible for registering users, user authentication and equipping users with proper credentials. What this means for digital business is that these technologies enable customers to buy items from an e-business by hiding their identity but proving certain facts, for example belonging to a role or group of users in possession of certain authorizations, having access to a certain bank account or having already paid in advance. This of course implies that the AAI is trusted to the organization relying on such services. Different types of AAIs and their use are surveyed in [17].

A different approach to privacy is the use of statistical databases. A statistical database is a data collection, for example all patients and the kind of information they asked for, but not revealing information that uniquely identifies the individuals. The value of such databases is the statistical information not the data itself. Therefore techniques are essential that can keep the statistics of the dataset valid while keeping the individuals' data itself private. Examples of such techniques are query size restriction (Only queries that retrain privacy are allowed.), data perturbation (Individual data is changed in a way that does not influence the statistics but makes the individual data useless.), or output restriction (Query results are altered in the case privacy is threatened). All these techniques have the disadvantage that they make the data less useful. Additionally it has been shown that by repeating slightly changing queries database trackers revealing individuals' privacy may be constructed.

3. Conclusions

Even though there are useful laws focusing on several aspects of trust, privacy and security, common agreements between the different countries are still missing. For the patient and the service provider engaged in e-health it should not make any difference, from a legal point of view, where the user, the provider and any intermediary service is geographically located. Such an effort must start with a common agreement and understanding leading to an all-encompassing legal and moral protection of patients' rights. In the past, legislators had to fight against specific violations as they appeared – resulting in a patchwork of various legal protections that only help to guard against isolated aspects of trust, privacy and security.

E-health service providers should better support for third-party services, trust infrastructure, privacy platforms and security solutions. Policies should clearly state in what countries the service is located and what laws do apply. They also should have a validity date and in case of changes should give the history of changes. Patients should more carefully choose the services based on statements related to privacy and security and on the existence of certified characteristics, such as privacy or site authentication seals. This would increase acceptance of the seals and put some additional pressure on providers to have their conformance with their published statements certified. However, privacy through organizational means does not actually enforce individual privacy. All approaches are only a help to guide the decision making process about whom to trust. This is only a first step; technologies are needed that also attempt to enforce the preservation of privacy.

Current technologies make a significant achievement to preserving the trust, privacy and security in e-health. However, more research is needed to perform this automatically (without user involvement) and with less involvement of trusted third parties. Finally there is a need to develop technologies that better fit the general security requirements. In today's world, strong anonymity is sometimes regarded as a potential risk to the security of the society or a country. Additional research is needed in order to understand how the two sets of conflicting requirements can be balanced and met under a single umbrella.

It appears, then, that we do know the way and we do have the technologies to solve many of the technical problems associated with securing e-health. If this was indeed the case, then all the real security breeches that we encounter everyday in e-health should not have been happening. What is, then, the problem?

The most usual problem is that, while everyone recognizes the need for securing e-health, what they do not know is that security is more than erecting physical and electronic barriers. According to Bruce Schneier, "*…the fundamental problems in computer security are no longer about technology; they're about applying technology*" [18]. The strongest encryption and most robust firewall are practically worthless without a set of organizational security measures, built around a security policy that articulates how these tools are to be used, managed and maintained. Such a policy concerns risks. It is high-level and technology neutral. Its purpose is to set directions and procedures, and to define penalties and countermeasures for non-compliance. An example of such a policy for HCEs can be found in [19].

References

[1]   Katsikas S, Lopez J and Pernul G. Trust, Privacy and Security in Digital Business. *Computer Science, Systems and Engineering*, 6 (2005), 391-399.

[2]   Kiountouzis E. Approaches to the security of information systems. In: Katsikas S, Gritzalis D and Gritzalis S (Edrs.) *Information Systems Security*. New Technologies Publications, Athens, Greece, 2004 (In Greek).

[3]   Arsenault A and Turner S. IETF PKIX WG, Internet draft, Internet X.509 Public Key Infrastructure PKIX Roadmap, March 10, 2000.

[4]   Lekkas D, Katsikas SK, Spinellis DD, Gladychev P and Patel A. User Requirements of Trusted Third Parties in Europe, in Proceedings, User identification and Privacy Protection Joint IFIP WG 8.5 and WG 9.6 Working Conference, 229-242, 1999.

[5]   Gritzalis S, Katsikas SK, Lekkas D, Moulinos K, Polydorou E. Securing the electronic market: The KEYSTONE Public Key Infrastructure Architecture. *Computers and Security*, 19, 8 (2000), 731-746.

[6]   Bhargava B, Lilien L, Rosenthal A, Winslett M, Sloman M, Dillon TS, Chang E, Hussain FK, Nejdl W, Olmedilla D, Kashyap V. The pudding of trust [intelligent systems] *IEEE Intelligent Systems*, 19, 5 (2004), 74-88.

[7]   Kini A, Choobineh J. Trust in Electronic Commerce: Definition and Theoretical Considerations. In: Proceedings of the Thirty-First Annual Hawaii International Conference on System Sciences-Volume 4, IEEE Press, 1998, 51-61.

[8]   Grandison T, Sloman M. A Survey of Trust in Internet Applications. IEEE Communications Surveys & Tutorials, Fourth Quarter 2000, http://www.comsoc.org/pubs/surveys.

[9]   Information Technology - Open systems interconnection - The Directory: Authentication Framework, ITU-T Recommendation X.509, June 1997.

[10] Information Technology - Open systems interconnection - The Directory: Public-key and attribute certificate frameworks, ITU-T Recommendation X.509, March 2000.

[11] Blaze M, Feigenbaum J, Lacy J. Decentralized Trust Management. In: Proceedings of the IEEE Symposium on Security and Privacy, IEEE Press, 1996, 164-173.

[12] Blaze M, Feigenbaum J, Ioannidis J, Keromytis A. The KeyNote Trust-Management System Version 2, RFC 2704, 1999, www.faqs.org/rfcs/rfc2704.html.

[13] Dillon TS, Chang E and Hussain FK. Managing the Dynamic Nature of Trust. *IEEE Intelligent Systems*, 19, 5 (2004), 79-82.

[14] Riedl B, Neubauer T, Goluch G, Boehm O, Reinauer G, Krumboeck A. A secure architecture for the pseudonymization of medical data. In: Proceedings of the Second International Conference on Availability, Reliability and Security (ARES'07), IEEE Computer Society, 2007, 318-324.

[15] Reiter MK, Rubin AD. Anonymous web transaction with Crowds. *Communications of the ACM*, 42, 2 (1999), 32-48.

[16] Chaum DL. Untraceable electronic mail, return address, and digital pseudonyms. *Communications of the ACM*, 24, 2 (1981), 84-90.

[17] Lopez J, Oppliger R, Pernul G. Authentication and Authorization Infrastructures (AAIs): A Comparative Survey. *Computers & Security*, 23, 7 (2004), 578-590.

[18] Schneier B, Economics and Information Security, June 29, 2006, http://www.schneier.com/blog/archives/2006/06/economics_and_i_1.html

[19] Katsikas SK and Gritzalis DG. The Need for a Security Policy in Health Care Institutions. *Int. J. of Biomedical Computing*, 35, Suppl. (1994), 73-81

New Sciences and Technologies

eHealth: Combining Health Telematics, Telemedicine, Biomedical Engineering and Bioinformatics to the Edge. Edited by B. Blobel, P. Pharow and M. Nerlich.
IOS Press, 2008

Technical Paradigms for Realizing Ubiquitous Care

Erich R. REINHARDT [1]
Siemens Medical Solutions, Erlangen, Germany

Abstract. Medical technology without coordination and without the right information available anywhere, any time, can only lead to results, that are inefficient, costly, and sometimes the wrong care for the patient. The most important lever to alter this situation is the use of healthcare information technology across the whole healthcare continuum: interoperable electronic records, electronic prescribing, clinical decision support, rules engines, workflow-based systems as well as a secure technical infrastructure. They are all a critical part of the solution and have the power to realize ubiquitous care. Together with the progress in medical technology, which provides for an earlier diagnosis and intervention, medical IT for process optimization will be the prerequisite to further improve the quality of care while reducing its costs.

Keywords. Healthcare-IT, Electronic Patient Record, efficiency in healthcare, optimizing workflows

1. Strategic Background

Global trends have a tremendous impact on healthcare – what is needed and how it is delivered. Our world population is increasing at a staggering rate. According to the median projection of the UN's Population Division, the current world population of 6.6 billion will grow by 1.3 billion until 2025, and 2.5 billion until 2050. And, with the population both aging (by 2050, there will be more people over the age of 60 than under the age of 14) and living longer, the demand and strain on healthcare systems will be unprecedented. On the one hand, the fact that we have conquered a number of previously fatal diseases and that we are able to live longer and with a better quality of life is a testament to innovations in medicine [1].

On the other hand, the challenge then becomes how to provide high quality care for an increasing number of people and to do so cost effectively and efficiently. According to PricewaterhouseCoopers (PWC), healthcare spending is expected to triple to $10 trillion by 2020 – comprising 20% of the U.S.'s GDP and 16% of the EU GDP [2]. Governments, payers, and consumer-driven organizations are putting strong pressure on the system to control costs and improve the quality of care.

This challenge is tough, yet definitely not impossible to master. To successfully open up the full potential in healthcare, we have to realize a high-quality, patient-centered medical care: highly efficient with the best and most effective processes. To

---

[1] Corresponding Author: Erich R. Reinhardt, PhD, Professor, Member of the Board of Siemens AG, President and CEO of Siemens Medical Solutions. Siemens Medical Solutions, Henkestraße 127, 91052 Erlangen, Germany; E-Mail: erich.reinhardt@siemens.com ; URL: http://www.siemens.com/medical

achieve this, one has to look at the entire system and understand the interdependencies of the individual components. It's necessary to include the complete continuum of care in our observations, that is, all steps in care, beginning with prevention and early detection, to diagnosis and therapy, to care.

We're therefore convinced that integrated IT solutions for optimizing clinical and administrative workflow are the keys to success. Important innovative trends in IT include knowledge-based decision support systems with an intense focus on combining multiple information sources and relying on annotated databases. In parallel to IT, molecular diagnostics – the use of in-vivo and in-vitro technologies including gene and protein analysis – is steadily gaining in importance, due to its many applications in individualized therapy and early disease detection.

2. Optimizing Workflows and the Decisive Role of IT in Healthcare

Optimizing the workflows in healthcare is critical to realize ubiquitous care. Workflow in this respect means all activities in conjunction with the care of a patient, in particular the temporal sequence and the information exchange among all participants. In fact, it is not very difficult to describe what makes an optimal process in healthcare. When a sick patient comes to the physician, the physician does everything to restore the patient's health as quickly as possible with as little burden to the patient as possible. Throughout the entire treatment, the physician is able access comprehensive information on the patient including also data from earlier examinations. He can call on specialists for an opinion and treatment as needed. Treatment is good and focused when all the parties involved work in concert.

Lack of information or lack of coordination can have far reaching and serious impact, e.g. resulting in needless mistakes, injuries or even loss of life, and staggering economic costs. In 2000, the landmark study 'To Err Is Human: Building a Safer Health System" brought this issue into world focus [3]. The paper reported the death of up to 90,000 patients due to treatment errors in the United States. Despite the worldwide outrage and advances, there is still more to be done. In fact, seven years later, the World Health Organization (WHO) estimates that one in ten patients is affected by some type of preventable medical mistake and identified nine solutions to improve the situation. Of the nine solutions, four are directly related to information technology.

"To Err is Human" is stating that many errors, such as medication-based mistakes like adverse drug events due to allergies or drug interactions could be prevented if the right information was only available at the right time. In fact, the report spurred the adoption of healthcare IT systems that manage the medication process and insure compliance with the five 'rights' of medication administration (right patient, medication, dose, route, time). It is obvious, that systems such as bar code monitoring for medication administration can have instant and positive effects. Overall, the idea is that if everyone can effortlessly do what needs to be done, when it needs to be done, without forgetting any steps, the entire enterprise will be more efficient and profitable.

Results achieved in different hospitals across the globe speak for themselves. By introducing Computerized Physician Order Entry (CPOE) systems – IT-supported prescription and dispensing systems – the number of hospital prescription errors dropped significantly – e.g., by 73% in Södersjukhuset, a hospital near Stockholm [4]. The time from medication prescription to dispensing was likewise substantially shortened, e.g., by 96% at Kingsbrook Jewish Medical Center in New York. Even implicating that the same nurse present during the prescription could be still on duty and thus could verify the patient was taking the appropriate medication.

3. Better Workflow – More than just Automation of Processes

Hospitals all over the world have acknowledged that workflow optimization is crucial to master the challenges lying ahead. In fact, the impact on clinical workflow was, according to an independent market study in the United States, named the no.1 or no.2 criterion for further purchasing decisions. But optimizing workflows holistically means of course more than just to automate processes like medication within a single hospital. In reality, patients are often treated by various healthcare providers, for example, a general practitioner, specialists in private practice, and a hospital. To ensure a smooth treatment without unnecessarily repeated examinations or search for relevant information, patient data has to be exchanged including information regarding treatments and therapies, diagnoses, and images.

In the words of IT, this means to create regional or even national networks enabling the smooth exchange of relevant information on a patient without breaks of media or hurdles. So called National Health Information Infrastructure Initiatives (NHII) are on the way in almost every developed nation to improve the overall care by bringing together all partners involved in the medical process. However, most initiatives cover yet only certain aspects of healthcare, like the prevention of diseases using IT-based screening programs; only a few projects have already a more comprehensive approach – like the telematics infrastructure to be built in Germany as well as the Electronic Health Record (EHR) initiatives, which are already implemented successfully in different parts of Scandinavia.

An excellent example for a successfully running screening project is the diabetic retinopathy screening for all diabetics in Scotland, initiated and managed by the NHS (National Health Service). Earlier, the country had too few ophthalmologists to perform all annually recommended exams of all diabetics – resulting in long waiting lists. Now, having implemented a screening process supported by Siemens' eHealth solutions, 300,000 patients can be examined annually at 73 remote locations all over the country. The images taken are analyzed and results are graded and quality assured in five regional centers. This allows the ophthalmologists to see only those patients that really require treatment. The Scottish Ministry of Health expects not only to entirely eliminate waiting lists, but also to reduce costs.

The Electronic Health Record (EHR) or Electronic Medical Record follows the same concept, but with a much broader scope. Once successfully implemented, informatics experts agree, the EHR will be at the core of creating effective, safe, and efficient healthcare systems worldwide. An EHR that is truly complete, transportable, and accessible across myriad healthcare settings and system boundaries will do much to solve that.

4. eHealth: IT-Based Cooperation Across the Healthcare Continuum

But, it is also time for the concept to move beyond simple replacement of ordinary paper records – an electronic file cabinet should not be our goal. The EHR must be a dynamic solution that is at the foundation – and not the end point – for coordination of care through sophisticated, workflow-driven systems that promote quality and effective care. Initial successes became visible today, for example, in Scandinavia. Several countries pursued the idea of the EHR to optimize clinical workflows establishing a nation-wide eHealth infrastructure. In Norway, for instance, more than 80% of patients already have an EHR. In Sweden, the regions have agreed on the content of a summary EHR, which will be introduced in 2008.

One of the largest projects worldwide is currently implemented at the Rhoen-Klinikum AG in Germany. In the future SOARIAN Integrated Care will support communication and data exchange between altogether 46 attached hospitals and other associated medical centers. Based on the agreement of the respective patient, relevant information – such as consiles, diagnostic images, and medical reports – can be easily digitally exchanged between all the physicians involved in the treatment. A web-based electronic patient record (webEPA) is at the core of the system. In its final setup the system will manage the medical data of more than one million patients annually. A specific Master-Patient-Index (MPI) guarantees that for each patient only one patient record exists – even if the patient registers in different hospitals of the network. An ingenious identity management provides for the protection of the patient's data, as only entitled persons get access to the data relevant for the treatment [5].

For a broad acceptance for such a comprehensive data and information exchange, data sovereignty must be always with the patient. Trendsetting IT systems today allow for that easily via a secure common network, enabling all participants to view the relevant information with a click of the mouse. The rollout of the electronic health card (eGK) in Austria shows how this can be successfully achieved. Today, the Austrian population shows a very high acceptance for the eGK after a relatively short time and the outcomes are convincing. Administrative patient data is now available digitally on the eGK, e.g. the patient is clearly identified in his current insurance status. The future possibility of digital prescriptions avoids breaks in the information flow as well as misunderstandings, e.g. due to badly readable writing of the prescription.

5. Monitoring the Chronically Ill

According to the WHO, more than 60% of healthcare expenditures go toward the chronically ill [6]. These illnesses require that the patients sufficiently understand the disease, coordinate treatment with the treating physicians, and monitor the course of the illness and compliance. Monitoring simply requires frequent, regular checks of usually only few and simple parameters to predict the near-term progression of the disease. Asthmatics, for example, blow into a tube to measure peak flow; patients with chronic heart failure check their weight daily. These values, monitored over time, indicate if the patient needs to be admitted to the hospital soon or whether he is in compliance and can continue a largely normal life. If the values point to hospitalization in the near future, an intervention with medication may prevent that. The results are a higher quality of life for the patient and lower costs for the healthcare system.

Therefore, the goal for efficient care programs for chronic diseases must be to remotely monitor critical values at short intervals and to respond quickly to changing circumstances [7]. If successful, savings can be substantial: E.g., recent studies from the US support that appropriate care plans for patients with chronic heart failure can reduce hospitalizations by up to 50%. Getting there sounds easy, but it doesn't always serve the interests of the healthcare system. Hospitals are reimbursed for patients treated, as are physicians' practices. No one gets paid if an acute case never happens. An example from the USA shows, however, how reimbursement below hospitalization cost for a certain disease, namely chronic heart failure, can initiate a business model resulting in better quality patient treatment and lower costs. Hospitalization for chronic heart failure involves on average 6 1/2 days in intensive care, the costs are around $8000. The hospital, however, is reimbursed $4000. In consequence, the hospital isn't really interested in treating these patients - they do so because they are contractually obliged – but rather in avoiding hospitalization. Using appropriate IT systems, the patients are trained and supported. They receive individual treatment plans and their own personal electronic patient record for regularly entering the values they measure. The physician, in turn, checks the figures and can intervene if they are worrisome, thereby avoiding a stay in the hospital. Both have benefits: The patient, who enjoys a higher quality of life, and the hospital, which preserves its financial resources. This kind of win-win situation needs to be found to benefit the patients and the healthcare system.

6. On the Way towards a Patient-centered Healthcare System

But, the vision of IT-enabled healthcare is even more revolutionary. Now, the medical industry is on the verge of the next phase of IT systems that capture and analyze knowledge to enable the most efficient and clinically effective care – patient-centric, personalized healthcare.

This is not a vision of the far-distant future – with advanced IT and medical technology innovation, all elements are in place today to improve care. Inefficient and incorrect care does not help the patient, and it also costs the healthcare system a tremendous amount of money. If physicians can accurately diagnose and characterize a patient's disease long before it impacts the patient's quality of life, and precisely treat the disease with limited side effects, there will be significant savings to the healthcare system, and immeasurable benefits to the patient.

Now imagine how IT systems in future can be leveraged to create knowledge: All of the information available in a patient's electronic record, captured over a lifetime, together with the images and test results, genetic history, and analysis of medical knowledge data bases, can help to predict – and possibly prevent – a disease before it occurs or at a very early stage. And, if a disease does develop, it can be treated more rapidly and with better outcomes. This is not intended to replace the physician as diagnostician and care provider, but it is simply not possible for the human mind to absorb and manage the vast, ever-growing body of clinical knowledge. Complementing and supporting the clinician, IT systems are designed to collect and analyze huge amounts of data and convert it into useful information.

This ability will become even more important if we take a look at the rapidly emerging field of molecular medicine. With in-vitro and in-vivo diagnostic tools, we now have the means to diagnose at a molecular level. And, only advanced IT systems are able to match and analyze all of the data and extract useful information and knowledge. There is nothing more discouraging and more costly than ineffective treatment. Therefore, the goal must be to combine all available information from multiple diagnostic modalities for achieving the most accurate diagnosis and selecting the most efficient therapy for every individual patient. Ultimately this will contribute to achieve the goals of cost-effectiveness and quality outcomes.

Through the mining of medical, clinical, and image information, the correlation of this to both workflows and outcomes enabled by analysis and knowledge, and the identification of new and improved, personalized means of care, healthcare will be fundamentally changed. As medical informatics experts, it is up to us to transform the use of healthcare information technology into a powerful medical tool. This is the vision we should all share. It is our goal and, together, we will achieve it.

Quite simply, IT holds the key for a potential quantum leap forward in the quality, safety, and cost of ubiquitous patient care – and for a fundamental transformation in the world of medicine.

References

[1]   UN Population Division (Edr.) World Population Prospects: The 2004 Revision Population Database.
[2]   PriceWaterhouseCoopers: Pharma 2020: The vision (2007).
[3]   Institute of Medicine (IOM). To Err Is Human: Building a Safer Health System (2000).
[4]   W. Baldauf-Sobez, et al. How Siemens computerized order entry systems helps prevent the human error. *electromedica* 71 (2003).
[5]   http://www2.rhoen-klinikum-ag.com/rka/cms/rka/eng/press/25975.html (2007).
[6]   Fishman P, von Korff M, Lozano P, Hecht J. Chronic care costs in managed care. Health Aff, Millwood, 1997.
[7]   Zahlmann G et al. Progress in Networked Disease Management and Screening Services. *electromedica* 69 (2001).

*eHealth: Combining Health Telematics, Telemedicine, Biomedical Engineering and
Bioinformatics to the Edge. Edited by B. Blobel, P. Pharow and M. Nerlich.
IOS Press, 2008*

Nanomanipulation and Nanotechnology for Future Diagnostics

Tadao SUGIURA [1], Megumi NAKAO, Tetsuo SATO and Kotaro MINATO
*Department of Genomics and Informatics,
Nara Institute of Science and Technology, Japan*

Abstract. Nanomanipulation is a technology to manipulate a small object sized in
nanometer to submicron scale. Optical tweezers is one of nanomanipulation
techniques, which can investigate pico-newton to femto-newton force exerted on
microscopic objects. We have developed a cell palpation system by use of optical
tweezers and performed palpation experiments on cells. With the cell palpation
system, an operator manipulates a probe particle to touch a certain location of a
cell and feels the strength of the cell by hand through a haptic device, which
displays force calculated and generated by a computer. We expect this technique
can be used in diagnostic purpose and utilized not only in research field but also in
daily medicine.

Keywords. Nanotechnology, nanomanipulation, optical tweezers, cell palpation

Introduction

Nanotechnology is desired to change people's life. Especially in medical field,
nanotechnology is expanding its field to various applications, such as drug delivery
systems, molecular imaging and also to field of nanomachine. Various types of
nanotechnology are now under development for medical applications.
Nanomanipulation is a technology to manipulate a small object sized in nanometer to
submicron scale. Nanomanipulation can be a powerful tool not only for manipulation
of micrometer-sized objects under an optical microscope but also for investigation of
pico-newton to femto-newton force exerted on such objects.

An optical microscope is widely used for research purpose in biology and medical
field and for diagnostic purpose in medicine. An optical microscope has many
advantages of cell investigation to other microscopy methods, like electron microscope
and atomic force microscope because observation with optical microscope can be done
under aqueous condition. Nanomanipulation for biological specimen under optical
microscope is desired. In such case manipulation of small object is become difficult.

Optical tweezers is a solution, which enables us to manipulate a small object under
an optical microscope. Optical tweezers utilizes a phenomenon called laser trapping
caused by radiation pressure force exerted by a laser beam. In laser trapping a small
object to be manipulated is irradiated by a strongly-focused laser beam, is pulled into a
laser beam spot by radiation force and is trapped in the spot. The trapped object can be

---

[1] Corresponding Author; Tadao Sugiura, PhD, Associate Professor, Graduate School of Information
Science, Nara Institute of Science and Technology, Takayama 8916-5, Ikoma, Nara 630-0192, Japan; E-mail.
sugiura@is.naist.jp

manipulated by changing the spot position of the laser beam. Ashkin first developed optical tweezers technology in 1986 [1]. Individual cells were manipulated by optical tweezers [2]. Block and coworkers performed to measure small force exerted by a single biomolecule [3, 4]. They succeeded to investigate pulling force onto a double strand DNA by a single RNA polymerase during polymerization process [5]. After their experiment, force measurement experiments under a single-molecular condition have been widely carried out by many researchers. Mechanical properties of DNA [6], force exertion by actin-miosin interaction [7] and microtubules and torque exertion by a rotating motor protein [8] are investigated by optical tweezers technique. Also binding force of single molecules was investigated. Rupture force between biotin and streptavidin [9] and binding energy of intra-molecular interactions in RNA are also measured. In such experiments, manipulation by optical tweezers was performed in nanometric accuracy even done under an optical microscope, which has a resolution of utmost 200 nm.

Nanomanipulation of a cell also will become more important. Individual cells have skeleton structure inside and outside on the cell to endure mechanical stress like blood pressure from outside. The structure consists of cytoskeleton, such as actin filaments and microtubules, and extra cellar matrix. Owing to the structure, a cell can hold its shape and stay at proper position. Nanomanipulation is expected to be used for investigation of mechanical property of skeleton structure of each cell. Mechanical property of individual cells is not fully investigated because there was no available method to measure forces on a cell. Nanomanipulation can be expected to reveal many unknown properties of cells by the measurement of mechanical property of a cell. Mechanical property of individual cells measured by nanomanipulation can be used as information for medical diagnostics.

In this manuscript nanomanipulation by light, which is recently developed by us, is described. Our final goal of nanomanipulation is diagnostic use for daily medicine, so we developed a palpation system, which produces feedback force from a cell and gives the tactile feeling (palpation) to an operator. By use of this system the operator can feel the elasticity of a specific cell and perform palpation. First principle of nanomanipulation by light is described, and then cell palpation system is described.

1. Weak Force Measurement by Nanomanipulation

In optical tweezers technique, dielectric particles [1] that has a diameter of submicron to several tens micron and also a nanoparticle like a single gold colloid of 40-nm diameter [10] and semiconductor nanoparticle of 200-nm diameter [11] can be manipulated. These particles are trapped in three dimensions so that the particle translated not only in lateral (x-y) directions but also in axial (z) direction. The translate motion of particles can be observed through an optical microscope, which is usually used for focusing a trapping laser beam. In a conventional optical microscope the particle position observed in submicron accuracy but by use of larger magnification of particle image the particle position can be determined till ~10-nm accuracy. When a quadrant detector, which has four sensing area on one chip, the accuracy can be enhanced till subnanometer [12]. Under its conditions the particle movement can be observed and sensitivity of force sensor is increased. Although these enhancement effect, still the special resolution, which is defined as a minimum resolving spread of two points in observed images, is limited utmost 200 nm because of diffraction limit of light.

On the optically trapped particle force exerts as the particle goes back to initial position of trapping if the particle displaces from an equilibrium position. Figure 1 shows the coordinate of the particle and the laser beam. The exerting force and trapped particle can be described as a spring - particle model. The exerting force by optical tweezers F_{trap} is described as

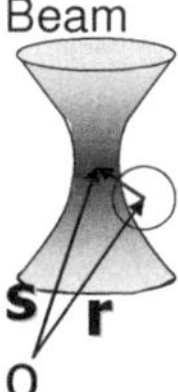

Figure 1. Principle of optical tweezers

$$\mathbf{F}_{trap} = K\,(\mathbf{r} - \mathbf{s}) \qquad (1)$$

where K is a spring constant of trapping. $\mathbf{r}$ and $\mathbf{s}$ represent position vectors of the particle and equilibrium position of trapping, respectively. When the particle manipulated in aqueous condition and touched to a cell, the kinetic equation of the system is given by

$$m\frac{\mathrm{d}^2\mathbf{r}}{\mathrm{d}t^2} + \mathbf{F}_{trap} + \mathbf{F}_{drag} + \mathbf{F}_{exter} = 0, \qquad (2)$$

where m is mass of the particle and other component that moves with the particle, F_{drag} is viscous drag force from liquid and F_{exter} is external force. In nanomanipulation condition, viscous phenomena can be described as Newtonian model because of small Reynolds number of the system. As a consequence the drug force is given by Stokes law as

$$\mathbf{F}_{drag} = 6\pi\eta a\frac{\mathrm{d}\mathbf{r}}{\mathrm{d}t} \qquad (3)$$

where I is coefficient of viscosity, a is radius of the particle. External force Fexter is represented as

$$\mathbf{F}_{exter} = \mathbf{F}_{Brown} + \mathbf{F}_{surf} + \mathbf{F}_{elast} + \dots \qquad (4)$$

where $\mathbf{F}_{Brown}$ is a force caused by collision of surrounding molecules (Brownian motion), $\mathbf{F}_{surf}$ is a force from cell surface and $\mathbf{F}_{elast}$ is a force caused by cell elasticity. Although there are some other interacting forces onto the particle, i.e. Coulomb force from charged surface and van der Waals forces, these are negligible in actual measurement.

In equation (2) the first term is from acceleration of particle. In general the effect of inertia of trapped particle is quite small compared to other forces. As a consequence the equation (2) is modified to

$$\mathbf{F}_{trap} = -\mathbf{F}_{drag} \quad \mathbf{F}_{exter} \qquad (5)$$

When the particle manipulated away from other obstacles, such as cells and surface of the sample cuvette, external force $\mathbf{F}_{exter}$ is negligible, so that equation (5) becomes $\mathbf{F}_{trap} = - \mathbf{F}_{drag}$. The magnitude of trapping force is equal to viscous force. From this relation the trapping force and spring constant of trapping K can be estimated from a result of viscous force - velocity dependence from an experiment.

External force appeared in equation (2) is investigated by applying force onto a sample slowly to reduce the effect the viscous force. The minimum force to be measured is determined by magnitude of spring constant K and the minimum measurable displacement of trapped particle. The spring constant of trapping is usually micro- to nano- N/m order in optical tweezers force measurement. This value is extremely small compared to other method, such as atomic force microscopy and surface force apparatus. This derives high sensitivity of force. This is an advantage of optical tweezers. The accuracy of particle displacement is described already. In case of ~20nm accuracy and 1micro Newton / m of spring constant, the minimum measurable force is around 20 fN. In our measurement, measurable force of 20 fN was achieved [13].

2. Cell palpation by Nanomanipulation

A cell is thought to have elastic characteristics like a piece of clay and also mechanical property mainly caused by cytoskeleton inside the cell. We expect these properties of a cell varies with its growth stage, protein content within the cell, gene expression and other inner status of the cell. So the measurement of mechanical property of a cell may give useful information for clinical diagnostics and for evaluating effect of medicine on the cell. Cell palpation, that is a novel concept ever heard before for us, is just like conventional palpation, which every medical doctor performs daily, and is for a cell as a target. With cell palpation, an operator manipulates a probe particle to touch a certain location of a cell and feels the strength of the cell through a haptic device, which displays force calculated and generated by a computer.

2.1. Cell palpation system

We have developed a cell palpation system to demonstrate our concept. Figure 2 shows the diagram of the cell palpation system. Optical tweezers is controlled by a computer which is connected with a haptic device.

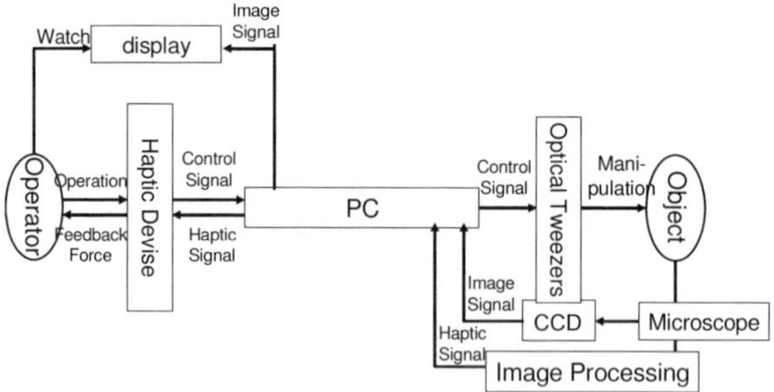

Figure 2. Diagram of cell palpation system

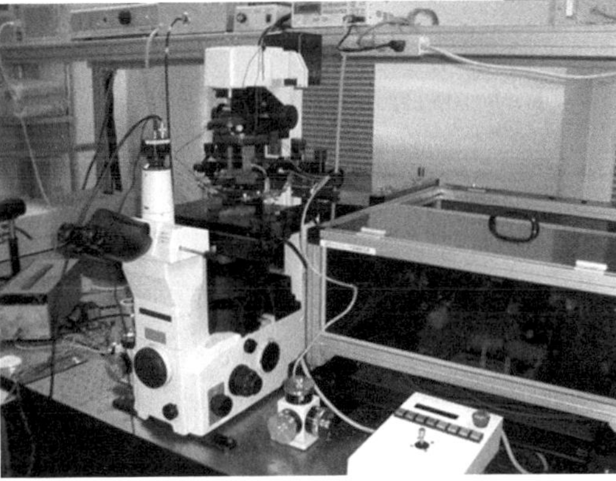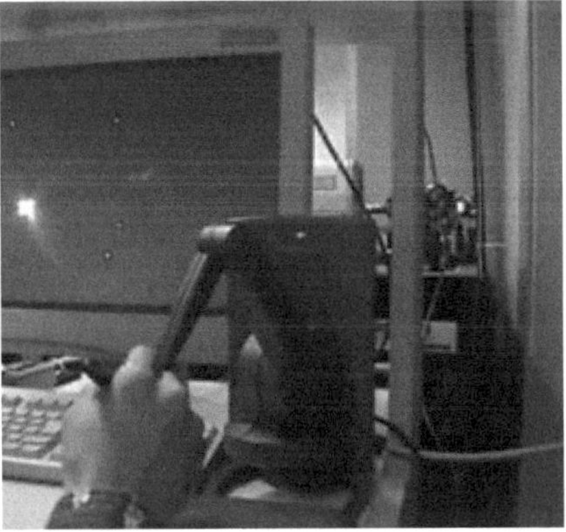

Figure 3. Optical tweezers system and haptic device

The haptic device gets the coordinate of the desired position pointed by the operator, then the computer controls the optical tweezers system as indicated by the operator.

Microscope images are taken through a CCD camera and are displayed on a monitor. Particle position on each image is estimated by image processing on the computer then the force exerting on the probe particle at each time is calculated from the displacement of particle position from the trapping position. The feedback force to the operator is displayed on the haptic device. According to the system above the operator locates the touch position on a cell and touches the cell with a probe particle, and then feels the feedback force from the cell. Hopefully this series of technique realizes palpation of a cell. To build up the system we use an optical tweezers system developed in our lab. The system is based on an invert microscope (Nikon, TE2000) with an objective (Nikon, PlanFluor WI, NA=1.20) to observe cells and to focus a laser beam. Spot position of the laser beam can be moved with two galvanomirrors. The laser for trapping is Nd:YVO$_4$ laser (wavelength of 1064 nm, maximum output power of 2 W). The haptic device to be used is commercial available one (PHANToM desktop, SensAble technology Inc.), which has a pen-type interface with 6 rotary encoders and can generate feedback force by 6 motors. The optical tweezers system is controlled by analog DC voltage output from a digital-to-analog converter (DA) board on a personal computer. Picture of whole system is shown in figure 3.

2.2. Palpation with non-surface modified probe particle

Figure 4 shows a view of a cell and probe particle under cell palpation experiment. The cell is mouse fibroblast cell Balb 3T3 cultured on a cover glass slip. The cell was adhered on the surface of cover glass. Probe particle was 3 micron diameter polystyrene particle. First the particle was trapped and manipulated to contact to the cell surface, then rubbed on the cell surface with circular motion. The movement of the particle and the relation between velocity and displacement are shown in Figure 5 (a) and (b), respectively.

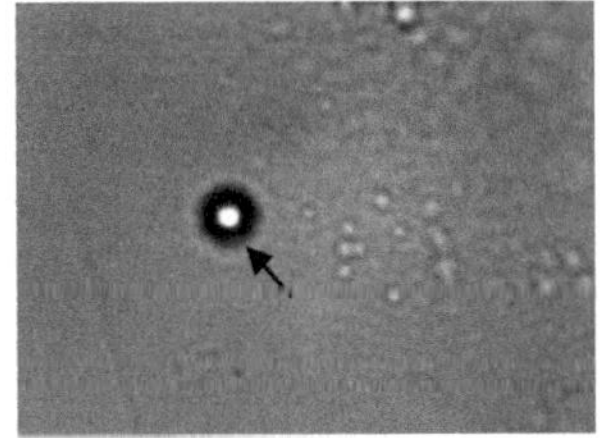

Figure 4. An image of cell palpation Particle is 3-micron diameter.

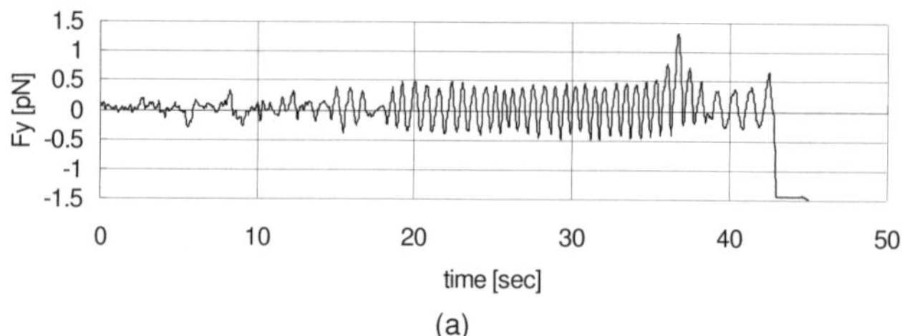

(a)

The particle movement has hysteresis characteristics, which is apparently different from ordinal. That is caused by friction on the cell surface. From these results friction coefficient can be estimated.

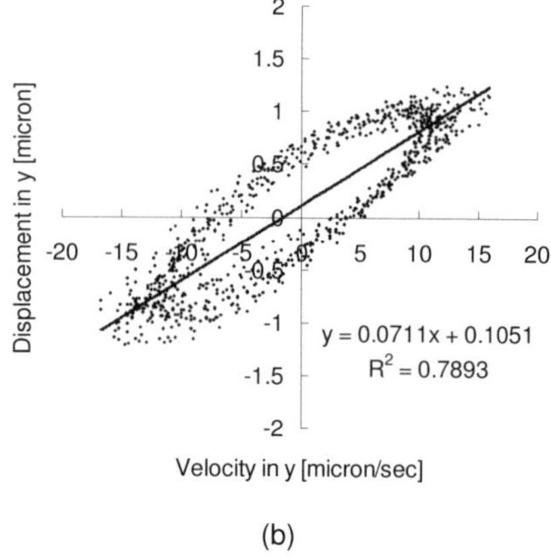

(b)

Figure 5. (a) Trajectory of probe particle during cell palpation, (b) relational plot of velocity and particle displacement. Particle touched on cell surface and friction force exerted on the particle. Particle is same as in Fig. 4.

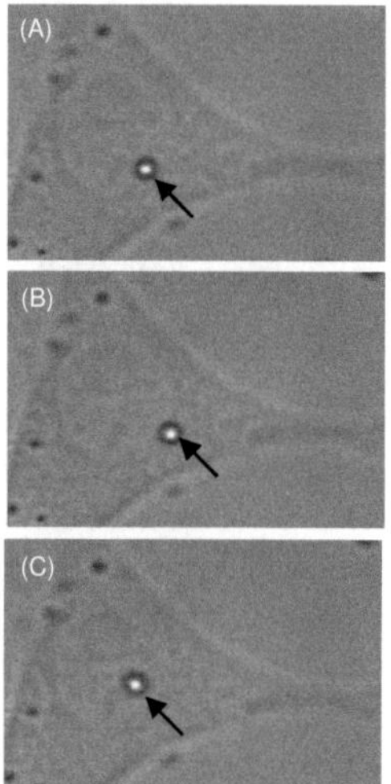

Figure 6. Cell palpation experiment with surface modified particle

2.3. Palpation with surface modified probe particle

We used a particle which has the surface modified by carboxylate. This particle easily adheres on a cell surface whereas the non-modified particle does not adhere on the surface. Figure 6 (left) shows a series of pictures during cell palpation with a surface-modified particle of 2 micron diameter.

At first the particle could be moved by changing laser spot position but suddenly the particle was fixed on the cell surface, and then the particle was forced to pull back toward the fixed position on the cell. Figure 7 shows the force exerted on the particle. A1 and A2 denote unstuck points of the particle from the cell surface. At these points, the

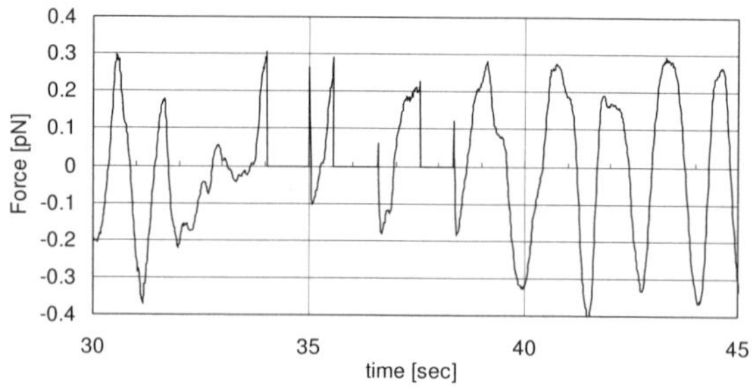

Figure 7. Force exerted on the probe particle during palpation experiment Particle was surface modified.

force on the particle are 0.3 pN, this value indicates the rupture force of particle to the cell.

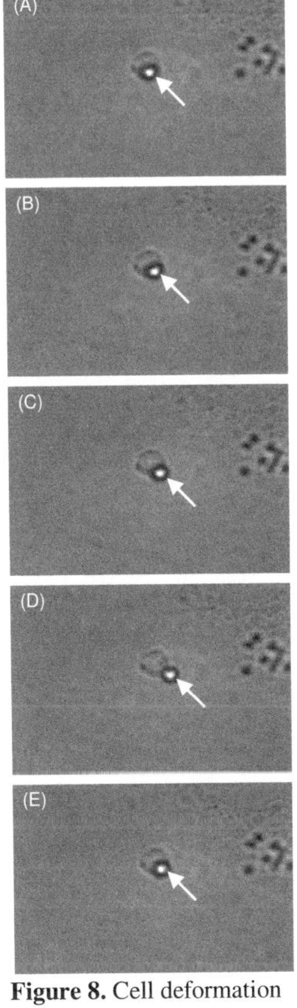

Figure 8. Cell deformation experiment; the particle indicated by arrows were fixed on a bump structure on a cell

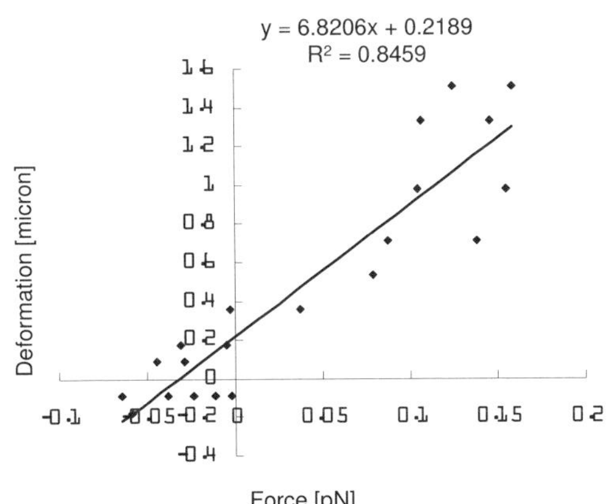

Figure 9. Relational plot of bump structure deformation and applied force

2.4. Cell deformation experiment

We demonstrated the deformation of small structure on a cell surface by radiation pressure force. Figure 8 shows a series of pictures taken a fixed particle on a bump structure and deform the structure. The probe particle gradually pulls the structure to the lower-right direction in the picture and the structure deforms little bit. The movement of the particle can be calculated and a mechanical property of the structure is achieved as shown in Figure 9. The graph represents the relation between applied force and deformation of the structure. The deformation is almost proportional to the applied force. From this result we may evaluate the elastic modulus of the bump structure.

3. Conclusions

We have developed a cell palpation system and performed palpation experiments on cells. In our current stage of this project, evaluation of deformation data has not been done yet. It is necessary to make cell palpation model as a kinetic equation and then estimate elastic properties as values. We hope this technique will be used in diagnostic purpose and utilized not only in research field but also in daily medicine.

References

[1] Ashkin A, Dziedzic JM, Bjorkholm JE, and Chu S. Observation of a single-beam gradient force optical trap for dielectric particles. *Opt. Lett.* 11, 5, 1986: pp. 288-290.

[2] Ashkin A, Dziedzic JM, Yamane T. Optical trapping and manipulation of single cells using infrared laser beams. *Nature* 330, 1987: pp. 769-771.

[3] Block SM, Goldstein LSB, and Schnapp BJ. Bead movement by single kinesin molecules studied with optical tweezers. *Nature* 348, 6299, 1990: pp. 348-352.

[4] Svoboda K, Schmidt CF, Schnapp BJ, Block SM. Direct observation of kinesin stepping by optical trapping interferometry. *Nature* 365, 6448, 1993: pp. 721-727.

[5] Yin H, Wang MD, Svoboda K, Landick R, Block SM, and Gelles J. Transcription against an applied force. *Science* 270, 1995: pp. 1653-1657.

[6] Smith SB, Cui Y, and Bustamante C. Overstretching B-DNA: the elastic response of individual double-stranded and single-stranded DNA molecules. *Science* 271, 1996: pp. 795-799.

[7] Tanaka H, Homma K, Iwane AH, Kitayama E, Ikebe R, Saito J, Yanagida T, and Ikebe M. The motor domain determines the large steps of myosin-V. *Nature* 415, 2002: pp. 192-195.

[8] Block SM, Blair DF, Berg HC. Compliance of bacterial flagella measured with optical tweezers. *Nature* 338, 1989: pp. 514-518.

[9] Ota T, Sugiura T, and Kawata S. Rupture-force measurement of biotin-streptavidin bonds using optical trapping. *Appl. Phys. Lett.* 87, 4, 2005: pp. 043901(1)-(3).

[10] Sugiura T, Okada T, Inouye Y, Nakamura O, and Kawata S. Gold-bead scanning near-field optical microscope with laser-force position control. *Opt. Lett.* 22, 22, 1997: pp. 1663-11665.

[11] Tanaka A, Sugiura T, Kawai T, Hasegawa Y. Three dimension optical trapping and arrangements of magnetic semiconductor EuS nano-aggregations. *Jpn. J. Appl. Phys.* 46, 11, 2007: pp.L259 - L261.

[12] Sugiura T and Okada T. Near-field scanning optical microscope with an optically trapped metallic rayleigh particle. *Proc. SPIE* Vol. 3260, Optical investigations of cells in vitro and in vivo, 1998: pp. 4-14.

[13] Ota T, Sugiura T, and Kawata S. Surface-force measurement with a laser-trapped microprobe in solution. *Appl. Phys. Lett.* 80, 18, 2002: pp. 3448-3450.

eHealth: Combining Health Telematics, Telemedicine, Biomedical Engineering and Bioinformatics to the Edge. Edited by B. Blobel, P. Pharow and M. Nerlich.
IOS Press, 2008

The Danubian Biobank Project

Gerd SCHMITZ [1], Charalampos ASLANIDIS, Gerhard LIEBISCH, Evelyn ORSÓ
Institute of Clinical Chemistry and Laboratory Medicine, University of Regensburg,
Regensburg, Germany

Abstract. The Danubian Biobank Consortium (www.danubianbiobank.de) was initiated in 2005 as a network of Danube Universities and associated partner universities between Ulm and Budapest, with a major focus on case/control studies of aging disorders like vascular and metabolic diseases, Type2-diabetes, and neurodegenerative diseases. Beyond case/control studies some centers also directly participate in longitudinal population based studies and population isolate studies or provide enabling technologies for these studies. The mission of the Danubian Biobank Consortium is to directly integrate biobanking into local and regional healthcare along the Danube through E-health portal structures and IT-based strategies. Biobanking as an integral part of the workflow of the healthcare process is considered as key element to generate qualified long term patient databases and health records. The major objective of the project is to generate a common central encrypted patient and sample information database to facilitate international research interactions, combined with local and regional biobanking facilities under common Good Practice (GP) and Standard Operating Procedure (SOP) conditions to move existing healthcare systems towards personalized healthcare. This process will be driven by local E-health portal implementation to network healthcare providers, industry, insurance companies, medical research and public healthcare in a Private Public Partnership (PPP) model to cover jointly the expenses. All information including patient recruitment, blood withdrawal and storage place of the samples will be saved in phase I as standardized processing procedures (SPP) to implement a central IT-based databank in phase II, which can be used in encrypted form for scientific project planning and investigations. In the local E-health portals the actionable health information will be also accessible for direct medical care for the authorized practitioner. In addition to local centers three regional DNA, plasma, and tissue banks in Regensburg, Vienna, and Budapest store samples and encrypted patient data for scientific purposes.

Key words. Biobank, Danubian, proteomic, lipidomic, genomic

1. Impact of Aging Disorders for European Healthcare Systems

Aging disorders are of major impact for the European healthcare systems. The fastest growing segment in the European population is over 65, a group which utilizes three to five times more healthcare services than their younger counterparts. Despite the major progress in reducing death rates from heart disease and stroke, their total impact has dramatically increased in the past decades. Risk factors such as diabetes have increased sharply, even for younger people. The epidemic of cardiovascular disease can be expected to continue, unless unprecedented public health efforts are made to stop it.

---

[1] Corresponding Author: Gerd Schmitz, MD, PhD, Professor, Institute of Clinical Chemistry and Laboratory Medicine, University of Regensburg, Medical Faculty, Franz-Josef-Strauss Allee 11, D-93042 Regensburg, Germany; Email: gerd.schmitz@klinik.uni-regensburg.de

The economic impact of these aging disorders rises each year. These costs include numbers of people requiring treatment of risk factors or early signs of disease, emergency treatment, efforts to reduce disability and to prevent recurrent episodes. Moreover, the non-productive time that increases labor costs must not to be forgotten.

2. Revolutionary Technologies and Information-based Medicine will Shape the Future of Personalized Healthcare

A comprehensive public health strategy must address these challenges. A preventive medicine has to push for a change of social and environmental conditions and to foster behavioral change. An important approach is risk factor detection and control. Potentially useful protein and genetic biomarkers should be applied in population studies and prevention programs. Epidemiological research is needed to understand how modifiable risk factors interact with genetic factors in progression of cardiovascular disease.

The development of novel preventive, diagnostic and therapeutic approaches is urgently needed to advance personalized healthcare in order to avoid adverse drug response, to ensure affordable and efficient healthcare for the aging population and to limit exploding healthcare costs. Personal healthcare will be achieved through a composite of scientific advances and new technology, and creative uses of information technology and human thought in the practice of medicine (Figure 1). Scientific advances and discoveries, as well as new technological capabilities, will be revolutionary. Innovation in the practice of medicine will be evolutionary. The combination of revolutionary technologies and evolutionary practices form information based medicine and will shape the future of personalized healthcare.

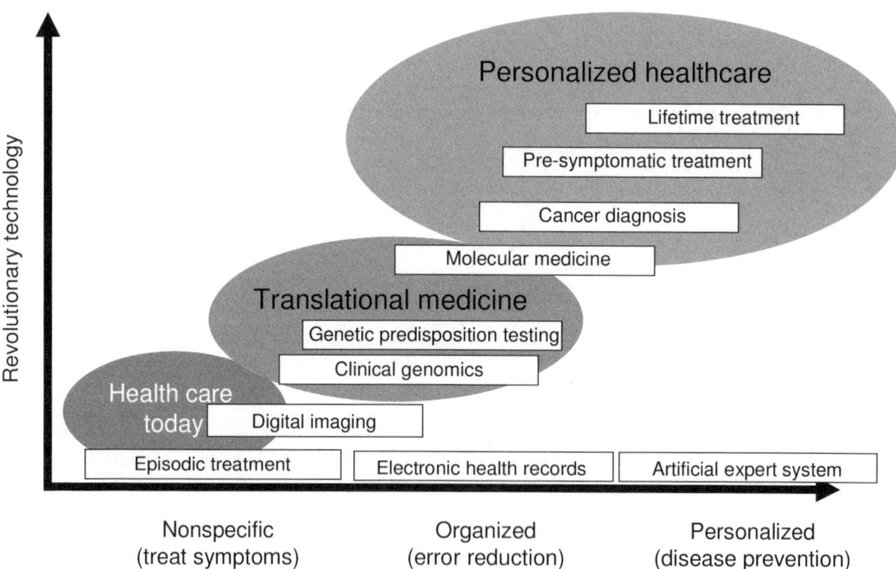

Figure 1. From today's healthcare to molecular medicine and personalized healthcare (Source: M. Hehenberger, IBM Healthcare and Life Sciences)

As more prospective patients enter the health market, pressures from consumers, employers, healthcare providers, payers and regulators will increase and drive the shift toward data integration and knowledge management in the development of diagnostics and therapeutics.

The identification of new diagnostic tools mainly depends on the correlation between genotype, phenotype and outcome, whereby accession to high quality, clinically well characterized samples will be the bottle neck in clinical research and development. The main challenges include the availability of large datasets for studying common diseases, the need for detailed phenotype data in order to classify patient subcategories as well as intelligent information technologies for data mining and analysis. The scientific discoveries, along with the new technological capabilities, will help finding and validation of targets. Adverse drug reactions or non-responders can be predicted. Based on a vast number of genetic effectors and their modifiers, each individual will be scored for precise determination of its disease probability. In the upcoming era suitable drugs can exactly be tailored to the needs of each person. This personalized medicine will become reality not until information technology will cope with the tremendous data masses. Last but not least the outlined strategy will save the resources of healthcare systems worldwide.

3. From Biobanking to Biomarkers

A key element in the process towards personalized healthcare and information-based medicine is the establishment of Biobanks that link disparate data and samples from different working units with already established workflow over time and space. This means the establishment of central DNA-, plasma- and tissue-banks together with the development of an IT-based infrastructure to support data integration, including electronic patient records, laboratory data, diagnostic imaging, genealogical records and the algorithms and tools required for analysis. No one individual, institution, or city can alone meet these challenges of biomedicine. Thus, formation of constant networks will be of outstanding importance and those countries and regions which are most successful in implementing biobanking structures will definitely be privileged in the competitive field of biomedicine. Pharmaceutical and diagnostic industry, healthcare providers and other stakeholders in the healthcare system will act as "customers" of such regional Biobanks. Thus, beside obvious scientific advantages for the participants, benefits will also include a continuous flow of industrial research funding, open the possibility for EU-funding and the provision of highly qualified jobs in the respective region. In return, biotechnology companies will reduce their labor costs and strengthen their international competitiveness by the use of such a large infrastructure.

4. "Private Public Partnership"- Networking of Science, Medicine, and Patients in E-health Portals

Modern European healthcare systems will be characterized by real-time integration of scientific results into practical medicine (Figure 2). New biomarkers and diagnostic methods for early detection of individual and regional disease risks will be developed.

Individualized drugs and strategies for health and individualized treatment of "better informed patients" will become available.

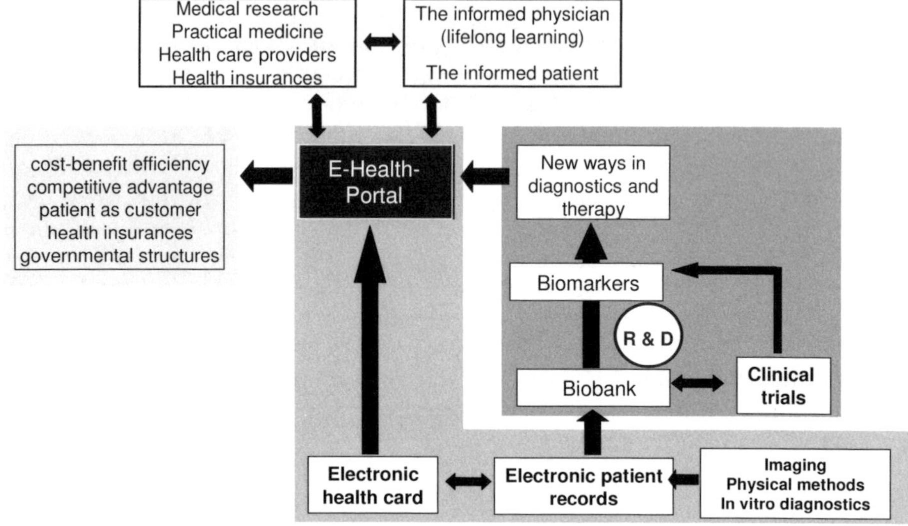

Figure 2. Real-time integration of scientific results into practical medicine via E-Health portals

An essential step is the customer-oriented networking of healthcare providers, insurance companies, public healthcare systems, and medical research. The expenses will be covered jointly by healthcare institutions, patients, and by pharmaceutical industry under the umbrella of „Private Public Partnerships" (PPPs). A key element in the process towards personalized healthcare is the establishment of integrated healthcare biobanks that link disparate data and samples from different working units allowing large multicenter trials and clustering of large enough disease entities. This is an efficient way to identify the genetic predisposition for early onset of aging disorders with a sufficient statistical power. Genetic diagnostic methods allow disease risk assessment facilitating individual prevention and early detection of patients at risk. The identification of such biomarkers results from the analysis of data related to personal health records, family history, physical examinations, in-vitro imaging techniques, and laboratory analyses.

The E-health portal shall give access to health information for patients, clinical assistants like nurses, and physicians in clinics and general practitioners or specialists. Information provided by the E-health portal can be subsequently converted into medical actions. Physicians can be informed not only at lower costs but also individual case-related ("on demand"), much faster and more comprehensively than by classical diversified training programs. The E-health portal offers practitioners a permanently updated information tool which allows life long E-learning. In turn, the patients get access to essential information on their state of health, individual risk factors, and special disease patterns and thus are able to discuss, in the dialog with their physician different possibilities of therapy and prevention. Electronic prescribing tools integrated into the E-health portal enable a physician to transmit a prescription electronically to a patient's pharmacy of choice. It decreases prescription errors and efficiently enables the process of checking for drug interactions and allergies.

5. The Danubian Biobank Consortium as an IT-based European Biobank Initiative

The Danubian Biobank Consortium has been established in 2005 as an integrated part of regional healthcare, connecting universities, associated teaching hospitals, primary prevention programs, and endpoint-related rehabilitation clinics along the Danube River and in neighboring regions (Figure 3).

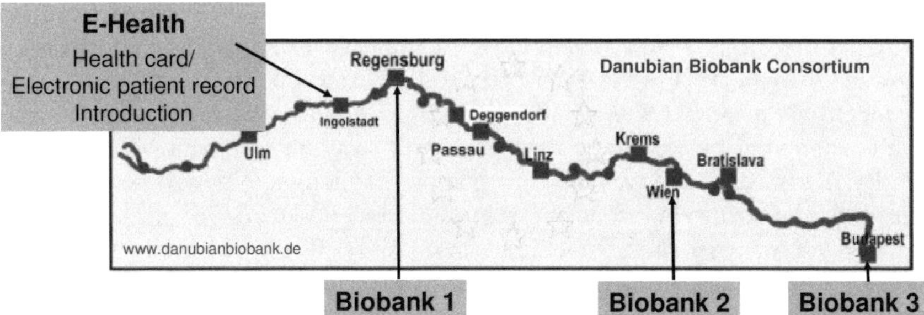

Figure 3. The Danubian Biobank Consortium – A Life Science Network of the Danubian Universities

The project will also integrate disease-specific patient organizations and self-care groups. The scientific network will address predominantly the field of non-cancer aging-disorders focusing on diabetes-related endpoints, including vascular disease, metabolic disease, and neurodegenerative disorders. Task forces will be constituted for the relevant topics of the biobank project including patient recruitment, sample and data management, public health, E-Health, epidemiology and genetics, enabling technologies, and research strategies. The project aims to select the most relevant and promising scientific targets utilizing the core competences developed in the individual partner institutions. During the integration process of the new EU partner countries, the Danubian Biobank Consortium will be transformed in the upcoming years to the „Danubian Biobank foundation for public utility in molecular medicine of aging disorders". The consortium is currently financed by local, regional and national projects and also funded by EU-grants (e.g. FP6-SSA018822; FP7-IP project LipidomicNet, project-no. 202272).

The long-term implementation of the Danubian Biobank relates to 5 work packages:

WP1: Networking, sample and data management logistic and IT issues of biobanking and generative of an interactive website
WP2: Standardization of clinical and diagnostic classification with definition of standards
WP3: Public health, epidemiology, and genetics, including integration of public health survey and population genomics into study design

WP4: Enabling technologies for structural on functional genomics, proteomics, metabolisms, lipid molecular species analysis and systems biology
WP5: The research strategy of the Danubian Biobank Consortium

6. WP1: Networking, Sample and Data Management Logistic and IT Issues of Biobanking and Interactive Website

Networking, bulk data management, sample handling, storage maintenance and retrieval are necessary preconditions for successful biobanking. The university-based diagnostic laboratories within this project provide these core competences. Unfortunately, insufficient sample and data handling due to the lack of GLP/GMP standards and TQM during acquisition and storage were drawbacks for many studies in the past. Therefore, one major objective is to improve sample/data acquisition and storage by strict application of GMP and GLP rules and to improve data/sample access by using electronic medical records and web-based communication. In addition, sample archiving is supported by electronic databases with strict enforcement of data privacy and security. By means of advanced information technologies, it will be possible to extract actionable health information from the tremendous flood of data, thereby turning the vision of personalized medicine into reality. In the upcoming era, suitable drugs will be targeted and tailored to the needs of each person. This process will result in a shared responsibility between pharmaceutical industry, physicians, and, last but not least, the patient.

The cluster of institutions responsible for Work Package 1 defines sample processing and sample handling and implement efficient quality control. One central data bank (Regensburg) and three geographically distributed local biobanks (Regensburg, Vienna, and Budapest) will be established as a first step. The Danubian Universities with the aid of IT companies, European projects and the P3G consortium is delineating a common IT architecture of the future network.

There are intensive ongoing activities at the centers in Regensburg and Vienna to implement health cards, E-health portals and biobanking into practical medicine. The E-health portal will provide access to health information for patients, clinical assistants like nurses, and physicians in clinics and general practitioners or specialists. The region between Erlangen/Nürnberg, Regensburg and Ingolstadt currently establishes as a PPP the European E-health Region Bavaria. A web-based patient health record study support system was implemented by the Danubian Biobank Consortium (www.danubianbiobank.de).

Recruitment of well-characterized patients is a cornerstone of biobanking and currently a two step approach is followed (Figure 4):

- Endpoint-oriented recruitment of e.g. patients with a cardiac event, obesity, manifestation of diabetes-associated complications etc.
- Recruitment via healthcare scenarios, e.g. screening programmes, self care groups etc.

The endpoint-oriented approach is mainly followed by the university and teaching hospitals or in collaboration with specialized practitioners. The common aim is to identify patients at high metabolic or vascular risk and their families. There are six recruitment areas in the field of preventive medicine which will generate data that are easily convertible to actionable health information. Using the knowledge of recent biobanking studies, the E-health portal will facilitate new high risk and preventive programs.

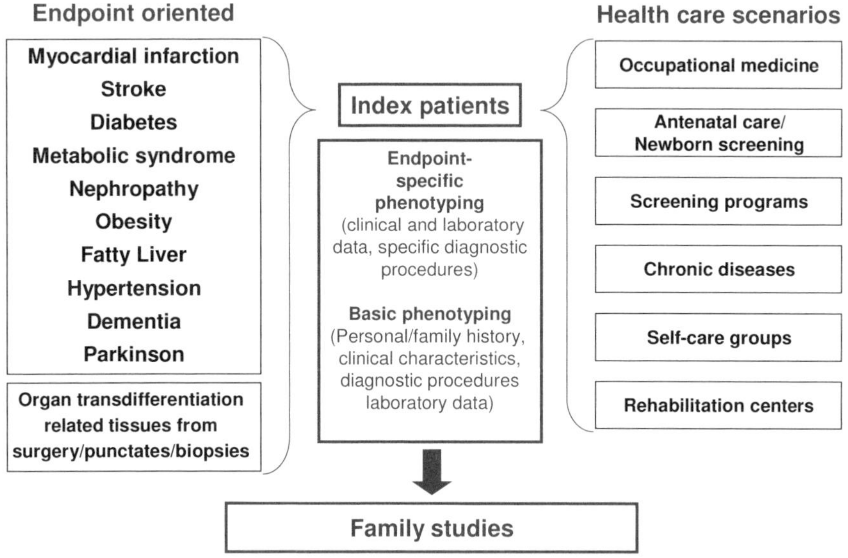

Figure 4. Endpoint and health scenario–based patient recruitment

7. WP2: Standardization of Clinical and Diagnostic Classification with Definition of Standards

As a prerequisite required for appropriate data analysis, anamnestic and pedigree information as well as clinical and diagnostic phenotyping have to be as complete and meaningful as possible. Clinical phenotyping includes family history, cognitive evaluation, and physical examination. In addition, endpoint-specific information complements clinical phenotyping. Regarding diagnostic phenotyping, basic profiles for in situ diagnostics, imaging data and in vitro laboratory diagnostics are used for all patients and, in addition, endpoint-specific profiles have been elaborated. The standards for optimised sample and data sets are defined in collaboration with the other European biobanking projects. Standardization will also encompass the precise characterization of control subjects. For that reason the Danubian Biobank is member of the P³G-consortium (Public Population Project in Genomics).

WP2 has developed the information content for the E-patient record and study support system operating already for all endpoints. In addition disease oriented sample materials and procedures have been defined to consider all preanalytical problems towards SOP establishment.

In collaboration with the Center for Clinical Studies at the university hospital in Regensburg (Koller), the Fraunhofer Institute for Toxicology and Experimental Medicine (ITEM) in Hannover (Borlak / Fröhlich) and the Fraunhofer Project group in Regensburg (Borlak / Schmitz) we are currently implementing the E-prescribing and Adverse Drug Reaction (ADR) software tool TheraOPT® (http://www.atheso.de/html/uber_uns.html) into the study support system.

Similarly the life style record software tool developed at the German Institute of Human Nutrition in Potsdam (Boeing) has been recently implemented into the Danubian Biobank Consortium study support system.

Improvement of patient phenotyping is a key issue and new strategies have been addressed to enhance information content and quality. New smart methods are under development to overcome the gap between collection of high content information and better stratification of patient subgroups in large cohorts. The idea of the "talking body" will cope with this challenge by integrating highly informative data from easy-to-use, non-invasive investigation into the biobanking database (Figure 5).

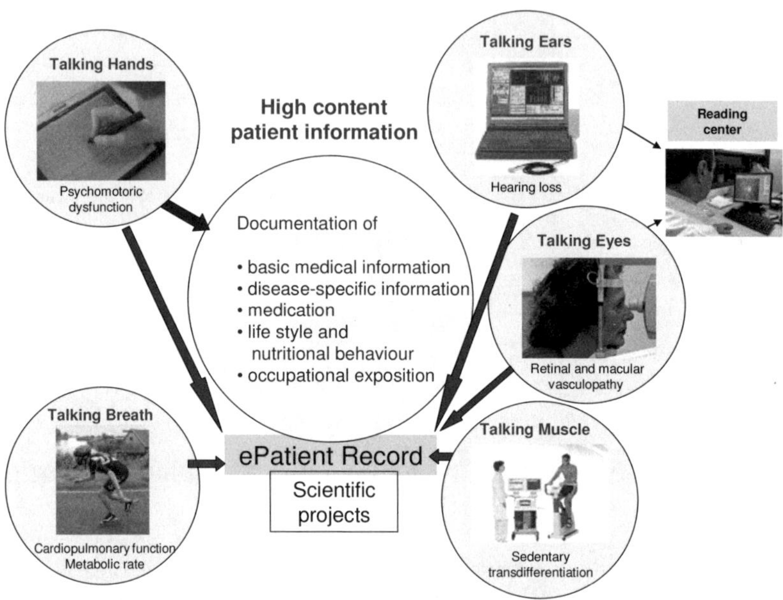

Figure 5. Talking devices in an E-Health environment

"Talking hands" as a combination of a smart multisensoric pen with tabletop technology is a suitable tool for documentation of basic medical and disease-specific information, but also for nutritional behaviour, medication, adverse drug responses and occupational exposition and life style. A questionnaire was established to get an overview for most important life style parameters influencing chronic diseases. Moreover, "Talking hands" is able to record hand movements reflecting cardiac sensomotoric and cognitive function. The exceptional MeDiPen developed by the University of Applied Sciences Regensburg is an ideal tool for this purpose since it enables recording of biometric and phenotypic data. "Talking Eyes" (EvoCare - Dr. Hein GmbH) is a quality-controlled screening enabling early detection of vascular diseases. "Talking Breath" (Viasys Healthcare Inc., Würzburg)offers a portfolio to test cardiopulmonary function, sedentary life style and metabolic status. "Talking Ears" (Otodynamics) allows screening of newborns and infants for sensory or conductive hearing loss, and can also be applied to premature vascular and metabolic aging. "Talking Muscle" allows the discrimination of trained muscle from sedentary transdifferentiation. "Talking Ears", "Talking Breath", "Talking Muscle" may become available as smart methods allowing to gain highly informative data for patient stratification. All instruments can be connected to a local network that, in turn, can be connected to a hospital information system via modern communication protocols like HL7.

8. WP3: Public Health, Epidemiology, and Genetics, including Integration of Public Health Survey and Population Genomics into Study Design

The scientific value of results depends on two crucial requirements, firstly, on a sufficient sample size to detect small gene effects and the application of appropriate statistical methods. Since the Danubian Biobank acts at a regional level, epidemiological analysis is a major component of our biobanking activities. The population-wide dimension also leads to the possibility to use genetic determinants for a public health strategy in the prevention, diagnosis and treatment of the diseases included in this study. In this context an important issue is to meet the patients' concerns about their right to privacy, and the fear of discrimination based on their personal and genotypic data (Tuomilehto, Finnland; Meitinger, Munich).

Experts in genetics/epidemiology define relevant project areas which are crucial from a genetic/epidemiological point of view. They ensure a high quality study design. Furthermore, Danubian Biobank develops policies to assure effective public health application.

This WP addresses all necessary control cohort issues relevant for the integrated healthcare case/control strategy of the Danubian Biobank Consortium.

9. WP4: Enabling Technologies for Genomics, Transcriptomics, Proteomics, Metabolomics Molecular Lipid Species Analysis

Rapidly evolving enabling technologies in the field of genomics, proteomics, metabolomics, and lipidomics are of major importance for sample analysis. Therefore, joining sample requirements and analytical technologies at the micro- and nano-scale are a major task of Danubian Biobank. The participating experts are defining strict sample preparation rules to meet the criteria of good practice.

The Danubian Biobank Consortium has developed multiple activities to implement novel technologies and SOPs for applications including:

1. Co-founding the European Lipidomics Initiative (SSA ELIfe, www.lipidomics.net; www.lipidomics-expertise.de) and establishment of the public domain, LipidomicNet method, data- and knowledgebase. The Danubian Biobank consortium established SOPs for lipidomics analysis based on mass spectrometry, HPTLC and HPLC methods that allow high-throughput analysis of all important lipid molecular species from minor sample volumes

2. Establishing the LipidomicNet knowledgebase.
   Rapidly evolving enabling technologies in the field of genomics, proteomics, metabolomics, and lipidomics are of major importance for sample analysis. Therefore, joining sample requirements and analytical technologies at the micro- and nano-scale are a major task of DanuBiobank.

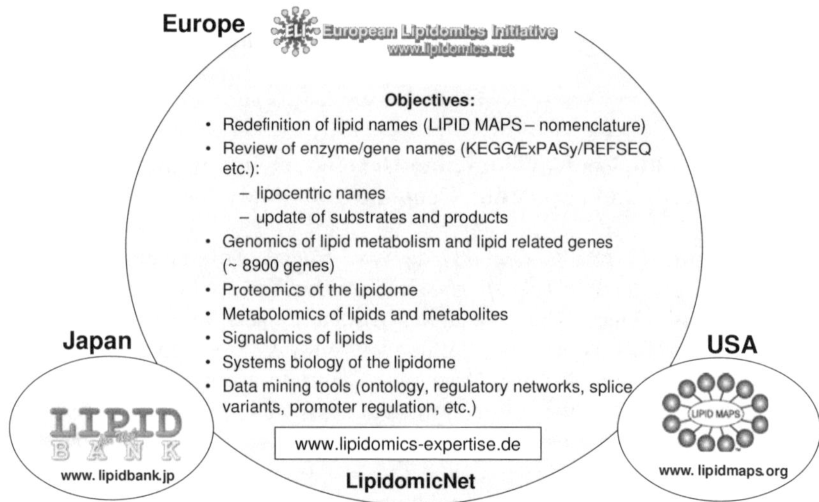

Figure 6. LipidomicNet initiative

The European Lipidomics Initiative (SSA ELIfe; www.lipidomics.net) consortium represents all European lipidomics experts and the Lipidomics Expertise Platform (www.lipidomics-expertise.de) is their scientific forum (Figure 6). The primary aim of this initiative was to mobilize and organize key stakeholders, researchers and end-users in the area of structural and functional genomics with emphasis on Lipidomics and proteomic research and to further define this field of research in terms of participants, scientific content and strength. ELIfe/LEP is creating a European technology and expertise platform bringing together technological know-how, science and industry and shaping the way in which metabolomic research and in particular lipidomic research is organized in Europe. ELIfe is collaborating with the NIH initiative LIPID MAPS - USA organization (www.lipidmaps.org) and the Japanese pendant Lipidbank of the RIKEN institute (www.lipidbank.jp).

Currently LEP serves as an information platform for lipidomics expertise, lipid standards and methods (Figure 7). As a future perspective this platform should help to standardize lipidome related nomenclatures and to establish and harmonize lipid metabolic pathways/tools in a worldwide effort together with the LIPID MAPS and the initiative Lipid Bank. The Danubian Biobank provides the patient samples for lipidomic biomarker validation, or originating from the LipidomicNet project funded by the Framework 7 (FP7) program.

3. Standard Operating Procedures (SOP) for EDTA-blood based cellular human monocyte and platelet analysis of parameters relevant for atherosclerosis have been established. Furthermore, also cytomics SOPs for preparative cell fractionation for genomic, proteomic and lipidomic analysis were introduced.

4. We introduced a new immuno-magnetic cell harvest system that needs no precentrifugation prior to magnetic bead separation (autoMACS™ Pro

Separator®; www.miltenyibiotec.com) and can be directly integrated into sample processing robotics.

5.　The other available in vitro technologies include high throughput genotyping, DNA-microarrays and Taqman PCR for genetic analysis and mass spectrometry and affinity binder technologies for proteomics.

6.　Imaging biomarkers and in vitro diagnostics
In vivo imaging technologies are expected to become indispensable tools for patient care. Imaging biomarkers will identify patients at risk at an early stage and in vivo imaging techniques will help to localize and characterize the underlying disorders in more detail. In contrast to this emerging approach, in vitro diagnostics are well established in clinical laboratories, with standardized technical specifications, systematic auditing for quality, and well defined metrics associated with disease.

Automation and integration are providing new opportunities for improving patient care. The recent availability of high content and high throughput platforms for genomics, proteomics, lipidomics, metabolomics, and cytomics are expected to provide deeper insights into mechanisms of disease pathology and provide direct actionable health data for clinical use. Through innovations in targeted chemistry, these insights will be transformed into novel biomarkers usable with both in vitro diagnostics and molecular imaging.

Despite rapid technological advances in imaging technologies, standardized use of quantitative imaging data in patient care is advancing slowly. The DICOM Committee has published the "Digital Imaging and Communications in Medicine" standard to begin the process of establishing a common standard for managing image data. Broad consensus on the DICOM standard has created a common foundation regarding image transfer and retrieval procedures, specification of a file format and regulations for media interchange, optimization of workflow within imaging departments, and general security enhancements. Imaging data, however, remains susceptible to operator variability and quantification of disease foci seems to be difficult. Nevertheless and despite these unresolved issues, localization of pathological processes remains the great strength of imaging.

The future of imaging biomarkers will not be limited by established *in vivo* imaging techniques. As a specific example, multiparametric flow cytometric analysis of the same markers in blood cells has the potential to replace time-consuming and expensive investigation with *in vivo* imaging analysis. Blood cells could function as probes for organ complications of metabolic, degenerative, or toxicological diseases. Using *in vivo* MRI, decreased μ-opioid receptor binding might be used to indicate alcohol abuse, personality disorders, reduced temperature regulation, physical and emotional stress or pain syndromes. Alternatively using calibrated multiparameter flow cytometry, the μ-opioid receptor could also be quantitated on peripheral blood mononuclear cells. In these applications, blood cells would function as indicators of vulnerability or resiliency factors in the assessment of a number of complex psychopathological diseases.

The combination of new enabling *in vitro* technologies, imaging biomarkers and the modern IT-based Danubian Biobank provides the opportunity to apply diagnostic tools to future curative and preventive medicine innovations. Linking the Danubian Biobank sampling strategy and patient informations with *in vivo* imaging and novel *in vitro* diagnostic biomarker validation will enable high-quality population-wide "Mega" trials. *In vitro* diagnostics clearly complement imaging biomarkers. In combination, the methods offer the potential to accelerate the advancement of individualized molecular medicine, with the potential to allow for direct patient monitoring of drug-target interactions in the near term and to detect life threatening disease before symptoms appear.

10. WP5: The Research Strategy of the Danubian Biobank Consortium

Researchers of the Danube universities have successfully developed core competences in vascular, metabolic and neurodegenerative disease endpoints. The Danubian Biobank project bundles existing activities and create a strategy that will fully leverage the biobank infrastructure. Firstly, we address vascular disease (e.g. stroke, myocardial infarction, peripheral artery disease, arterial thrombosis, kidney failure), secondly metabolic disease (e.g. obesity, metabolic syndrome), and thirdly neurodegenerative disorders (e.g. dementia, Parkinsonism). Lastly, the strongest partners cooperate on the most promising scientific topics.

As a common denominator blood monocytes were selected as a target for biomarker development. Blood monocytes are at the interface of metabolic organ diseases ("monocyte-integrator hypothesis") which relate to metabolic overload dependent transdifferentiation of liver, adipose, heart and skeletal muscle tissues. Figure 7 shows diseases in which the blood monocyte that harbors relevant disease candidate genes, adopts a crucial role by extravasation and differentiation into specialized tissue macrophages.

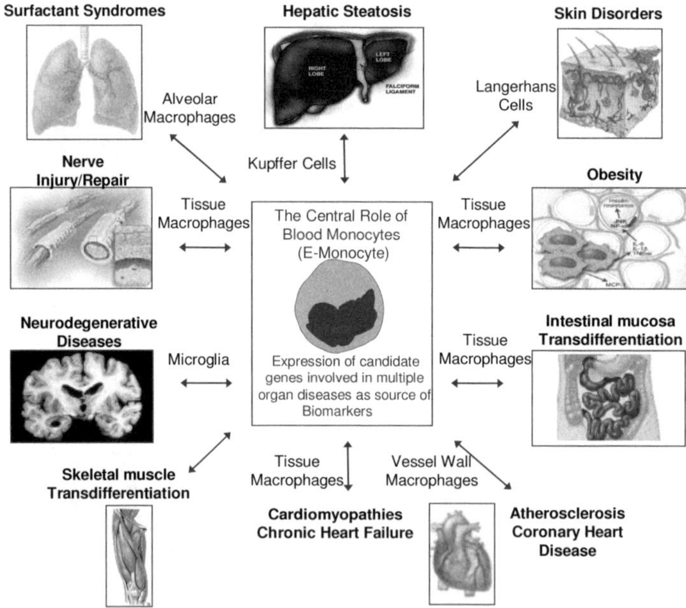

Figure 7. The central role of the blood monocyte as a potential source of biomarkers for organ diseases

The clinical manifestations and endpoints of metabolic and vascular diseases are variable depending on both the individual genetic predisposition and environmental components. Recent findings support the view that metabolic learning processes (Figure 7) induce organ transdifferentiation in several tissues and organ cell types important for the metabolic syndrome. Organ transdifferentiation targets the intestine (enterocytes), adipose tissue (omental and subcutaneous adipose tissue), liver (hepatocytes, stellate cells, Kupffer cells), pancreas (beta-cells, pancreatic islands), muscle (skeletal and cardiac myocytes), vascular wall (endothelial cells and SMC) and the monocyte/macrophage system. Transcription factor networks and their target gene clusters are pivotal for initiating and maintaining organ transdifferentiation. Functional genomic analysis of transcriptional regulatory networks and the identification of master switch transcription factors for cell differentiation programs will shed light on the regulatory networks involved in diseases integrated by the blood monocyte. We are currently applying this strategy to monocytes related to atherosclerosis and metabolic disorders (Figure 7) including vascular diseases, obesity and metabolic syndrome (Atherosystems), to monocytes involved in acute and chronic systemic inflammation and autoimmunity (Immunosystems) and to monocytes as microglia orthologues relevant for neurodegeneration (Neurosystems). This functional approach allows the comparison of the patient's monocyte response with that of the virtual n-dimensional control monocyte regulatory network, which we term the *E-monocyte*, to rapidly identify disease relevant aberrations and to generate actionable health information (Figure 8A).

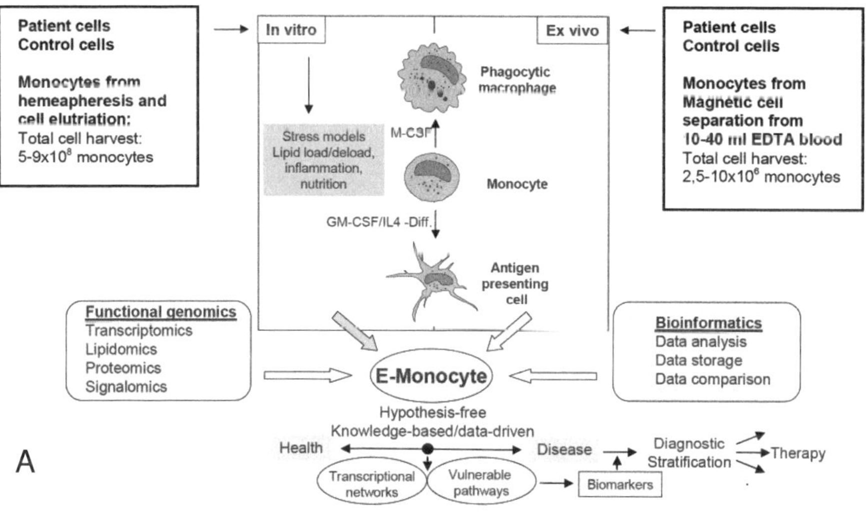

Figure 8A. Experimental strategy

The E-monocyte is a step towards systems biology that requires simultaneous investigation of multiple interacting components and use of quantitative high-throughput technologies such as DNA-microarray analysis, Taqman Low-Density Arrays in a Microfluidic Card format or Expression Sequencing, ESI-MS/MS and MALDI-TOF analysis, affinity binder assays and multiparameter flow cytometry. Computational biology and bioinformatic approaches are also applied to handle and interpret the volumes of data necessary to define these complex biological systems. In a mapping-and-arraying strategy (Figure 8B) which includes "disease-related mini-genomes" consisting of all genes within published scored genome loci intervals related to the metabolic syndrome complex, strictly stratified patients with extreme phenotypes and verified monogenetic defects are selected for in depth analysis including whole genome transcriptomic profiling and lipidomic analysis of ex-vivo monocytes exposed to an in-vitro stress panel and plasma lipid species analysis and proteomics of apolipoproteins and their sialoforms, along with already available genome-wide linkage and polymorphism data.

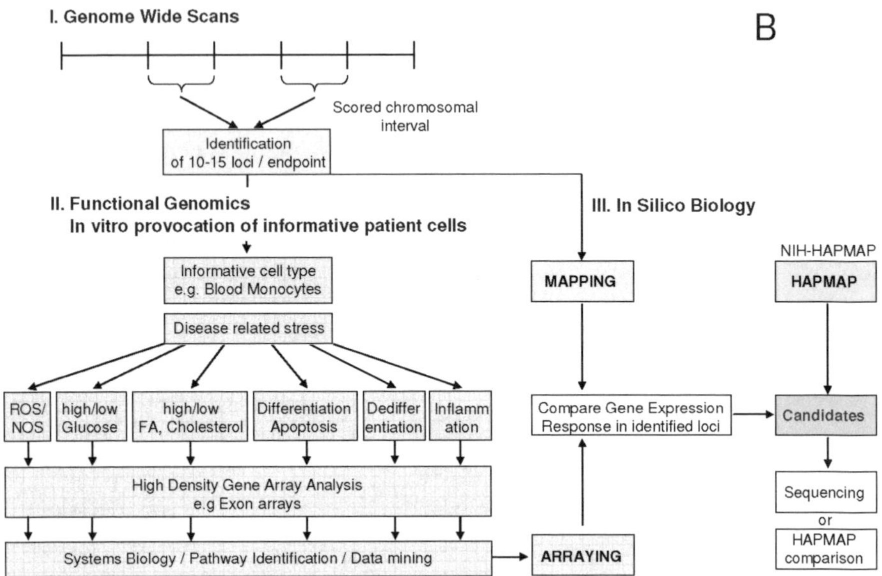

Figure 8B. Mapping and arraying approach using informative patient cells

11. Adipose Tissue as an Endocrine Organ

Adipose tissue has long been regarded as a passive type of connective tissue that stores energy as triglycerides and releases energy as free fatty acids, however, this point of view has now changed. Anatomic, metabolic and biochemical characteristics of visceral adipose tissue (VAT) indicate its importance for metabolic and inflammatory diseases. The discovery that numerous hormones, proteins, peptides, complement factors, cytokines, enzymes and receptors - collectively known as adipokines (Shimomura et al., 1996) - are expressed in and secreted by adipocytes redefined the total adipose tissue mass as a real endocrine organ at the interlink between energy metabolism and defence (Ahima and Flier, 2000).

Contributing to endocrine, paracrine and autocrine mechanisms, adipokines are involved in regulating energy homeostasis, neuroendocrine, autonomic, immune, hematologic, angiogenic, vascular and endothelial functions. Adipokine secretion differs greatly among mature adipocytes, preadipocytes, adipose tissue matrix, stroma-vascular cell fraction or simply total adipose tissue (Fain et al., 2004), which complicates the interpretation of basic and clinical research studies addressing the role of the adipose tissue in obesity, metabolism and immune function.

12. Obesity, Inflammation and the Role of the Adipose Tissue as an Immunological Organ

It has become evident that the adipose tissue connects energy metabolism with immune function and host defence (Lyon et al., 2003).

Obese adipose tissue is characterised by progressive infiltration of macrophages as obesity develops (Weisberg et al., 2003; Xu et al., 2003) . In obesity, adipocytes begin to secrete low levels of TNF-α which stimulates preadipocytes to produce MCP-1.

Similary endothelial cells also secrete MCP-1 in response to cytokines. Increased secretion of leptin and/or decreased production of adiponectin by adipocytes may also contribute to macrophage accumulation in adipose tissue which is even higher in omental adipose tissue as compared to subcutaneous adipose tissue from the same individual. Later in obesity macrophages may be the major culprits for IL-6, IL-1B, and TNF-α secretion thereby contributing via NFκB/JNK activation to the development of insulin resistance in adipocytes. Recent gene expression analysis identified that the largest class of genes (~ 30%) significantly regulated in obesity consists of macrophage and inflammatory genes in white adipose tissue (Curat et al., 2004; Weisberg et al., 2003).

Transplantation studies revealed that most of the adipose tissue macrophages develop from bone marrow-derived precursor (Weisberg et al., 2003). Due to the expression of a wide variety of complement factors, hormones, classical cytokines and adipokines and components of the renin-angiotensin system (RAA), it is suggested that the adipose tissue functions as part of the immune system.

13. The Cellular Crosstalk in Human Subcutaneous and Omental Adipose Tissue in Obesity and Insulin Resistance Syndromes

Our work aims to identify a similar cross talk between adipocytes, vascular endothelial cells, myofibroblastic elements, and adipose tissue macrophages as established for hepatic parenchymal cells (HPC), sinus endothelial cells (SEC), hepatic stellate cells (HSC), and Kupffer cells (KC) in the liver (Figure 9 B,C).

Transdifferentiation of the normal brown liver to a yellowish fatty liver and induction of fibrosis related to obesity, insulin resistance, type2 diabetes and metabolic syndrome involves the dysregulation of the interplay between hepatocytes, retinoid storing hepatic stellate cells (HSC) and monocyte-derived Kupffer cells (Figure 9 A, B). HSC are pericytes of sinusoidal endothelial cells (SEC) and are kept in a quiescent adipogenic phenotype with an excessive storage of retinoids by the threshold activity of the transcription factor PPARγ. Loss of this influence, increased inflammation or remodeling activity associated with increase in TNFα, TGFα/ß, PDGF released either from Kupffer cells, tissue macrophages or SEC, leads to activation of HSC and the conversion to myofibroblastic cells.

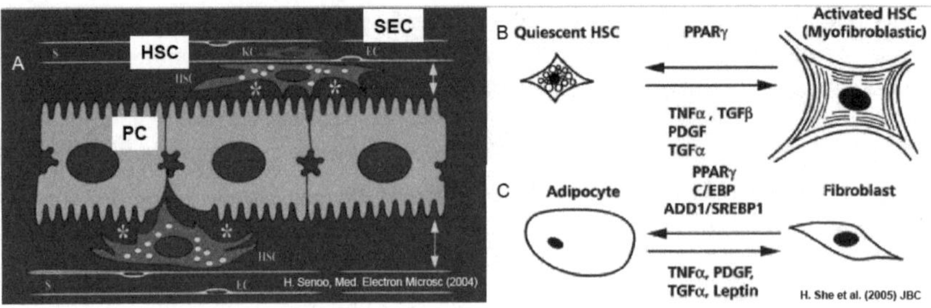

Figure 9. Cellular crosstalk in liver (Panel A: Senoo H., Med. Electron. Microsc. 2004, Panel B) and adipose tissue (Panel C: She H. et al. JBC, 2005). PC = Parenchymal Cell (Hepatocyte), HSC = Hepatic stellate cell; SEC = Sinusoidal endothelial cell

By analogy to the liver, adipogenic differentiation from mesenchymal progenitors is promoted by the master transcription factors PPARγ, C/EBP, ADD1 / SREBP1c and inhibited by TNFα, PDGF, TGFα, and leptin (Figure 9C).

The following five research modules of WP5 also reflect the patient recruitment strategy from screening programs and preventive medicine areas:

Research module 1: Transdifferentiation and pathomechanisms of organ dysfunction in the metabolic syndrome complex

Research module 2: Metabolic effects on the development of chronic diseases in ex hormone-sensitive organs

Research module 3: Atherogenic vascular disease and blood compartment interactions

Research module 4: Genetic background of chronic renal insufficiency and kidney transplantation

Research module 5: Molecular pathomechanisms of neurodegenerative disorders. Integration of international neurodegenerative biobank and networking activity into the Danubian Biobank Consortium.

Research module 1-4 reflects the vascular and metabolic disease complex. Research module 5 aims to integrate and combine existing networks of "local" neurodegenerative disease biobank activities in Germany (Ulm, Regensburg, Dresden), Austria (Linz, Vienna), Hungary (Budapest, Kecskemet, Baja, Gyula). Currently, 5150 stored biological samples (blood, liquor, DNA, etc.) of patients with neurodegenerative diseases (Dementia, Parkinson, Huntington, motoneuron diseases, Ataxia, essential tremor, Restless legs, Vascular encephalopathy and Stroke) are available, and about 8000 patient per year are seen by the cooperating clinics that can be integrated into a joint network biobank activity. The overall scientific approach is to correlate general metabolic, genetic, and environmental factors, both with specific disease entities and with aggravating or protective factors for neurodegeneration in general.

14. Future Perspectives

The major goal of the Danubian Biobank Consortium is to provide proof of concept and feasibility studies as a model for the development of translational medicine towards personalized healthcare.

References

Ahima RS and Flier JS. Adipose tissue as an endocrine organ. *Trends Endocrinol. Metab* 11 (2000), 327-332.
Curat CA, Miranville A, Sengenes C, Diehl M, Tonus C, Busse R, and Bouloumie A. From blood monocytes to adipose tissue-resident macrophages: induction of diapedesis by human mature adipocytes. *Diabetes* 53 (2004a), 1285-1292.
Fain JN, Madan AK, Hiler ML, Cheema P, and Bahouth SW. Comparison of the release of adipokines by adipose tissue, adipose tissue matrix, and adipocytes from visceral and subcutaneous abdominal adipose tissues of obese humans. *Endocrinology* 145 (2004), 2273-2282.
Lyon CJ, Law RE, and Hsueh WA. Minireview: adiposity, inflammation, and atherogenesis. *Endocrinology* 144 (2003), 2195-2200.
Shimomura I, Funahashi T, Takahashi M, Maeda K, Kotani K, Nakamura T, Yamashita S, Miura M, Fukuda Y, Takemura K, Tokunaga K, and Matsuzawa Y. Enhanced expression of PAI-1 in visceral fat: possible contributor to vascular disease in obesity. *Nat. Med.* 2 (1996), 800-803.
She H, Xiong S, Hazra S, Tsukamoto H. Adipogenic transcriptional regulation of hepatic stellate cells. *J Biol Chem.* 2005 Feb 11;280(6):4959-67
Senoo H. Structure and function of hepatic stellate cells. *Med Electron Microsc.* Mar;37(1) 2004:3-15. Review
Weisberg SP, McCann D, Desai M, Rosenbaum M, Leibel RL, and Ferrante AW Jr. Obesity is associated with macrophage accumulation in adipose tissue. *J. Clin. Invest* 112 (2003), 1796-1808.
Xu H, Barnes GT, Yang Q, Tan G, Yang D, Chou CJ, Sole J, Nichols A, Ross JS, Tartaglia LA, and Chen H. Chronic inflammation in fat plays a crucial role in the development of obesity-related insulin resistance. *J. Clin. Invest* 112 (2003), 1821-1830.

eHealth from Dream to Reality

eHealth in Europe: from Vision to Reality

Ilias IAKOVIDIS [1] and Octavian PURCAREA
European Commission, Directorate General Information Society and Media,
Unit ICT for Health, Brussels, Belgium

Abstract. It is now 20 years that the European Union supports research and development of information and communication technologies based tools for healthcare (eHealth). From 1989 till today, funding has continually been increased, initiating new research, complementing Member State initiatives, strengthening European industrial competitiveness, and tackling new health and social problems related to the free movement of people in the EU. By now, many of the earlier visions and dreams have been realised or are close to wider implementation. Accordingly, the European Commission is now providing strong support also for market validation and implementation of eHealth solutions and services, and at the health policy level. Examples are the recent eHealth Action Plan, annual High Level Ministerial Conferences, an upcoming Recommendation on European eHealth Interoperability, or the Member States-led Large Scale Pilot on a pan-European core patient summary and ePrescribing. This will be complemented by a Lead Market Initiative identifying eHealth as a core future innovation field. Growing cooperation with counterparts in the USA and elsewhere underline that eHealth is becoming a global reality. A more than 40 year old vision is now closer to global reality for the better of all citizens.

Keywords. eHealth, European Commission, ICT for Health R&D, eHealth Strategy, interoperability, eHealth deployment

1. eHealth in Europe - the Early Days

The European Commission (EC) R&D Programmes have been supporting ICT for Health (eHealth) by now for more than 20 years resulting in over 450 projects worth more than € 1 billion. All of these activities have contributed to the emergence of standardised eHealth solutions such as electronic health records and a health knowledge infostructure that was only possible through the projects on EU level. They also included various promotion activities such as the eHealth Ministerial Conferences. The EC was one of the first international funding agencies to support research and development (R&D) in eHealth (in areas such as medical informatics, health telematics and biomedical informatics) at a larger scale, and has invested over € 650 million in eHealth research projects alone during this time period. The goal that has underpinned the EC's R&D policy in eHealth has been the development of tools for continuity of care. These have included electronic health record systems, regional health information networks that connect all the points of care (i.e., hospitals, primary care, labs,

---

[1] Corresponding Author: Ilias Iakovidis, PhD, Deputy Head of Unit, ICT for Health Unit, DG INFSO, European Commission, B-1049 Brussels, Belgium; Email: Ilias.Iakovidis@ec.europa.eu

pharmacies, and homes), and support to all stages of prevention, diagnosis, treatment and follow-up.

2. Supporting eHealth Today and Tomorrow – Realising the Vision

By now, many of the earlier visions and dreams have been realised or are close to wider implementation. Accordingly, since FP6 and in the context of other activities, the EC has provided strong support not only for R&D activities, but also for market validation and implementation of eHealth solutions and services, and at the eHealth policy level.

2.1. Continuing Support for R&D

Currently, in the context of the new 7th Framework programme (FP7), the emphasis of the EC's eHealth R&D programme is on personal health systems that transform each patient into a "node" of local and regional health information networks. Continuous health status management, disease prevention and patient education are enhanced and enabled. The importance of eHealth and its achievements have been appropriately recognised at the highest levels. As a result, the EC's budget for eHealth R&D has been doubled over the next two-year period to € 100 million a year. Other research topics include ICT for patient safety and support to predictive medicine. Patient-specific models are being developed to assist in safer medical operations, alongside the development of personalised treatments and safer drugs [1]. Predictive medicine brings together the medical and bioinformatics communities to collaborate on molecular medicine, where disease and physiology aspects are integrated from the level of molecule and cell to the levels of organs and systems [2].

In the area of patient safety the European Commission supports R&D in advanced information systems that can demonstrate beneficial impact on patient safety and risk assessment through the prediction, detection and monitoring of adverse (drug) events using novel integration and data mining methods and tools.

2.2. eHealth Policy Support

2.2.1. eHealth Action Plan

Since 2004, the EC has also taken a lead in coordinating eHealth policy development and applications deployment by adopting a European eHealth Action plan [3]. Strategic objectives include:

- Provide integrated, interoperable and secure Health information networks and online services supporting online services for better quality and personalised care;
- Enable citizens to access quality health knowledge on-line and enable access to patients to their health record;
- Stimulate national and regional implementation plans and investment and beneficial deployment of eHealth solutions across Europe;
- Facilitate transparency and growth of an innovation friendly eHealth market.

The *activities* under the eHealth Action Plan are expected to:

- Support Member States in developing deployment roadmaps and investment in eHealth;
- Stimulate investment and beneficial deployment of eHealth solutions;
- Accelerate the development of interoperable solutions;
- Facilitate labelling, certification and accreditation of eHealth systems;
- Provide more legal certainty in using and managing eHealth systems and services;
- Facilitate the growth and transparency of the eHealth market;
- Address the fragmentation of the eHealth landscape across Europe.

This eHealth Action Plan is imbedded in the wider context of realising the EU *Lisbon Strategy* [4], and the consequent EU and Member State activities. The creation of a European eHealth area [5], free patient mobility [6] and empowering the citizen through eHealth tools and services [7] are now key policy objectives of the Union, which are also firmly embedded within the framework of the i2010 Initiative [8].

2.2.2. eHealth Ministerial Conferences

These developments also illustrate the recognition by policy makers across the European Union Member States of the enabling value of eHealth solutions in ensuring the highest possible health level for their citizens. Since 2003, annual High Level Ministerial eHealth Conferences have strongly supported these aims [9]. E.g., in the conclusions to the High Level eHealth Conference 2006 in Malaga, Spain, the participants, policy makers on EU and national ministerial level, as well as CEO level industry representatives and distinguished researchers and experts, acknowledged that [10]: "Europe can benefit from eHealth that focuses on ensuring better:

- *Prevention of diseases*
- *Prediction of diseases*
- *Personalisation of healthcare*
- *Participation of Europe's citizens in their own healthcare improvement*
- *Increased patient safety throughout all stages of the healthcare process*
- *Productivity and performance of Europe's healthcare systems, and of Europe's third healthcare industrial pillar*
- *Monitoring of indicators and production of regular data and reports on health status.*

eHealth can also underscore and underpin other current concerns of healthcare authorities throughout Europe, such as:

- *Providing support to health professionals by making up-to-date information available on disease prevention and management*
- *Assessing means of cross-border healthcare purchasing and provision*
- *Understanding and monitoring of health professionals' mobility*
- *Creating interaction and organisational links among the public health community in Europe*
- *Creating a network of health impact assessment and health systems*
- *Creating an operational network of Member States' patient safety contact points."*

In April 2007, the Member States and the European Commission made a common declaration summing up the *conclusions of the 2007 eHealth Conference in Berlin,* therein "stressing the following key issues:

1) National well-organised eHealth infrastructures are pre-requisite for cross-border solutions;

2) European standardisation will open up market opportunities;
3) Existing National roadmaps must be taken into account;
4) Implementation of eHealth services require greater synergies with research and education;
5) Agreement on common standards by all EU Member States is essential;
6) The eHealth industry and other stakeholders must be involved."

Interoperability and electronic health records have entered explicitly the cooperation plans of Member States: "There will be an increased focus on the deployment of eHealth systems, setting up of targets for interoperability, use of electronic health records, and reimbursement of eHealth services" [11].

2.3. eHealth Deployment

2.3.1. Towards European eHealth Interoperability

The lack of interoperability in systems and services has long been identified as one of the major challenges to the wider implementation of the Union's eHealth applications. The opportunities and positive benefits of achieving interoperability in eHealth are ultimately considerable, whereas various barriers and challenges continue to act as impediments. In order to provide support to addressing these challenges and based on the activities described above, the EC services issued in September 2006 a report *"Connected Health: Quality and Safety for European Citizens"* [12], which provided a framework for the work leading to a milestone by the end of 2007 in the form of guidelines and recommendations to EU Member States for ensuring near future basic interoperability of eHealth systems. Furthermore, the Commission is working on a *Recommendation* that "supports the premise that connecting people, systems, and services is vital for the provision of good healthcare in Europe, and significantly contributes to the establishment and functioning of the internal market by ensuring the free flow of patients, eHealth products and services" [13]. Interoperability is desirable for all citizens to have the capability of receiving healthcare services, regardless of the way they are delivered, having regard to technological neutrality and future technological progress.

The ultimate goal of European eHealth interoperability is to enable access to a patient's summary and emergency data from any place in Europe, respecting data privacy and security. The Recommendation seeks to allot various responsibilities to both the European Commission and to the Member States. For example, standardisation plays an integral part in the European Union's policies to increase the competitiveness of companies and to remove trade barriers. In the area of eHealth, the 2005 Report from the European Committee for Standardization [14] (CEN) emphasised that health information standards are essential to achieving the goals of eHealth in Europe. In particular, the Member States are invited to undertake actions at five levels:

- At the political/legal level: To build a political platform that is aimed at setting up the necessary legal and regulatory environment so as to render eHealth infrastructure and services interoperable. This could involve more effective coordination, and harmonisation – where necessary, of the Member States' legislations.
- At the organisational level: To agree on an organisational framework for interoperability that recognises the autonomy of each Member State in what concerns the development of the relevant eHealth infrastructure and services

but creates a common domain with the necessary interfaces to enable the national domains to interact.

- At the technical (including architectural) level: To promote the use of technical standards and architectures, and the establishment of common interoperability platforms.
- At the semantic level: To coordinate efforts towards semantic activities by agreeing on common priorities, initially (through agreed, high-priority use cases) and to share these results and experiences.
- At the level of evaluation, monitoring, and education: To evaluate, monitor, analyse, and reflect on all the intended developments and possible others in the eHealth interoperability field, and to consider various education mechanisms.

2.3.2. Towards Large Scale Pan-European Implementations of eHealth Solutions

Acknowledging the increasing mobility of European citizens, EU Member States (MSs) with support form the EC are expected to start implementing a so-called Large Scale [eHealth] Pilot (LSP) in 2008. Already at the High Level Health Conference in April, 2007, in Berlin they concluded:

"Large Scale Pilots will test the application of improved patient summaries in different health contexts such as medical emergencies and prescription dispensing. [...] As part of this joint initiative, progress will be made in relation to improving interoperability; use of electronic health records; deployment of research results; and development and coordination of eHealth standards essential to cross-border applications." [15]

A project proposal by 12 Member States has been submitted to the EC Competitiveness and Innovation Programme (CIP) [16] which directly addresses this specific pan-European policy goal and targets two eHealth application fields – a core patient summary useful in case of an unexpected, initial encounter between a European citizen and a doctor from a country different from the patient's country of origin, and (pan-European) ePrescribing.

2.3.3. eHealth Products and Services as a Market Leader in Europe

Recently, eHealth products and services have also been recognised as a potential global market leader in which Europe should invest. [4] The 2006 *Aho Report* [17], "Creating an Innovative Europe", identified eHealth as an example of a key area, where a market for innovations and their wide diffusion can flourish, and public policy should have a significant role in fostering its further development. The EC subsequently proposed a *Lead Market Initiative (LMI)* [18] to facilitate the creation and marketing of innovative products and services. One of the four key areas targeted for action concerns the support for eHealth as a lead market.

The views developed in this article are those of the authors and do not necessarily reflect the position of the European Commission.

References

[1] Stroetmann VN, Stroetmann KA, Thierry JP, Purcarea O. Advanced ICT for patient safety and quality of care. In: International Hospital Equipment & Solutions, V. 32, No. 8 (Dec. 2006), pp. 12-13, eHealth for Safety - Impact of ICT on Patient Safety and Risk Management. Veli N. Stroetmann, Jean-Pierre Thierry, Karl A. Stroetmann, Alexander Dobrev: European Commission. eHealth for Safety Report, October 2007. Luxembourg, Office for Official Publications of the European Communities, 2007 (70 pp. - ISBN-13 978-92-79-06841-6) http://www.ehealth-for-safety.org/news/documents/eHealth-safety-report-final.pdf

[2] Iakovidis I: eHealth Matters. Deputy Head, ICT for Health, European Commission, DG Information Society and Media, in World of Health IT Conference 2006, Geneva, Switzerland

[3] Communication on "eHealth - making healthcare better for European citizens: An action plan for a European eHealth Area", COM (2004) 356 final. See http://europa.eu.int/information_society/activities/health/policy_action_plan/index_en.htm

[4] Presidency Conclusions of the Lisbon European Council, 22-24 March 2000.

[5] Commission of the European Communities - COM (2004) 356: e-Health - making health care better for European citizens: An action plan for a European e-Health Area, Brussels, 2004-04-30.

[6] CEC (2004): Follow-up to the high level reflection process on patient mobility and health care developments in the European Union. COM (204) 301 final, Brussels, 20.04.2004.

[7] Wilson, P., Leitner, Ch. and Moussalli, A. (2004): Mapping the Potential of eHealth, Empowering the citizen through eHealth tools and services. Maastricht: European Institute of Public Administration. This was the overriding topic of the 2004 European Presidency eHealth conference in Cork, Ireland, in May 2004.

[8] Commission of the European Communities – COM (2005) 229: Communication from the Commission to the Council, the European Parliament, the European Economic and Social Committee and the Committee of the Regions: "i2010 – A European Information Society for growth and employment", Brussels, 1.6.2005

[9] eHealth conferences: 2003 in Brussels, Belgium, 2004 in Cork, Ireland, 2005 in Tromsø, Norway.

[10] Draft Final Conference conclusions – High Level eHealth Conference 2006, Málaga, Spain; http://www.ehealthconference2006.org/images/stories/Conclusions.pdf

[11] eHealth Conference 2007, Final Declaration of Member States and the European Commission, 17 April 2007:

[12] http://europa.eu.int/information_society/activities/health/docs/policy/connected-health_final-covers18092006.pdf

[13] Draft Recommendation on eHealth Interoperability, for informal public consultation, http://ec.europa.eu/information_society/newsroom/cf/itemdetail.cfm?item_id=3540

[14] Report from the CEN/ISSS eHealth Standardization Focus Group: Current and future standardization issues in the e-Health domain: Achieving interoperability, Final version, March 2005

[15] ibid.

[16] Competitiveness and Innovation Programme, Information Communication Technology Policy Support Programme Call, http://ec.europa.eu/information_society/activities/ ict_psp/index_en.htm

[17] Aho E (2006): Creating an Innovative Europe: Report of the Independent Expert Group on R+D and Innovation Appointed Following the Hampton Court Summit, available at: http://ec.europa.eu/invest-in-research/pdf/download_en/aho_report.pdf

[18] Commission of the European Communities - Communication from the Commission to the Council, the European Parliament, the European Economic and Social Committee and the Committee of the Regions of 13 September 2006 "Putting knowledge into practice: A broad-based innovation strategy for the EU" [COM(2006) 502 final], www.europe-innova.org/exportedcontent/docs/6/6206/en/EN%20502%20-%20original.doc

eHealth: Combining Health Telematics, Telemedicine, Biomedical Engineering and Bioinformatics to the Edge. Edited by B. Blobel, P. Pharow and M. Nerlich.
IOS Press, 2008

eHealth: Connecting Health Care and Public Health

E. Andrew BALAS [a,1], Santosh KRISHNA [b], Tsigeweini A. TESSEMA [a]
[a] *College of Health Sciences, Old Dominion University, Norfolk, Virginia, USA*
[b] *School of Public Health, Saint Louis University, St. Louis, Missouri, USA*

Abstract. Reducing risks and improving benefits to the patients are requirements health professionals are faced with in their daily work. Furthermore, cuts in health funds and the competition for budgets require to enhancing efficacy and efficiency of health services. For meeting both challenges, adequate information and knowledge is needed, which can be gathered from documentation systems such as Electronic Health Records or Personal Health Records (PHRs), but also by performing dedicated clinical studies such as randomized controlled trials (RCTs) or cohort studies. Based on a literature analysis, quality of, and benefits from, RCTs have been analyzed. The benefits from connecting public health and PHRs are discussed in some details.

Keywords. Effectiveness research, randomized controlled trials, personal health records, public health

Introduction

In daily practice professionals make critical decisions that involve risks and benefits. Correct decision is closely related to having adequate information and knowledge available in an accessible manner at the right time. This can only be affordable by making a system that can gather routine data and make it available and accessible when needed. This is rather a realistic optimism for our times because the great advancements in information technology (IT) can be utilized in balancing the demands and needs for the benefit of public health.

Beyond its use in improving communication in healthcare programs, IT is critical for transforming the overall healthcare quality. Namely IT will be able to integrate complex information from different sources that can facilitate providers' access to relevant public health data as well as enabling patients' to be better involved in personal health decisions.

American health care is viewed as one of the most advanced but most expensive systems in the world. Over the past four decades Medicare's and Medicaid's costs per beneficiary have increased about 2.5% points faster per year than has per capita gross domestic product [1]. If these costs continue growing at a similar rate, for the next four decades federal spending will likely rise to 20% by 2050. Despite the increasing spending, a growing proportion of the population reports being unable to obtain needed

---

[1] Corresponding Author: E. Andrew Balas, MD, PhD, Professor, College of Health Sciences, Old Dominion University, Norfolk, Norfolk, VA 23529, USA; Email: abalas@odu.edu

medical care due to cost [2]. Life expectancy is shorter and infant mortality rate is higher for the United States than for many other industrial countries [3]. Moreover an increasing proportion of the US population reports being unable to obtain needed medical care due to cost [2].

Much of these inequalities are related to the lack of proper knowledge management in public health so far. This points out to using public health data for evaluating relative effectiveness between available health care choices. In this regard proper utilization of IT will accelerate and transform the healthcare system by allowing proper data gathering, storage, analysis and exchange between care givers and users both for routine care as well as for research and policy processes. This will rapidly transfer innovative research outcome into practice that ultimately lead to a healthier society.

At present the healthcare system is affected by several factors that are interconnected to one another. The following sections highlight the problems inherited in the healthcare services and practices. In addition the sections discuss a better design for connecting healthcare to public health and thus to bring improved quality and value to healthcare and self care.

1. Unnecessary Procedures: A Burden of Public Health

The escalating cost of health care has had an enormous impact on the national economy. Growth in pharmaceutical expenses, duplication procedures, unnecessary procedures, over utilization and misuse of technology have been identified as cost drivers in health care [4, 5]. Our purpose was to provide an overview of the literature on unnecessary procedures performed by clinicians.

Electronic databases were searched for eligible studies by using MEDLINE (1966-2004), PubMed, Cochran Review, CINAHL, and ACP databases. Search was conducted on only English language publications by using phrases like unnecessary procedures, inappropriate procedures, duplicate procedures, redundant procedures, needless procedures, pointless procedures, unwarranted procedures, outdated procedures and medical necessity. Subsequently, we calculated the estimated cost of an unnecessary procedure by using HCUP and CMS databases based on ICD-9 codes. The cost of a procedure was obtained using the Health Care Utilization Project developed and maintained by the Agency for Healthcare Research and Quality (AHRQ).

Among 1037 articles retrieved by the search, only 30 met the eligibility criteria and they were either randomized controlled trials (RCTs) or cohort studies. The resulting unnecessary procedures were performed across different medical specialties in the United States. Broadly, these procedures have been divided into four categories, 1) general surgery, 2) obstetrics and gynecology, 3) subspecialties, 4) non-therapeutic and miscellaneous procedures. Outcomes and conclusions of the study are summarized below.

1.1. General Surgery

Approximately 20% (57,848) of the estimated number of appendectomies (289,742) performed were said to be unnecessary procedure [6], especially in patients with abdominal pain of unknown etiology. In certain groups such as women of reproductive ages, the rate of this unnecessary procedure may be as high as 26%. With a cost of

$13,479 for each appendectomy procedure, the estimated total cost of unnecessary procedures (20%) can be approaching $779.73 millions per year.

1.2. Hysterectomy

Hysterectomy is the second most common OB/GYN surgical operation. An estimated 2.3 hysterectomies were done per 1000 population in 2000 [7], resulting in a total number of 650,000 procedures performed annually in the United States. Of these numbers, 76% procedures were without appropriate prior diagnostic evaluation and in some cases no consideration was given to alternative options [8]. The 487,500 hysterectomies represent potentially unnecessary procedures, resulting in a total cost of $7.6 billion for unnecessary procedures at a rate of $15,607 per procedure [9].

1.3. Subspecialty Surgery

Tonsillectomy is performed frequently among US children with an annual total of 287,000 procedures (National Survey of Ambulatory Surgery, 1996). In a study by Spinou et al [10] eighteen (38%) did not have symptom of sore throats at all. The occurrence of malignancy in children with unilateral tonsillar enlargement is very low. Therefore, tonsillectomy is an unnecessary procedure in a case of unilateral tonsillar enlargement without any other clinical findings suggestive of malignancy. Again based on the on an estimated cost of $9,052 per procedure [7] these patients incurred estimated total costs of $425,444 as a result of unnecessary procedures.

1.4. Non-therapeutic and Miscellaneous Procedures

In several cases, routine radiograph investigation appears to serve only as a protection against malpractice claims. A knee radiograph is routinely performed to identify fractures in acute knee injuries. An estimated 1.3 million patients visit US emergency departments with acute knee injuries each year. However in a study by Stiell et al [11], only 6% (60,000) of such patients actually had fracture, while the results were negative in over 92% of cases. The study reported, a set of five clinical criteria were used to identify 100% of the cases that had fractures. These included 1) aged 55 years or older, 2) tenderness at head of fibula, 3) isolated tenderness of patella, 4) inability to flex to 90°, 5) inability to bear weight both immediately and in the emergency department. A knee radiograph was appropriate for patient with one or more of the above clinical findings. Per knee radiograph procedure, the cost is $49.26 [12], while the total costs of unnecessary knee radiograph is around $46,624,000. The unnecessary knee radiograph could have been avoided with the proven use of clinical judgment prior to investigation.

In summary, evidence suggests that clinicians continue to perform unnecessary procedures. Several factors have been attributed to the increase in the numbers of unnecessary procedures and rise in health care costs in the country, which include lack of consensus among clinicians on the effectiveness of some procedures or medical services, variability in medical practice across different states, lack of information and knowledge on the effectiveness of new and expensive technologies, unavailable criteria or standards to help clinicians make a decision on the appropriateness of procedures, and the practice of defensive medicine [13]. The large numbers of unnecessary procedures are in part responsible for the high health care costs.

2. Promise of Comparative Effectiveness Research

One obviously visible obstacle in the current healthcare system is the lack of sufficient evidence about relative effectiveness of available therapies and intervention methods. Comparative effectiveness is simply a measure of what works best in healthcare. Depending on the goal of the comparison, outcomes may be interpreted in terms of risks, cost effectiveness and benefits, and length of time. In this regard comparative effectiveness research is an essential step and a scientific tool for addressing the challenges and growing gaps in healthcare quality and value. Unfortunately the interest in technology assessment that has emerged during the mid 1990s has often shown little progress and impact on this issue.

Research methodologies like RCTs can be used for many purposes such as evaluating new drugs and new tests of new healthcare and medical care technologies. Trials can also be used to assess new programs for screening and health early detection, or new ways of organizing and delivering health services. RCTs are considered gold standard in measuring the efficacy of new therapies because of their ability to reliably detect moderate differences in clinical outcomes and thus limit the uncertainty related to estimating the efficacy and efficiency of a specific therapy. Moreover RCTs are less subject to confounding and bias for the evaluation of effectiveness and thus provide the strongest evidence to make recommendations based on outcomes.

Clinicians are taught that RCTs provide the most robust evidence in medicine. Therefore as clinicians aim at balancing benefit and risk of therapies every day, they extrapolate evidence from RCTs to their own patient population believing that their patients will benefit from an equally large effect.

Basically, presumed benefits of large publicly funded controlled clinical studies include (i) forceful highlighting of a perceived important needs; (ii) promise of definitive and unbiased answers to important questions; (iii) focused application of all available resources and talents; (iv) multiple publications from a most carefully collected, large sample; and (v) source of pride for funding agencies. However when looking closely to the spectrum of recent comparative studies, questions are arising.

For example, the antihypertensive and Lipid-Lowering Treatment to Prevent Heart Attack Trial (ALLHAT) multi-center study needed $120 million government support to follow 42,218 Americans for five years. The study concluded that older thiazide-type diuretics (as opposed to newer patented drugs) should be the drugs of choice for first-step antihypertensive therapy.

Another study, the multi-center Multiple Risk Factor Trial (MRFIT) screened 350,000 middle-aged men. Researchers selected close to 13,000 believed to be at greater risk and were divided into a treatment and control groups. After ten years and $115 million in expenses, the treatment group substantially achieved their objectives but fared no differently from controls.

Another trial was launched by the National Institutes of Health, Women's Health Initiative (WHI) in 1993. Over 14 years, this $625 million study involved 160,000 women at 45 clinical centers and thousands more in community studies. The Clinical Trial component was the most expensive and complex, and involved 63,000 post-menopausal women. The trial investigators concluded that the low-fat, high-starch diet as reflected by the USDA food guide pyramid is outdated. However, women in the study only modestly lowered their fat levels, from 38% to 29% i.e., failed to reach the trial's target of 20%. From the beginning, the Institute of Medicine raised several concerns about the structure and budgeting of the WHI.

One additional example in this category is the Clinical Antipsychotic Trials in Intervention Effectiveness (CATIE) where early results raised rather questions about reimbursement policies for antipsychotic medications, the fourth largest group of medications prescribed in the United States. The New England Journal of Medicine report by the CATIE research team concluded that older medication, perphenazine, was as well tolerated as the newer compounds and as effective as three of the four newer drugs. However, controversies surrounding the early conclusions forced NIMH to release a note of caution about the use of results from this $42 million trial to inform reimbursement policy.

Based on these and other case studies, the leading particular risks of large clinical trials for comparative effectiveness are summarized below

2.1. A Large RCT is Uncontrolled Investigation

The only possible way to provide a scientific outcome is by proving the reproducibility of the outcomes under similar conditions. This process requires re-conducting the study and therefore will demand additional resources for covering expenses related to the re-trial. However the expenditure on a large clinical trial is huge in the first place and therefore re-funding for replication of the study is unthinkable. Due to this limiting factor, outcomes of large RCT are readily adopted without re-conducting the investigation and thus in the absence of replicable results.

2.2. Large RCT Closes Doors for New Inventions

The average NIH funding for a single non-RCT grant proposal is about 1.5 million USD, less than 1% of the budget for a single large RCT. Therefore when funding a large RCT, the process is limiting the opportunity for many other apparently small but more scientific researches that could result in new innovations and advancements for the future.

2.3. Large RCT Constitute an Overpowered Population Size

Clinical trials study whether two or more interventions are the same or different in producing the outcome of interest. In this case what is required is the minimum sample size needed to detect a worthwhile benefit signified by statistical power. As the sample size increases beyond a certain level, the study gets a statistical power that can detect negligible differences in the outcome of interest. In this sense, large RCTs can reveal statistically significant but practically irrelevant differences.

2.4. Large RCTs Tend to Test Old and Outdated Therapies

The process to conduct a single large RCT, from planning to execution, is time consuming. Such a lengthy process can take more than three decades. By the time of approval, the investigated therapies are probably outdated. However since RCT is considered a gold standard, outcomes are likely to be adopted by policy makers and practitioners without negotiation. Therefore, this process limits the potential benefit from other new and probably improved generations of therapies.

2.5. Large RCT Aim at Assessing Risks

The goal in conducting RCTs is to reliably detect moderate differences in clinical outcomes and to limit the uncertainty related to estimating the efficacy and efficiency of a specific therapy. Also immediate risks that appear during the time of intervention are evaluated and followed up in the process. However long term risks are not known until the intervention is applied across a wide range of patients for a longer period of time. Therefore increasing the size and duration of RCT for the sake of evaluating risks is probably unethical because the basic principle of randomizing persons is meant only for assessing benefits but not risks. In fact the best way to assess risks linked to therapies is addressed by retrospective studies.

3. Connecting Public Health and Personal Health Records

The use of electronic personal health records is spreading in the United States and worldwide. In a 1998 concept paper, the National Committee on Vital and Health Statistics (NCVHS) described three types of computer-based health records: patient (clinical), personal, and population health records. With the advancement of web-based technologies and interest in making records accessible to patients, the number of services available and the number of actual personal record users is rapidly increasing. Besides their promises for self-care, electronic personal health records also have a tremendous public health potential.

Public health routinely relies on data about individual health in an aggregate format. Epidemiologic surveillance uses birth and death statistics, disease specific information about nationally notifiable infectious diseases (e.g., AIDS, tuberculosis, botulism, poliomyelitis, giardiasis and others). In addition to such conventional reports, CDC collects data on blood testing from organizations such as the American Red Cross (e.g. hepatitis B and C, Chagas disease, West Nile Virus and others). The CDC BioSense project further expands the data collection from health care providers that agreed on Data Sharing (e.g., the Department of Defense and Veterans Administration, LabCorp, or the American Association of Poison Control Centers).

3.1. Twelve Essential Health Information Rights

To live a healthy and successful life, we need timely and trustworthy information about issues important to our health. As citizens, we have many rights including important rights to essential health information. The following points summarize these rights that appear to be essential:

Risks to our health
1. Advance warning about environmental, occupational, nutritional, and other hazards to our health
2. Freedom from irrelevant, unsubstantiated, and unsolicited messages about health risks that are either negligible or non-existent

Information about therapies
3. Access to the latest scientific information that can help to protect or regain citizens' health
4. Freedom from misinformation about therapies that have never been reliably linked to better outcomes

Availability and safeguarding of personal health information
5.　An easy and complete access to any health information in our personal record
6.　Based on your authorization, easy access to your records by your caregiver
7.　Confidentiality and privacy protection of your health information
Informed patient participation in health care decision-making
8.　Right to be heard in the process of patient care and clinical decision-making
9.　Freedom to make informed decisions without feeling pressurized
10.　Choices and information about outcomes of procedures and providers

Health education for effective self-care
11.　Right to get disease specific, individually tailored patient education
12.　Right to get reimbursed health education when it can improve outcomes

3.2. Personal Health Records

Today, electronic personal health records offer the potential for new information source. A personal health record (PHR) is typically a health record that is initiated and maintained by an individual. PHR can include a wide variety of important information such as medications, allergies, surgeries, immunizations, laboratory tests, contact information, basic providers and insurance. Concerning these important aspects, the current PHRs have various limitations namely, lack of online input from diagnostic and other services and also difficulties in sharing such records.

With the spread and increased sophistication of PHRs, their public health and clinical research significance is likely to increase rapidly. Using PHRs as clinical patient records and also as a resource for public health purposes will offer (i) a major new source of important health information; (ii) increased information about otherwise hard to obtain records (e.g., symptoms and syndromes); and (iii) an opportunity for individuals to support public health and bio-defense.

The history of widespread use credit cards offers some projections for the future potential of PHRs in health information exchange. The idea of a card for purchases was invented in 1887 by Edward Bellamy in his utopian novel Looking Backward, set in the year 2000. He used the term "Credit Card" eleven times in his novel. In 1958, Bank of America created the BankAmericard that eventually evolved into the Visa system. In 1966, a group of 14 US banks formed Interlink, a processing association to exchange information on credit card transactions. The widespread use of credit cards depends on the banking system being perceived as reliable for banking purposes. The Truth in Lending Act (TILA) of 1968 and the Fair Credit Billing Act of 1986 represented important Congressional contributions to the accelerated use of credit cards in consumer transactions.

Coming back to public health, the following particular measures could accelerate the use of PHRs and their implementation in public health and research:
1.　Coalition and standards for digital clinical data sharing into PHR
2.　Encouraging privacy and confidentiality protection for PHR providers
3.　Provider and patient incentives for using and sharing PHRs
4.　Regulation supporting PHR availability for public health surveillance
5.　Incentives for offering stored PHR information for health research

In conclusion, Personal Health Records could and probably should be recognized as a major public health information asset. Such records offer an unparalleled opportunity and power to reveal relevant information of public health significance.

References

[1] Congressional Budget Office. The Long-Term Budget Outlook (December 2005), pp 6-7 and 31-32.
[2] Obtaining needed medical care. Early release of selected estimates based on data from the 2007 national health interview survey. National Center for Health Statistics. Center for Diseases Control and Prevention. available at http://www.cdc.gov/nchs/about/major/nhis/released200703.htm
[3] International cooperation at a crossroads: Aid, trade and security in an unequal world. Human development report 2005. available at http://hdr.undp.org/reports/global/2005/
[4] Beever C, Burns H, Karbe M. U.S. Health care's technology cost crisis. available from:http://www.strategy-business.com/enewsarticle/enews033104?pg=0 (accessed: October 2004)
[5] Agency for healthcare Research and Quality (AHRQ). Health care costs: Why do they increase? What can we do? available at http://www.ahrq.gov/news/ulp/costs/ulpcosts.htm (accessed: October 2004)
[6] Flum DR, Koepsell T. The clinical and economic correlates of misdiagnosed appendicitis. Arch Surg. 2002; 137:799-804.
[7] Owings MF, Kozak LJ. Ambulatory and inpatient procedures in the United States, 1996. Vital and health statistics. Series 13. No. 139. Hyattsville, Md.: National Center for Health Statistics, November 1998. (DHHS publication no. (PHS) 99-1710).
[8] Broader MS, Kanouse DE, Mittman BS, Berstein SJ. The appropriateness of recommendations for hysterectomy. *Obstet Gynecol.* 2000; 95:199-205.
[9] HCUPnet, Healthcare Cost and Utilization Project. Agency for Healthcare Research and Quality, Rockville, MD. available from: http://www.ahrq.gov/data/hcup/hcupnet.htm. (accessed: October 2004)
[10] Spinou E, Kubba H, Konstantinidis I, Johnston A. Tonsillectomy for biopsy in children with unilateral tonsillar enlargement. *Int J Pediatr Otorhinolarygol.* 2002; 63:15-7.
[11] Stiell IG, Greeberg G, Well GA, McDowell I, Cwinn AA, Smith NA, Cacciotti TF, Sivilotti ML. Prospective validation of a decision rule for the use of radiography in acute knee injuries. *JAMA.* 1996; 275:611-615.
[12] Centers for Medicare & Medicaid Services (CMS). available from: http://www.cms.hhs.gov/default.asp? (accessed: October 2004)
[13] Eisenberg JM. Evaluation science & our health care system. available from: http://www.hhs.gov/asl/testify/ t970417a.html. (accessed: October 2004)

177

ICW eHealth Framework

Karsten KLEIN [1], Astrid C. WOLFF, Oliver ZIEBOLD and Thomas LIEBSCHER
InterComponentWare AG, Germany

Abstract. The ICW eHealth Framework (eHF) is a powerful infrastructure and platform for the development of service-oriented solutions in the health care business. It is the culmination of many years of experience of ICW in the development and use of in-house health care solutions and represents the foundation of ICW product developments based on the Java Enterprise Edition (Java EE). The ICW eHealth Framework has been leveraged to allow development by external partners – enabling adopters a straightforward integration into ICW solutions. The ICW eHealth Framework consists of reusable software components, development tools, architectural guidelines and conventions defining a full software-development and product lifecycle. From the perspective of a partner, the framework provides services and infrastructure capabilities for integrating applications within an eHF-based solution. This article introduces the ICW eHealth Framework's basic architectural concepts and technologies. It provides an overview of its module and component model, describes the development platform that supports the complete software development lifecycle of health care applications and outlines technological aspects, mainly focusing on application development frameworks and open standards.

Keywords. eHealth, electronic health record, model driven software development

Introduction

The ICW eHealth Framework consists of a solution platform and a development environment. The solution platform contains modules that provide application programming interface (API) functionality, which can be used by health care applications or add-on modules. Modules can expose web service interfaces that can participate in an orchestrated service-oriented architecture (SOA).

The foundation of the ICW eHealth Framework is a flexible and high-quality development environment. Application developers can use the development environment and its tools to enhance their productivity in health care software projects. A key element is the Code Generator, which is able to generate code and configuration artifacts from a UML (Unified Modeling Language) domain model. It allows a very flexible evolution of the overall platform architecture and the modules based upon it as new requirements arise.

The central strength of the eHealth Framework is its holistic approach. The ICW eHealth Framework offers a development, deployment and maintenance infrastructure that supports to efficiently develop, release and maintain applications or to integrate developments by partners with existing solutions. In combination with excessive documentation, tutorials, guidelines and best-practices covering the utilized technologies the

---

[1] Corresponding Author: Karsten Klein, InterComponentWare AG, Industriestraße 41, 69190 Walldorf (Baden), Germany; E-mail: karsten.klein@icw.de

ICW eHealth Framework offers a kick-start advantage in a demanding health care software market.

1. Architecture

1.1. Primary Objectives of the ICW eHealth Framework

Security: Enterprise-class authentication and authorization mechanisms ensure a very high level of security for sensitive medical and personal data.

Data Protection: In addition to application level security protection on transport and database level is of central importance.

Extensibility and Integration: The architecture supports the fast and efficient development of new application modules and services by ICW or its partners. The architecture eases an integration of eHF services into heterogeneous existing health care environments and higher-level business processes.

Modularity: The chosen architecture encourages and promotes the reuse of modules and services, and thus supports a distributed, loosely-coupled development of application modules by ICW and its partners. This leads to a significant increase in speed, and enhanced flexibility, as well as a decrease in complexity, overall costs, and time-to-market.

Layered Architecture: To separate vertical concerns, different abstraction layers are introduced that have well-defined and controllable access to other layers of the system while isolating technical details of adjacent layers. A layered architecture enables the replacement of technologies used in an individual layer without affecting others.

Separation of Concerns: In addition to architectural layers, general so-called cross-cutting concerns are addressed using aspect-oriented programming (AOP) methods. In other words, business logic should be strictly separated from concerns, such as security logic or transaction management. This allows a better reusability of application components and easier maintainability.

Scalability and High Availability: The architecture scales from small user groups to several million users. The system can be deployed to support high availability. This means that the system is not dependent on any single-point-of-failure and that maintenance of the application will not affect availability.

Testability: The application architecture supports fully-automated module and service testing. This enables to include acceptance and regression tests in automated test suits in order to monitor and report quality metrics.

Portability: The architecture of the ICW eHealth Framework eases porting between different Java EE containers. Portability is promoted by orientation towards a *Plain Old Java Objects (POJOs)* programming model.

Standard Technology: The ICW eHealth Framework is based on open source frameworks widely accepted in industry and can therefore benefit from the experience and skills of a growing community.

Serviceability/Maintainability: Software in a productive environment has to satisfy strong service level agreements and the derived non-functional requirements. The ICW eHealth Framework defines standard procedures and tools for operating, maintaining and managing an eHF-based product.

1.2. Module and Component Model

An important architectural objective of the ICW eHealth Framework is the realization of a modular approach. At the highest abstraction level, it is composed of modules, which consist of more fine-grained business, presentation and integration components. Modules are either *business service modules* or *library modules*. A *business service module* implements a business service interface and maintains a separate database schema[2]. A *library module* is a framework or a set of abstract base classes with well-defined extension points that provide a common implementation basis for other modules. It may define service interfaces specified in the context of a framework, or may offer other service APIs encapsulating the implementation of its library functions.

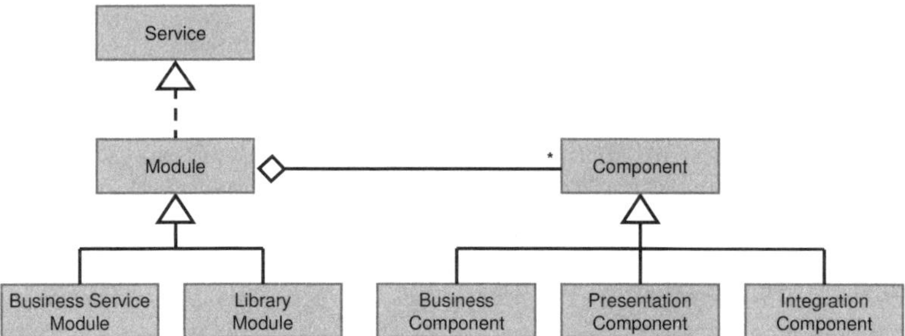

Figure 1. Module and Component Meta Model

Modules within the ICW eHealth Framework either interact synchronously via procedure calls (request-response) or asynchronously via one-way messages. Message-based interactions are primarily used to communicate application events. Messages are sent via messaging services provided by the application platform.

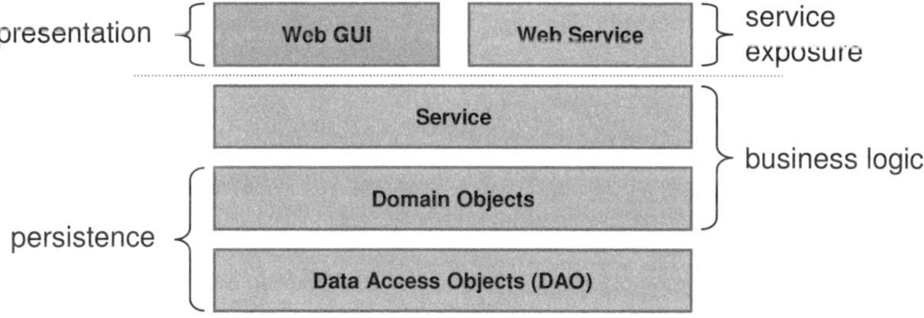

Figure 2. eHF Business Service Module Layered Architecture

The **Persistence** layer is an abstraction layer to internal data sources. It maps domain objects of the business layer to the representation constituting the persistence layer of the module. Modules may choose their own persistence mechanism. The actual access to the data sources is encapsulated using the DAO (Data Access Object) pattern.

The **Service** layer implements the business logic of an ICW eHealth Framework Business Service module. It aggregates the business logic in a central place, which pro-

---

[2] Each module can be configured to store its data in physically separate database.

motes consistent behavior across different applications. It hides complex logic from application clients ensuring an easier, faster and less error-prone development.

The ICW eHealth Framework Business Service modules may optionally contain a browser-based graphical user interface (Web GUI), as well as a web service interface.

The **Web Service** layer allows external systems (service consumers) to access the eHF Business Service module's business logic in a programmatic fashion.

The **Web GUI** layer is accessible by standard web browsers. It interacts with the service layer for executing business logic. The eHF modules do not provide any Web GUI layers. They are currently added by customers adopting the ICW eHealth Framework by contributing Web GUI dedicated library modules.

2. Development Environment

The ICW eHealth Framework provides both a runtime environment for health care solutions and an application development platform that can be used for the development of new and the extension of existing modules. Since it supports and accompanies the full software development lifecycle the modules provided by the framework itself have been developed using this development environment. The ICW eHealth Framework supports agile and iterative development methodologies. This approach, when applied consistently, will result in the creation of lean, high-quality, robust and sophisticated health care applications while enhancing the productivity of the development team.

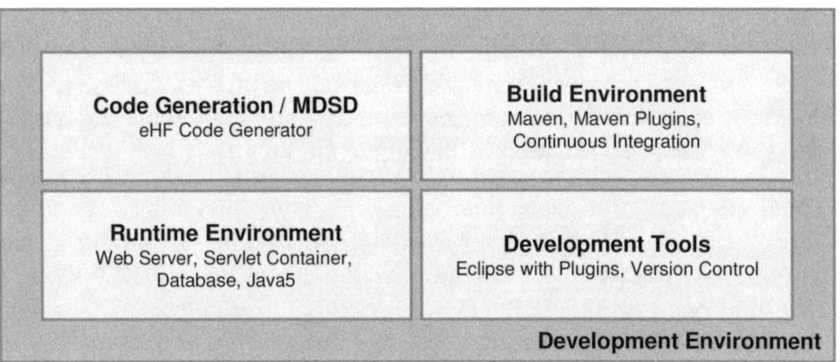

Figure 3. ICW eHealth Framework Development Environment

2.1. Repetitive Tasks and Continuous Integration

Module development requires a significant amount of repetitive routine tasks, which can easily be automated. The ICW eHealth Framework supports such automated tasks in its development environment. I.e. (to list a few):

- Generation Process
  - *Code Generator* performs model-to-code transformations
  - *Hibernate tool* for generating schema creation scripts
- Database Handling
  - *Database lifecycle*, e.g. starting and stopping the development database

- *Database bootstrap and test data import* for initializing the database with bootstrap and test data
- *Database upgrade,* for testing the upgrade procedure
- Quality Assurance Reports and Documentation
    - *Source code analysis* for control of code consistency
    - *Unit tests* to perform module unit tests
    - *Regression Tests* to perform functionality regression testing
    - *Test Coverage* to report test coverage metrics
    - *JavaDoc* to obtain complete module API documentation
- Product Build
    - *Assembly* to integrate several modules into a distributable artifact
    - *Deployment* to deploy an assembly artifact on a target system

The ICW eHealth Framework provides tools and guidelines which enable partners to easily implement a fully automated **Continuous Build and Integration** process. By utilizing the toolkit CruiseControl, the version control system is constantly monitored for changes, any change triggers the build process including the execution of all tests (JUnit). Consequently, the continuous integration process runs several times a day, detecting and reporting errors as early as possible.

Model-Driven Software Development (MDSD) [1], [2] is the backbone of the ICW eHealth Framework's development lifecycle support. The *Code Generator* is based on the openArchitectureWare open source generator framework and is able to generate a significant amount of configuration, code and other module-specific artifacts. The main generator input is a UML domain model. From this model a full-fledged and ready-to-use skeleton of the module can be generated, which covers all required architectural layers and reusable artifacts. It automates the creation of the full persistence data model, the appropriate service layers and the integration layers. Custom service methods can be added as required. The generator approach abstracts from the technical details of the architecture, emphasizing the domain model, the accompanying business logic and services. It is highly configurable and can be customized to meet specific needs.

2.2. Runtime Environment

A mature **Runtime Environment** is necessary in order to enforce an efficient development lifecycle for health care applications. For the ICW eHealth Framework, a reference deployment infrastructure based on open source components that utilizes the Apache HTTP server is used. For development purposes, this web server acts as Secure Socket Layer (SSL) endpoint for secure communication. A Tomcat Server with a special security configuration is used as servlet container during the development process.

The ICW eHealth Framework development environment uses a lightweight Hypersonic SQL (HSQLDB) database engine providing persistence functionality.

2.3. Development Tools

The ICW eHealth Framework supports **Version Control** of source code in a versioning system. The eHF modules are maintained by a Subversion (SVN) repository. Other systems, such as Concurrent Versions System (CVS), are supported as well.

The ICW eHealth Framework is complemented by an **Integrated Development Environment** (IDE). It covers all relevant aspects for the fast and successful development of eHF modules, as well as the assembly of completed health care applications. Based on the popular Eclipse project and equipped with useful plug-ins, it eases and improves the development process. As well as Eclipse's common capabilities, several plug-ins are provided to facilitate interoperability with other frameworks and components used within the ICW eHealth Framework. The most important plug-ins are:

- *Spring IDE*: Graphical user interface for Spring configuration files.
- *AspectJ Development Tools (AJDT)* [3]*:* Tools support for AspectJ within the IDE.
- *Subversive*: Allows version control using SVN within the IDE.
- *Database Plug-ins:* Integrate SQL clients to access SQL-compliant databases.
- *Checkstyle Plug-in and configuration*: Ensures eHF checkstyle conformity.
- *JUnit Plug-in*: Allows the execution of JUnit tests within the IDE.

3. eHF Module Description

The business service modules and library modules of the ICW eHealth Framework are built on top of industry-standard application frameworks and can be deployed on any J2EE 1.4-compliant application server. The modules are organized into four categories:

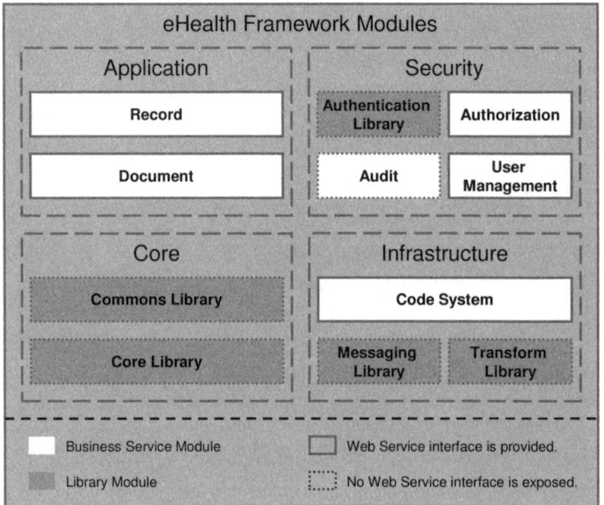

Figure 4. ICW eHealth Framework Modules

- *Core* - represents the core platform for other modules and provide basic functionalities which are used as a basis by individual business service modules
- *Infrastructure* - enables the interaction between different modules and with 3rd party systems

- *Security* - sophisticated security modules providing components and services to control access to sensitive data, such as medical information.
- *Application* - allows the maintenance of medical information

Each set of module services is defined by a separate Web Service Description Language (WSDL) document, which describes the supported message exchange patterns and formats.

3.1. Core Modules

The **Commons** library module is the central library module providing a sophisticated base infrastructure and functionality. It includes definitions of generic components and interfaces, which are used or enhanced by the dependent modules:

- Axis web service infrastructure with backward compatibility extension
- Abstract Domain Object class hierarchy
- Processor definitions for bootstrapping and importing data
- Code and Code System infrastructure
- Generic implementation of Hibernate Data Access Objects (DAOs)
- Exception class hierarchy
- Domain object validation infrastructure
- Persistence layer extensions
- Result paging infrastructure
- Standard API definitions
- Classes for handling and converting date and time objects
- General infrastructure components and utility classes

The **Core** library module hosts a general domain model, which is used throughout the framework in order to prevent duplication of models and associated logic. This simplifies and encourages reuse. The domain model is enriched with domain-specific logic to further enhance the usage of these central model elements. The Core Library module does not provide a persistence mechanism of its own, the actual persistence of the data is performed by the modules using the respective domain object. Typical members of the Core Library module are:

- Participants – e.g. Person, Address, Device, Organization
- Terms – e.g. Date, Time, Time Interval
- Codes – e.g. Code System, Code, Annotated Code, Unit Code
- Identifiers and Qualifiers – e.g. Reference, Instance Identifier

3.2. Infrastructure Modules

Many terms, nomenclatures, dictionaries, controlled vocabularies and classification systems have been introduced by standardization organizations. Within the ICW eHealth Framework they are summarized as so-called *code systems*. Code systems strongly supplement the expressiveness of the domain models, and may include domain specific code systems to describe administrative data, such as gender, country codes and medical codes (e.g. diagnosis and encounter type), as well as system-level code systems, such as error codes or validation messages.

The **Code System** module manages code systems to enables health care applications to use and localize these standardized terms, or to ultimately handle, validate, and resolve codes in different languages. The module offers dedicated flexibility to manage code systems and enables other eHF modules to address code-based tasks.

Code-based validation of the data model instances ensures the consistency of the overall information stored in the system and supports specific demands regarding internationalization and localization through customized code systems. The module furthermore supports the integration of external catalogues or terminology services. The code systems provided by ICW eHealth Framework are described in an XML format and can be imported into the database as part of the standard build or deployment procedure.

The **Messaging** library module provides a messaging infrastructure API. Message-based communication among modules decouples the dependencies and enhances their potential for reuse. It supports 3rd party Java Messaging Service (JMS) solutions and provides a lightweight in-memory message server. A dedicated set of adapters is provided for the supported messaging technologies. An adapter translates between the Messaging API and technology-specific APIs.

The ability of applications to react to new use-cases depends on the coupling of the components constituting the application. Messaging infrastructures can be used to build event-driven architectures to decouple components and thereby increase flexibility.

The **Transform** library module offers a generalized infrastructure for the conversion of objects between different data models. The transformations are declaratively described by configuration files, avoiding the need to write any additional Java code.

3.3. Security Modules

In order to ensure the security of web-based systems, it is essential to verify the identity of interacting users. This applies to both human users and external systems. The **Authentication** library module verifies the identities of users that are authenticated either with the help of a username and password, of a secure PIN (personal identification number), or of a valid X.509 client certificate using standard public key infrastructure (PKI) mechanisms. Only authenticated users are allowed to perform business operations.

Table 1. Login Filters

Filter Type	Description/Usage
Form Login	Performs username and password authentication. Credentials are provided by standard HTML web forms.
BASIC Login	Performs username and password authentication as well. Uses the browser's HTTP BASIC authentication capabilities.
Client Certificate Login	Requires an X.509 certificate. Incoming certificates are validated against the server's truststore. Client certificates login can be configured to support authentication with health professional cards (HPC) and electronic health cards (EHC).
PIN Login	Authenticates users providing a secure PIN. The user's PIN is requested by a standard HTML web form.

The module can easily be extended with additional authentication methods. Authentication methods are enforced via servlet filters (login filters). They delegate the validation of supplied user credentials to an authentication. An adapter interface allows for the integration with various user stores (e.g. the Lightweight Directory Access Protocol (LDAP) or legacy user management systems) to compare user data to supplied credentials. The module provides filters for all required authentication methods by the Servlet 2.4 specification, including additional proprietary filters. Login filters are not restricted to browser-based access and can also be applied to web service requests.

Information stored in health care applications must be strictly access controlled. The **Authorization** module implements a hierarchical role-based access control model. Roles usually define responsibilities within organizations. Responsibilities imply certain permissions, which can be assigned to roles. Roles can have parent roles, from which they inherit permissions. Users are granted permissions by assigning them to one or more roles. In addition to role-based permission assignments, the eHF security services also support the direct assignment of permissions to users and groups. Furthermore, the Authorization module supports a user-driven management of permissions: A user, who has administration permissions for a dedicated security domain, is enabled by the module to assign specific permissions of this domain to other users. The user can grant or revoke fine-grained permissions within this domain down to the level of single instances, and optionally limit the validity of permissions to a certain period of time. The delegation of administration rights to other users is also possible. The other user may further assign these permissions, depending on the amount of granted rights. Additional permission management primitives, such as predefined permission profiles, black lists and white lists, are supported as well. Permissions can be managed via a Java interface and web service interface. The permissions are stored in the database.

The Authorization module provides an *Access Decision* service. A health care application can use this service to ensure that only authenticated and authorized users can access the application data. In order to put this into practice, a health care application creates an access decision request, containing information on the data access request. This request is then submitted to the access decision service provided by the Authorization module. If the current user has sufficient permissions to access the requested resources, the access decision service gives a positive access decision response to the health care application for further processing. The client is informed if the user does not have sufficient permissions to access the requested resources. To separate the access decision logic from the actual business logic, calls to the access decision service are implemented using AOP interceptors.

The **User Management** module can be used by a health care application to manage the lifecycle of its user-specific information. The module provides a set of interrelated services for managing the lifecycle of user accounts, and for the administration of role hierarchies and organization hierarchies. In its current implementation, the module stores user management data in the database. Since application modules can only access user management functionality via the module's interfaces, persistence mechanisms can easily be exchanged. The *User Account Service* allows the customer registration process of a health care application to create and manage user accounts. User account data includes user identifiers, personal data, contact data and payment information. Password management functionality allows users to change their passwords and administrators to reset passwords. Policies control password lifecycles and ensure that trivial passwords cannot be created. User searches can be performed via flexible query interfaces. The *Role Service* provides the basis for role based access control mechanisms. It supports role lifecycle management and the organization of roles into role hierarchies. Organizational structures are represented by group hierarchies. A group, for example, may represent an organization's department and define the context or scope for roles. The *Organization Service* supports the management of groups and their structuring into hierarchies[3]. Users can be assigned membership to one or more groups.

The **Audit** module implements means to store audit information of security relevant actions like authentication attempts, changes in permission settings, user management activities or any access to medical information in a file or a relational database. The auditing of events is critical for satisfying specific regional data security requirements. Each log entry captures the user that caused the security relevant event, the operation that was invoked, the resource concerned, and the time the event occurred. Message-based communication between application modules and the Audit module decouples these components from auditing concerns. Transformers in the event message stream convert application event messages into audit entries.

3.4. Application Modules

The **eHF Record** Module delivers the basic foundation for an electronic health record, describing the central information in a medical system. This information is exposed by appropriate services that provide access to the following data:

- **Administrative Data** comprises data on the subject of the record, medical contacts (e.g. the family doctor or the primary pharmacy), emergency contacts and insurance.

- **Basic Medical Data** primarily defines a common basic data types for medical information that is intended to be stored in a structured way within an electronic health record. The general data structures of Basic Medical Data are based on the HL7 v3 RIM (Health Level 7, version 3 Reference Information Model) [4]. They currently cover encounters, observations (including measurements of different types, diagnoses, health risks and allergies) and substance administration (including medication and vaccination).

This module provides Create, Read, Update and Delete (CRUD) services for data access, and other services like calculation, filtering and validation for GUI and external web service consumers. The eHF Record module comprises components which are dedicated to one of the previously mentioned data domains. An additional feature is the support of links amongst basic medical data and external references to objects from other modules (e.g. documents). The domain objects in this module are equipped with the standard persistence mechanisms created by the eHF Code Generator. The Record module is composed of two sub modules separating the administrative from the medical data. This enables to physically divide the storage of the persisted information and supports central data protection and pseudonymization considerations.

The **Document** Module represents the central document storage of the ICW eHealth Framework. It enables the storage of arbitrary content that can be in a binary format (e.g. pictures) or may be of textual nature, such as plain text or XML files. The module supports a specialized versioning mechanism and provides two basic methods for uploading and downloading documents: The *upload method* stores a given docu-

---

[3] The support for organizations is limited to role management. An extension of the user management organization functionality is subject to future development.

ment or a composition of documents with associated meta information in the system. If the document does not exist as an entry in the system, a new entry is created. Otherwise, the existing document is updated and its version number is incremented. The *download method* provides the functionality to download documents and document compositions. Updating a document results in a new version of the document or document composition, leaving previous versions unaltered.

3.5. Usage Scenario

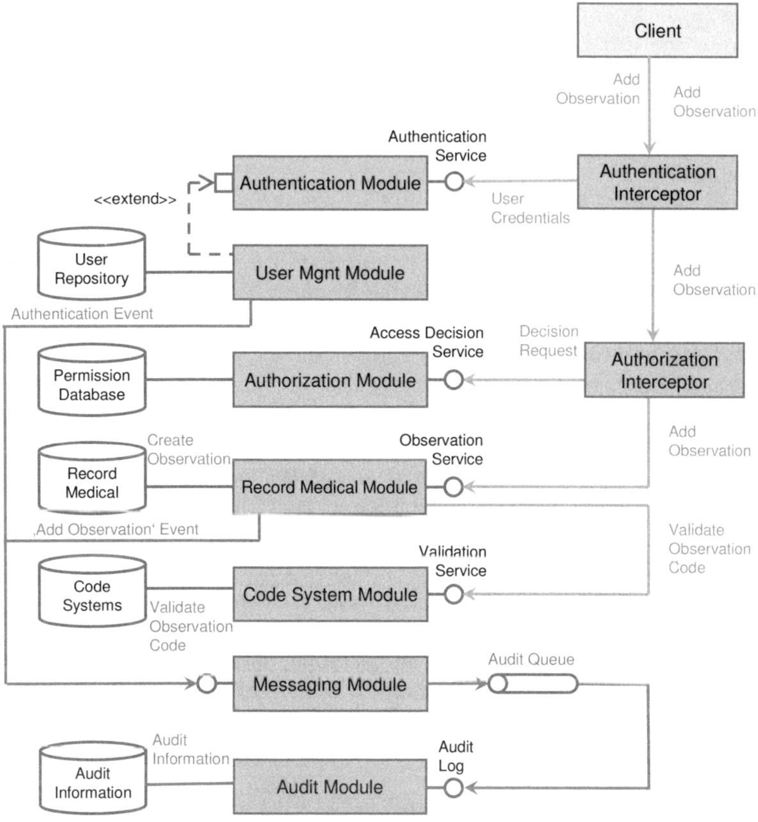

Figure 5. Usage Scenario

This section describes a usage scenario for the ICW eHealth Framework in a web application environment in order to demonstrate how the different modules interact with each other. A client application, e.g. a browser or a web service, sends a request to an application built with the ICW eHealth Framework. In this example the intention of the request is to add a new observation (e.g. a blood pressure value) to a health record. Security logic is applied to business components by using AOP interceptors. Authentication interceptors ensure that all external requests are properly authenticated. They enforce user authentication by validating credentials contained in the request, against data obtained from the User Management module. Regardless of the authentication result, the User Management module generates a security authentication event and uses the infrastructure functionality of the Messaging module to publish the event. Components, such as the Audit module, can use one of the provided adapters of the Messaging module to receive and process events of interest. After the events are consumed by the Audit module, they are removed from the message queue.

Authorization interceptors use the Authorization module to check whether or not the authenticated user has sufficient privileges to access the requested resource. An authorized user request is forwarded to the intended service, in the case of this usage scenario the observation service of the Record module. The Record module uses the Code System module to dynamically validate coded information. The code system, which lists the supported observation types, is queried and the result matched with the observation type. After the coded information was successfully validated the Record module stores the observation domain object in the database. A respective security-relevant creation event is emitted und processed by the audit module.

4. Technology

This section provides technical information on the development environment of the ICW eHealth Framework, and on the runtime platform it uses. A health care application that uses the ICW eHealth Framework requires at least a J2EE 1.4-compliant servlet container to operate (e.g. Tomcat 6 or BEA WebLogic Server 9.2). A Java Platform Standard Edition 5 virtual machine is required, since the ICW eHealth Framework uses Java 5 language features such as annotations, enumerations and generics.

Hibernate is a sophisticated **Object-Relational Mapping** (ORM) framework for persisting domain objects in a relational database. ICW eHealth Framework domain objects are enriched with JPA (Java Persistence API) annotations, based on Hibernate's JPA support. Furthermore, ICW eHealth Framework domain objects are realized as POJOs, improving their testability outside of a container. Spring is a widely used framework with Inversion of Control (IoC) and Aspect Oriented Programming (AOP) support. It encourages the use of POJOs. In general, any database supported by Hibernate 3.2.4 can be used with the ICW eHealth Framework. However certain exceptions determined by the capabilities and limitations on the database level exist. Off the shelf the ICW eHealth Framework offers support for HSQLDB and Oracle.

The ICW eHealth Framework uses **Aspect-Oriented Programming** (AOP) methods to enable clean encapsulation of cross-cutting concerns, such as access decision, transaction management, error handling or monitoring. Cross-cutting concerns are functional and technical aspects of an application, which apply to many of its components or units. Instead of directly hard-wiring cross-cutting concerns into these units, AOP enables the developer to apply such aspects in a declarative way, without having to modify existing code. Spring AOP is used to apply aspects to Spring-managed components. In case this approach cannot be applied, AspectJ is used as an alternative.

Apache Axis is the web service engine of the ICW eHealth Framework. It exposes the services of a business service module through web service interfaces which comply with WSDL 1.1 (Web Service Description Language) and SOAP 1.1 (Simple Object Access Protocol).

The Security Modules of the ICW eHealth Framework are based on the **Java 2 Security Architecture** and on the **Java Authentication and Authorization Service** (JAAS). They provide implementations for standard Java authentication and authorization service provider interfaces (SPI). Health care applications can invoke ICW eHealth Framework Security Services via standard application programming interfaces offered by the Java SDK. The ICW eHealth Framework provides a standard JAAS policy provider, and can thus be used for extending the security mechanisms of application servers that comply with the *Java Authorization Contract for Containers* (JACC). The ICW eHealth Framework Security complements Java EE Security (J2EE 1.4 and Java EE 5) with hierarchical role-based access control mechanisms and instance-based access control. It allows for more than one authentication method per web application.

5. Outlook

ICW's objective is to provide a state-of-the-art eHealth development framework. This section is intended to list ongoing activities and future plans concerning the development of the ICW eHealth Framework.

Significant efforts are made to define **Health IT Standards** for communicating and storing medical information. The requirements concerning security aspects in particular and information protection in general are of utmost importance, and can vary between regions or countries, depending on the applicable legislation. ICW continuously evaluates the latest trends in technology and actively participates in this definition process, for example through the German HL7 User Group or through its involvement in the IHE (Integrating the Health care Enterprise) initiative. The ICW eHealth Framework modules have adopted the HL7 RIM model in their domain models and will continue to incorporate modifications. The future development of the ICW eHealth Framework will support a native HL7 v3 messaging interface, so that applications using the framework can interact with other HL7 v3 message based systems.

The **MDSD Approach** will be further pursued, extended and improved. It offers substantial flexibility for application developers and allows for the evolutionary development of the underlying platform. This can be achieved transparently for in-house developers and external partners, and enables a variety of possibilities in the context of porting an application to different platforms. The approach will be further enriched with best practices and the knowledge of domain experts.

Future development of the ICW eHealth Framework will support the main **Single-Sign-On** (SSO) authentication scenarios. First, a user can connect to multiple eHF-based applications and authenticate only once. Second, a user can authenticate to an eHF-based application and use the obtained credentials to connect transparently to another application which is not eHF-based, or vice versa. These can be addressed using different technical approaches ranging from a tight integration of specific authentication modules from different vendors to allow for SSO between a defined set of applications all the way to supporting cross-domain identity federation based on circles of trust between different application providers. Several interesting standards in this area such as SAML (Security Assertion Markup Language) and Liberty are well established in the marketplace and are investigated by ICW.

Web Services: ICW closely observes current technology trends and considers incorporating valuable emerging technologies into the ICW eHealth Framework. One example in the **Web Services** area is support for Web Services Security (WS-S). The use of WS-Security will offer many advantages such as providing end-to-end security (whereas the use of Transport Layer Security (TLS) via HTTPS only ensures point-to-point security).

Federated Record: Health records are typically stored in heterogeneous, distributed health care systems. In order to provide an integrated view of patient data from these systems, the future development of the ICW eHealth Framework will emphasize aggregation and federation aspects. The end-consumer will benefit from the fact that all the patient related data of these distributed health care systems will be presented in a single view.

Integration: Future releases of the ICW eHealth Framework will also incorporate an Enterprise Service Bus (ESB) infrastructure to address various important integration scenarios. Examples of such scenarios are the IHE-XDS [5] and IHE-XPHR [6] profiles.

6. Conclusion

The ICW eHealth Framework provides the technological platform for several of ICW's own eHealth applications. External developers have the freedom to choose in which manner they intend to use the ICW eHealth Framework to develop their own eHealth solutions:

- Applications can be built directly on top of the ICW eHealth Framework and can use and extend the provided services, for example services related to the electronic health record.
- Using the ICW eHealth Framework developers do not have to worry about standard tasks such as persistence, access control, authorization, and auditing. Therefore they can fully focus their development efforts on the implementation of their specific business logic. Costs and development time are reduced and the time to market for products is shortened while product quality is increased.
- New applications can be integrated via open interfaces with ICW's own applications or with other applications based on the ICW eHealth Framework. This helps to ensure the efficient exchange of data between heterogeneous health information systems focusing on different health care sectors.
- ICW solutions can be expanded with value-added offerings, for example by integrating disease-specific additional packages into the personal health record LifeSensor.

References

[1]	Stahl T, Völter M., *Model-driven Software Development: Technology, Engineering, Management*, John Wiley Sons, New Jersey, 2006.
[2]	e. Evans, *Domain-Driven DESIGN: Tackling Complexity in the Heart of Software*, Addison-Wesley Longman, Amsterdam, 2003.
[3]	A. Colyer, A. Clement, G. Harley, *Eclipse AspectJ: Aspect-Oriented Programming with Aspectj and the Eclipse Aspectj Development Tools*, Addison-Wesley Longman, Amsterdam, 2005.
[4]	A. Hinchley, *Understanding Version 3: A primer on the HL7 Version 3 Communication Standard*, Mönch, 2005
[5]	*IHE IT Infrastructure Technical Framework:*, Revision 4.0, ACC/HIMSS/RSNA, 2007
[6]	*IHE Patient Care Coordination Technical Framework*, Revision 3.0, for trial implementation, ACC/HIMSS/RSNA, 2007

National eHealth Strategies and Implementations

eHealth: Combining Health Telematics, Telemedicine, Biomedical Engineering and Bioinformatics to the Edge. Edited by B. Blobel, P. Pharow and M. Nerlich.
IOS Press, 2008

193

Bavaria – Motor and Partner for Advanced Health Services

Gerhard KNORR [1]

Bavarian State Ministry of Labour and Social Affairs, Family and Women, Hospital Department, Munich, Germany

Abstract. What has long since been everyday practice in consumer electronics, office communications and in the private sector, meaning the use of information and communications technologies and the Internet, is still not routine procedure for public health services. The State of Bavaria was very quick to recognize the importance of telematics in public health for better health care and for Bavaria as an economy location. Ever since 1995, we have been promoting innovative and forward-looking pilot projects in the field of telemedicine to ensure that all patients – in a state like Bavaria – can have state-wide access to a wide range of telemedical applications. While innovative IT applications that network doctors in private practice, patients and clinics and hence reduce friction losses at the interfaces of the classic sectors – in-patient treatment, out-patient care as well as rehabilitation and nursing care – are gaining ground in the health market, there is still much to be done to bring our public health system up to the latest IT state of the art. A key factor on the road towards digital medical care will be the introduction of the electronic health card in Germany. It is expected in 2008.

Keywords. Health service provision, Bavaria, health policy

Introduction

When it comes to telecommunications applications in medicine, the terms "telemedicine", "eHealth" or "telematics in public health" are used as synonyms. In the field of project initiation and promotion in Bavaria, the term "telemedicine" has established itself. It covers the use of information and communications technologies, electronic data processing (EDP) and networking in the public health sector. Telemedicine is a vital instrument for improving the quality of public health care, it enables us to examine, monitor and treat patients over long distances and gives us online access to information and second opinions from experts.

For more than 10 years, the State of Bavaria has been supporting many telemedical projects with different focal points and using funding that so far totals close on € 9 million. These funds were raised from the technology development programs of the State of Bavaria, "BayernOnline" and the "High-Tech-Offensive" as well as the "Social Fund". Under these programs, the Bavarian Ministry of Social Affairs has so far promoted 32 telemedical projects and given substantial support to other projects.

---

[1] Corresponding Author: Gerhard Knorr, Ministerialdirigent Dr., Head of the Hospital Department in the Bavarian State Ministry of Labour and Social Affairs, Family and Women, Munich, Bavaria, Germany; Email: Gerhard.Knorr@stmas.bayern.de

The projects are multifarious and cover a wide variety of telemedical applications. Support has been granted to projects for teleconsultations, teleradiology, telemonitoring, teletherapy, electronic patients' cards for diabetics, the electronic Health Professional Card, electronic patients' records and expert systems. Superordinate topics, like data protection, also played an important role in specific projects. Currently, a matter of central importance is the project setting up Ingolstadt as a test region to test the electronic health card in a telematics infrastructure before its nationwide introduction and to prepare for its routine use.

As examples of telemedicine applications, some projects promoted by the Bavarian State Ministry of Labour and Social Affairs, Family and Women are presented, in which the benefit of the new technologies for hospital care can be excellently demonstrated.

1. Successful Telemedicine in Bavaria

Bavaria has started a series of telemedicine projects with high expectations in terms of quality of diagnosis and treatment. First of all, some telemedical stroke projects, where the overarching goal was to improve stroke care throughout Bavaria, in other words to eliminate the existing divide in health care between on the one hand conurbations with specialised Stroke Units and, on the other, rural regions not having any neurological clinics.

1.1 Project for Integrated Stroke Care in the Region of South-East Bavaria

The "Telemedical Pilot Project for Integrated Stroke Care in the Region of South-East Bavaria, TEMPiS" was implemented by the stroke centers in Munich-Harlaching Municipal Hospital and the District Medical Centre (Bezirksklinikum) of Regensburg in collaboration with twelve partner clinics in South-Eastern Bavaria. To extend the range of diagnostic facilities, several neurosurgery departments were also integrated into the project. A major feature of TEMPiS are structural and organizational measures, such as, for example, the concentration of stroke treatment by building up specialized units including so-called stroke teams in the regional hospitals, continuing professional development and further training of all employees, quality control by the centers and the standardization of treatment procedures.

In particular, however, use is made of state-of-the-art information and communications technology to facilitate rapid diagnosis and therapy. The centers and the participating hospitals are equipped with efficient video-conference systems that enable images to be transmitted digitally (CT, MRT, X-ray and ultrasonic images) while the neurological examination is in progress. Teleconsultations are carried out round the clock.

The results of an efficiency analysis supporting the project convinced the health insurance funds, so that the TEMPiS services could be adopted as standard procedures and financed by the health funds.

Similar projects to TEMPiS are also being implemented in Swabia;

- TESS: Use of telemedicine for the widespread care of stroke patients in Central Swabia (originally as the first pilot project in this field) and
- SARA: Stroke Initiative in the Augsburg region and the Allgäu.

1.2 Stroke Network with Telemedicine in Northern Bavaria

Another network currently being developed in the North of Bavaria is the "Stroke Network with Telemedicine in Northern Bavaria – STENO Network". 11 regional hospitals are networked with three neurological centres – Erlangen University Clinic, Nuremberg Clinic, Bayreuth Hohe Warte Hospital – to improve the acute care of stroke patients. For the neurological telemedical consultations with video examination and diagnosis, a modular system specially developed for medical use and tested by Erlangen Neurocenter is used to transmit video, audio, image and text data. The telesupport system is IP-based and can access a variety of data formats (DICOM, JPEG, HTML), so that it can be combined with other IT applications. A wide range of patient data can thus be brought together. Appropriate connections and networks linking the telemedicine partners guarantee the online transmission of various forms of data to a good image quality. The use and updating of a special software program control the telemedical workflow in the stroke network and support the data management. Development and operating procedures, treatment and quality assurance in the acute phase of stroke care are carried out in line with the TEMPiS concept.

The telemedical network for the acute care of stroke patients in the North of Bavaria closes another geographical gap in acute stroke care. For the patients affected, this is of inestimable value for preventing or at least reducing any lasting disability, but it is also of the utmost importance to the national economy.

In future, other decentralized hospitals and medical institutions with stroke units are to be networked telemedically and the material concept of TEMPiS taken over with a view to closing any care gaps still existing in Bavaria.

1.3 Digital Global Tumour Documentation System

The third project to be presented is the "digital global tumor documentation system", which excellently highlights the bandwidth of telemedicine.

In order to facilitate the universal identification and assessment of tumor diseases of all kinds within the scope of the cross-sectoral care of patients, a documentation system was developed in Regensburg Tumor Centre that could be used for all 51 forms of cancer (tumor entities). The further developed system was based on the "OnkoSuite" digital documentation prepared for the mamma carcinoma. The digital documentation system can replace the previously paper-bound documentation, which is very time-consuming for the doctors supplying the data as well as for the documentation assistants engaged in saving the data in the Tumor Centre and also involves the risk of transmission errors. What is more, statistical analyses can be made on the basis of the documented data to standardized quality criteria, which allow conclusions to be drawn as to the effectiveness of selected forms of therapy and thus contribute to a scientifically sound further development of tumor treatment for the benefit of the patients.

The system can take over data from hospital information and medical practice management systems as well as from the health-insurance card and in future from the electronic health card. It supports disease management programs and is consistent with the generally accepted standards of the German Federal Office for Quality Assurance (Bundesgeschäftsstelle für Qualitätssicherung). It also allows data to be analyzed according to the parameters of the German Cancer Society (Deutsche

Krebsgesellschaft) and the German Society of Senology (Deutsche Gesellschaft für Senologie) as well as to independently definable criteria.

In the near future, the Regensburg Tumor Center plans to extend use of the system to include electronic tumor documentation and to link up with the proposed telematics platform for the public health service.

2. Lessons Learned for Telemedicine Projects

In previous project promotion schemes, the main concern was to use telemedicine mainly to raise the quality of patient care so that the patient can directly benefit from of the new technology. While in future we will continue to look for innovative, quality-oriented telemedical developments, we will also give more support to widespread applications and networking.

Not only telemedicine, the digitization of medicine and medical technology have triggered increased demand for communication, process optimization in diagnostics, therapy and aftercare are also directly related to electronic communication and the quality of medical care. At the latest with the German Law governing the Modernization of the Statutory Health Insurance (GMG), which came into force in 2004 and stipulated the introduction of an electronic health card as well as the legal principles for creating a telematics infrastructure, the signal was sent for the entry into the digital age in the public health sector.

3. Expectations for the Future

The electronic health card will enable emergency data, prescriptions, medical reports and patients' records to be saved and exchanged in digital form. To this end, a total of some 80 million cards will have to be issued in Germany and more than 185,000 doctors and dentists in private practice, nearly 22,000 pharmacies, some 2,200 hospitals and about 238 health insurance funds will have to be networked. A gigantic project that is currently being tested in miniature in 7 selected states in Germany for its efficiency and compatibility with the telematics infrastructure.

Bavaria is not only well placed with the test region of Ingolstadt, but also directly involved in the work to introduce the electronic health card. The tests are currently in progress in the test states under real conditions of use and with real data. In the Ingolstadt test region the user tests have been successfully completed. The field tests with up to 10,000 insured persons, 31 doctors in 15 practices, 15 pharmacies and 2 hospitals (Ingolstadt Clinic, Kösching/Eichstätt Hospital) have already started. During the tests, the electronic health card will be used alongside the health-insurance card. Electronic prescriptions and emergency data will be tested by the offline method, in other words by saving the data on the card. Pre-tests with individual electronic health cards, which had been carried out before the cards were supplied to the participating insured persons, have gone exceptionally well. All in all, initial reactions to the test measures in Bavaria are very satisfactory, including from the care providers.

Following nationwide introduction of the basic form of the electronic health card (probably in April 2008) we will not lose sight of our real goal: to network all the players in the public health sector and set up online applications with the electronic health card – electronic prescription, electronic medical report and electronic patient's records. Because only with these comprehensive online functions can medical care be improved, while also making further economies. And these steps promise the hoped-for added value for the public health sector.

4. Discussion and Conclusions

A short overview of "Telemedicine in Bavaria" and on the "Introduction of the electronic health card" has been given. The goals for the Bavarian State's continued support of telemedicine and eHealth projects will not change dramatically. In particular, it is intended

- to facilitate manifold telemedical services in all the regions of Bavaria,
- to promote networking with centers of excellence
- and to speed up the launch of the electronic health card as a key feature of the electronic exchange of data in the public health service and the use of all possible functions of the card.

As the State of Bavaria was very quick to recognize and support the importance of telemedicine and its economic potential, not only medical technology but also telematics in public health are contributing to the great economic prosperity of our State. By using a wide variety of telematics applications in public health, it is possible to not only step up the quality of health care for the population and save costs, but also to boost economic strength in one of the largest economic sectors in Germany – public health – and to create jobs. This is an aspect not to be underestimated in the social and employment policy of a state.

In particular the introduction of the electronic health card is an exceptionally ambitious project that will revolutionize the information and communications technology of the public health system and might be copied by others.

At the moment electronic communications, health care and the public health industry are not only being talked about on all sides, but in a country like Germany with few natural resources they are also major economic and political instruments. Imagination and ingenuity are the only raw material this country has. It must make full use of it.

*eHealth: Combining Health Telematics, Telemedicine, Biomedical Engineering and
Bioinformatics to the Edge. Edited by B. Blobel, P. Pharow and M. Nerlich.
IOS Press, 2008*

Current Status of National eHealth and Telemedicine Development in Finland

Jarmo REPONEN [a,1], Ilkka WINBLAD [b] and Päivi HÄMÄLÄINEN [c]

[a] *FinnTelemedicum, University of Oulu and Raahe Hospital, Finland*
[b] *FinnTelemedicum, University of Oulu, Finland*
[c] *STAKES (National Research Centre for Welfare and Health), Finland*

Abstact. This eHealth paper shows the results of a survey produced by
FinnTelemedicum, Centre of Excellence for Telehealth at the University of Oulu
and STAKES (National Research and Development Centre for Welfare and Health
development in Finland) under assignment of the Finnish Ministry of Social
Affairs and Health. The survey shows the status and trends of the usage of eHealth
applications in the Finnish health care in 2005. The results are compared to an
earlier survey made in 2003. The 2005 survey included all service providers in
public and private medical services: hospital districts or central hospitals for
secondary/tertiary care, primary health care centers and a sample of private sector
service providers. The results show that the usage of eHealth applications has
greatly progressed throughout the entire health care delivery system. The current
wide utilization of the eHealth applications in Finnish health care forms a solid
basis for developing future eHealth services. Finland has taken the initiative to
build a national archive for electronic health data with citizen access by 2011.

Keywords. Health information systems, Electronic Patient Record, eHealth,
telemedicine

Introduction

Finland is a large and sparsely populated country of 5.3 million inhabitants, who live in
an area of 338,000 square kilometers. In the eastern and the northern parts of the
country the population density is especially low and distances are great. Health care
services in Finland cover all people living in Finland. The constitution states that public
authorities shall guarantee for everyone, as provided in more detail by an Act of
Parliament, adequate social, health and medical services and the promotion of the
health of the population.

According to a recent report by OECD on Finland [1] the Finnish health system
performs well. Finnish people are more satisfied with their healthcare than people in
many other OECD countries. Health spending is low-cost compared with the GDP
(7.4% in 2004). Many indicators of health care performance are good. Deaths from
heart attacks and strokes have dropped sharply over the past 30 years and the delivery
of quality medical care includes high rates of screening for cancer, a high rate of kidney
transplants in proportion to patients with renal failure, and a high rate in the rapid
treatment of broken hips. However, there are inequalities in access to services of a

---

¹ Corresponding Author: Jarmo Reponen, MD, PhD, Professor, FinnTelemedicum, University of Oulu,
c/o KTTYL, P.O. Box 5000, FIN-90014 Oulu, Finland; E-mail: jarmo.Reponen@oulu.fi.

general practitioner. Until recently, many patients faced long waiting times to see a doctor at a health care centre, and there were long waiting lists for elective surgery. However, the introduction of waiting-time targets by the government in March 2005, has somewhat improved the situation. The Finnish health care system, like in so many other countries, now faces severe challenges. These challenges include: technological changes, which are increasing the costs of hospital services and prescribed medicines; rising patient expectations; and a rate of an ageing population, which will be much more rapid than in other European countries between 2010 and 2020.

Every one of the 251 Finnish primary health care centers is owned by a single municipality or by several municipalities together. A health care centre can be defined as a functional unit or as an organization that provides primary curative, preventive, and public health care services to its populace. The number and type of personnel in each health care centre depends on the size of the population it serves and on local circumstances. The staff consists of general practitioners, sometimes medical specialists, nurses, public health nurses, midwives, social workers, dentists, physiotherapists, psychologists, administrative personnel. All are employed by the municipality or the municipalities. The number of inhabitants per health care centre doctor varies, averaging at 1500-2000.

Each municipality belongs to a particular hospital district, containing a central hospital. Of the central hospitals, five are university hospitals that provide specialized tertiary levels of treatment. Each hospital district organizes and provides specialized hospital care for the population in its area. Finland is divided into 20 hospital districts. In addition, the semi-autonomous province of Ahvenanmaa forms its own district. A hospital district is an administrative entity. In different hospital districts the central hospital may operate in more than one location and there may be supporting regional hospitals as well. The over all number of hospitals is about 70. This includes the five university hospitals, 16 central hospitals and over 40 smaller specialized hospitals. Hospitals have out-patient and in-patient departments. The range of specialized care varies according to the type of hospital. Federations of municipalities, i.e. hospital districts, own all the hospitals. The population of hospital districts varies between 70,000 and 1,300,000 inhabitants.

Private health care in Finland mainly comprises of out-patient care, which is available mostly in the larger cities. Physicians can run a practice within a private company, the number of which was 1000 in 2005; or as a stand-alone practice. The majority of doctors working in the private sector are specialists, whose full-time job is at a public hospital or at a health care centre. Patients do not need a referral to visit private specialists at private clinics. Physicians working at private clinics are allowed to send patients with a referral either to public or private hospitals. There are only a few private hospitals, providing less than 5% of the bed days in the country [2].

The Finnish Ministry of Social Affairs and Health has regularly instructed and followed the implementation of information and communication technology (ICT) or eHealth development in health care. Under an assignment of the Ministry the authors conducted a comprehensive survey on the implementation and the use of ICT in 2003 and 2005 [3], [4], [5].The first survey showed the prevailing situation right before the National Project for Securing the Future of Health Care had began. The second 2005 survey shows what has happened halfway through the project. The purpose of the study section presented here is to record what is the development stage in electronic health care domain before introduction of a nation wide electronic health record archive. The Finnish approach was to select an electronic patient record (EPR) as a backbone, which carries all other services [6]. The position of EPR is strong because there is a long tradition of a uniform, structured patient record already in paper domain. There is also well controlled use of a unique patient identifier. The latter part of the paper then describes the legal actions and development path that has been planned.

1. Methods of the 2003 and 2005 surveys

The structured web-based questionnaire was distributed by e-mail to all public health service providers or hospital districts and health care centers, and to a sampling of private health care providers. The survey was conducted by the present authors for the first time in 2003 [3] and repeated in 2005. In this paper we present mainly the year 2005 data and use the year 2003 data as a comparison. The questionnaire comprised of: the identification of the responding organization and the respondent; questions about the adaptation of electronic patient records systems; systems or applications to transfer/exchange patient information between organizations during care processes and the standards in use for the migration of patient information; methods of authentication, identification, and informed consent of patients; the usage of different e-Education systems for staff education; the types of human and material resources needed; systems supporting quality control and service delivery; and the adaptation of different e-Services for patients.

The total number of the questions was 97. Most of which also included further questions on how old the system or application concerned was, and the intensity of use. The questions for hospitals, health care centers, and private health care providers differed to some extent, depending on the nature of the services they provided.

The intensity of use told the amount (%) of the action or function being carried out by electronic means. For example, if a service provider used EPR for the documentation of patient data in half of the cases and a paper-based record for the others, the intensity of use of the EPR was 50%. Several of the questions in the survey were copies of questions from the FinnTelemedicum survey of late 2003, using the same web-based data collection methods.

The questionnaire was emailed between October and November 2005 to all public service providers. That is to 21 hospital districts and 251 health care centers. The questionnaire was also emailed to a sample of 65 private health care service providers including 30 of the largest service providers, and 35 who had responded to the 2003 survey. Additional information was obtained by telephone interviews.

A full report with a detailed description of the method and all the findings of the survey has been published in June 2006 in Finnish [4]. An English version with edited information was published in February 2007 [5].

2. Results of the 2003 and 2005 surveys

2.1. Coverage

Responses to the questionnaire were obtained from all the hospital districts (100 %, n=21). A total of 179 (71.3 %) of 251 health care centers responded to the questionnaire. The responses covered 88.2 % of the whole population of Finland.

Additional data was also obtained from 27 health care centers, which had not responded to the present survey, but had to the 2003 survey.

Results were obtained from 28 private service providers, about half (n=13) from the biggest private service providers and about half (n=15) from those companies that had responded to the 2003 survey. The private providers included enterprises, from conglomerates with hospital and operative services, to small part-time general practices. Because the private providers are a heterogeneous group, the results concerning them can only be regarded as indicative.

The health care centers which did not respond were smaller in size than those who did, covering only 12 % of the population of the country. Therefore, the answers obtained can be regarded as representative in terms of primary and secondary health care. Because the public sector covers 85 % of all health services, the results can be regarded as representative for the whole country.

2.2. Results of Local Services

2.2.1. Electronic Patient Record

In *specialized health care* EPR was in use in all but one of the 21 hospital districts. One hospital district had the EPR at a planning stage at the end of 2005. Among the 17 of the 20 users of the EPR the intensity of use was over 90 %. One hospital district had the intensity of 50-90 %, and two between 25-49 % Compared to the data from the 2003 survey, there is a very strong progress both in the coverage in various medical specialties and in the intensity of use. Because of the complexity of secondary care (hospital) medical records, the coverage aspect is an important indicator of EPR penetration.

In *primary health care centers* EPR was in use in 240 (95,6 %) of the 251 health care centers, three of them had it at a testing stage, and eight at a planning stage. Compared to the 2003 results, a coverage of 93,6 % means that it is near saturation point. The 11 health care centers lacking EPR were small and remote, and some of them were planning on converging with a larger neighboring health care centre. The intensity of use was very high: Among 91 % of the EPR using health care centers, the rate was over 90 %, while among the rest it was 50-90 %.

Among the 28 responders of the *private health care service providers*, 25 (89 %) used EPR. Compared to the 2003 surveys the figures seem to be similar. The intensity of use was high: three out of four providers had an intensity of use of over 90 %.

2.2.2. Picture Archiving and Communication Systems

The results of the PACS survey for secondary care (hospital districts) are represented in Table 1. The progress has been fast during the past two years. 15 out of 21 hospital districts had a PACS in production in 2005. What is more important is that they were practically filmless (over 90% of the medical images were utilized only in digital form). The rest of the hospitals planned to have their PACS in production towards the end of year 2007. After that, all the hospital districts are totally filmless.

Table 1. PACS installations in 21 Finnish hospital districts in 2003 and 2005.

Measure:	2003	2005
PACS in production phase	10/21	15/21
PACS in pilot phase	1/21	2/21
PACS in installation phase	10/21	4/21
PACS usage > 90%	6/21	15/21
PACS usage 50 - 90%	3/21	1/21
PACS usage < 50%	4/21	1/21

In the primary health care centers, the current trend is not to have a PACS of their own, but to combine their efforts with a local regional hospital or with a larger hospital district. There are many innovative solutions available. E.g. in the most northern hospital district all those primary health care centers that produce x-rays are fully digitized and store their images at the central hospital. Those images can be accessed directly from their physician's desktop through an electronic patient record (EPR) interface. In some areas small regional hospitals have a combined image archive and distribution system together with the primary health care centers.

According to the current survey, in year 2005 full picture archiving and communication systems or system components are in use in 95 out of 179 primary health care centers (53%) based on the information provided by the vendors. In the previous survey in year 2003 the PACS usage information was obtained directly from the primary health care centers and they then announced that PACS components were used in 27 (17%) primary health care centers. Even though the methodology is different, this information reveals that the use of PACS at the primary health care level has increased in Finland.

2.3. Results of Regional Services

The exchange of electronic patient information between providers of health services necessitates the use of networks with high data security, which can be actualized through different kinds of intranet solutions or secure internet connections. This inter-organizational data exchange is increasing rapidly in Finland. This is because digital data depositories in individual health care institutions are in active clinical use, and protected data connections enable the communication of electronic patient information.

Before discussing many different and yet at the same time partially overlapping forms of data exchange, a couple of definitions are needed. *Electronic referrals* are basically sent to another institution in order to transfer the responsibility of patient care. Electronic discharge letters are then returned to the sending institution once the patient's treatment is finished. The referral can evolve to an *electronic consultation letter*, if neither responsibility for the patient, nor the actual patient is transferred, but professional advice for treatment is sought or professional opinions are given. There are special cases like *teleradiology* which can be used for consultation but also for information distribution, the same applies also to the *telelaboratory*. *Regional patient data repositories* or *exchanges* can serve many purposes: they can provide a source of reference information for past treatment, a basis for current patient data distribution in a geographically distributed health care environment, as well as a data depository for consultation services and workload distribution. In a normal medical practice, the various forms of data distribution complement each other.

For collaboration between primary and specialized health care, the most important messages are referral letters, consultation letters, and feedback or discharge letters. In addition to a narrative text, the letters can include results of laboratory tests and radiological examinations.

2.3.1. e-Referral and e-Discharge Letters

The e-Referral letter signifies a course of action by which the referring physician, usually a general practitioner, draws up a message with an intention to transfer a patient and the responsibility of care to a hospital. The role of hospitals in this kind of collaboration with health care centers is to receive referral letters, and provide a letter showing the treatment, and to give feedback through a discharge letter.

This service is presently provided by 16 of the 21 hospital districts. Rapid progress has been made during the last couple of years, when in 2003 the service was available in about half of the hospital districts, in 2005 three fourths used such systems.

2.3.2. Electronic and Remote Consultations

Electronic consultation was provided by 11 of the 21 hospital districts, and it was at a testing or planning stage in the rest of the hospital districts, except in one hospital district.

About one third (36 %) of the 174 health care centers purchased electronic consultations from hospitals. Another third had said to be planning it or having even tested it. The health care centers purchasing electronic consultations seemed to be very active with its use: among 70 % of the 49 health care centers which answered the question it was their principal mode for consultation.

Consultations by televideo conferencing between health care centers and hospitals takes place according to the following procedure: at the health care centre the patient, the general practitioner, and the nurse attend the video session. In the hospital a specialist accompanied by a nurse gives the consultation. This service has increased in hospitals since 2003 and 10 of the 21 provide it regularly while five were in testing or piloting phase.

Among 179 health care centers which answered the questionnaire, 21 (12 %) purchased video conferencing in order to consult a specialist of a hospital. In addition, ten health care centers had been planning or were testing it. Although specialist consultations by video conferencing were now being provided by more hospitals than earlier, the number of health care centers purchasing the service had not increased from 21 in 2003.

2.3.3. Regional Data Exchange Systems

Due to a well developed public communications network, investing in creating a closed, healthcare dedicated network was not deemed necessary. The demands of healthcare telecommunication have been served through the use of commercial high speed public data networks and virtual private network (VPN) tunnels over the public network.

Regional patient data repositories are equally used by many health care organizations and institutions for the exchanging of data. According to this survey, nine out of 21 hospital districts have a regional patient data repository in clinical use and six districts are running pilot projects

2.3.4. Teleradiology and Image Distribution through a Regional Archive

Teleradiology has been one of the first applications of telemedicine in Finland. The first experiments were made already in 1969 and real implementation started at the beginning of the 1990's. In 1994 all the five university hospitals had teleradiology services [7]. The regular service started in the sparsely populated northern areas, but has then spread all around the country.

The boarder line between teleradiology and image distribution through a regional archive is gradually vanishing with certain services. In the current survey, we investigated all the methods used for a regional image transfer service. For a regional service, the basic assumption was that a hospital should have a local PACS installed. Then, the technical infrastructure behind the implementation of a regional image distribution could differ. In some areas, image viewing is through a regional reference database. In other areas there is a dedicated common regional radiological database ("regional PACS"). A third solution is to view images through regional access to an EPR archive, which contains also images.

The results of 2003 and 2005 on teleradiology and regional image distribution/archive services for secondary care (hospital districts) are presented in Table 2. Also the usage percentage is given, if available. Since teleradiology services could be independent of local PACS or a regional archive, a combined look at image transfer services is given. The key information is that 18 out of 21 (86%) hospital districts utilize some form of electronic distribution of radiological images.

Table 2. Teleradiology and regional image distribution services in hospital districts in 2003 and 2005.

Measure:	**2003**	**2005**
Teleradiology in production phase	13/21	16/21
Teleradiology in pilot phase	4/21	2/21
Teleradiology usage > 90%	2/21	5/21
Regional archive in production	3/21	10/21
Regional archive in pilot phase	0/21	3/21
Regional archive usage > 90%	0/21	3/21
Either teleradiology or regional archive in use	13/21	18/21

In the primary health care sector, the combined results show that 52 primary health care centers out of 179 (29%) had some method of teleradiological image delivery in production. This is a remarkable increase compared to 2003, when 15 primary health care centers were using teleradiological image delivery.

2.3.5. Telelaboratory

Regional distribution of laboratory results through a regional archive was utilized by 11 out of 21 Finnish hospital districts, one was at the pilot-project stage and three were planning to provide such a service in the near future. In addition, 16 out of 21 hospital districts utilized some other form of electronic transmission of laboratory results to the primary health care centers in their region. These other services partially overlapped with the usage of the regional archives. The combined results showed that a total of 19 out of 21 (90%) hospital districts had some method for the electronic distribution of laboratory results in 2005. This figure has nearly doubled from 2003 when 10 hospital districts used telelaboratory services.

In the primary health care sector, 48 health care centers out of 179 (27%) informed that they received daily laboratory results electronically through a regional database and 71 informed that they are either at a testing or planning stage. This means that those dealing with primary care will accept new services like receiving telelaboratory data as soon as the hospital districts can provide it.

2.3.6. ePrescribing

In Finland a national *e-Prescribing* pilot-project was launched in 2002. The pilot-project ran from 2004-2006. The system was tested in two hospital districts and in a couple of health care centers. Finland opted for a system based on a national prescription database. In the pilot-project system, a doctor creates a prescription with a legacy system, signs it with a strong electronic signature, and sends the secured message to the national prescriptions database. The patient goes to a pharmacy, where the pharmacist accesses the database with the pharmacy's system. The pharmacist makes the required changes and marks the dispensing information on the electronic prescription, signs the markings with a personal smart card, and saves the markings to the prescription in the database. The medicine is then dispensed to the patient [8]. The further development is covered later in this paper.

2.4. Information Exchange between Health Care Organizations and Patients

20 hospital districts and 79 % of all the health care centers maintained their own websites. The hospital district and a half of the health care centers who still did not have an individual website were running pilot-projects or were planning the implementation of their own website.

Information exchange with patients by SMS messaging was used by one and tested by three of the hospital districts. It was used by nine (5 %) health care centers and tested by 11 (6 %) of the 179 health care centers. With private providers information exchange with patients by SMS was used by three (11%) and tested by five (18%) of the 28 private providers.

Only one health care centre used secure e-mails in information networks, but 15% of them used conventional e-mail. Remote browsing of EPR by the patient was not in use anywhere, but was planned to be implemented by two hospital districts, three health care centers, and one private care provider.

3. New Legislation on eArchive and ePrescription

3.1. National EPR and Other Patient Information Archiving System

The Government has decided that for reasons dealing with the practicality and economy, the information management structure of Finland be at least in part organized on the national, instead of the regional level. The core of the national Finnish ICT infrastructure for social and health care will reside in a national digital archive for patient documents. In addition, there will be one logical connectivity centre for eHealth communication. Exchanging data between organizations will be conducted on a national and not a regional level. The service will be maintained by the Social Insurance Institution (KELA). The legislature will obligate all health organizations to participate in the construction of a national IT architecture for health - a project that is expected to be finished by the end of 2011. It will include a national public key infrastructure (PKI) system for health care professionals. The system will be administered by the National Authority for Medico-legal Affairs. The legislation dealing with the creation of a national level IT infrastructure for health was received by parliament in October 2006, accepted in December 2006 and finally come into effect in July 2007.

Technical planning and defining has started and the vendor consortium has been selected. All the public care providers must join in. Private care providers can choose between the national archive and paper archiving. Moreover, all those regional patient record projects that receive governmental financial support should obey the technical connection requirements by the end of 2009. The original legal archive copy will reside in the national archive; the institutions can have their everyday operational copies in their own patient record systems. The index to the document archive is a link directory, which can be seen with an oral consent. Patients can refuse publishing of their records in the directory. Retrieval of actual data is only by strong authentication and electronically transmitted permission.

It has been planned that the National EPR Archive will offer citizens a chance to browse selected personal health information - namely, reference information for the use of services, referral and discharge letters, certificates, statements and results of examinations, and access log data about the visits to the to the personal patient record.

3.2. National ePrescription

At present, permanent e-Prescription legislation has been given to the parliament and has been accepted in December 2006. The system described in the draft legislation is based on the experiences of the pilot-project. A national e-Prescription database hosted by the Social Insurance Institution (KELA) will be created and strong authentication and a smart ID-card for professionals with an e-signature systems and SSL-secured messages from health care providers and pharmacies to the database will be used. The Finnish ePrescribing is aimed to be fully integrated with the different EPRs and a centralized receipt data file, to cover all pharmacies, and to contain continuously updated knowledge about all prescribed drugs of the patients, all using highly secured networks. The application to be built offers an usable platform for decision support for the drug safety. The legislation come into effect in April 2007 and service piloting should start already in 2008.

4. Discussion

Present study is part of a continuing survey, which follows the implementation of Finnish national eHealth roadmap. The ideas are based on the European eHealth action plan, like citizen-centered and patient-centered services, the full continuum of care and well-informed patient. This series of studies reveals data for administration and planning and even for international benchmarking.

The electronic patient record is the most important tool for health professionals in acquiring and documenting information about patient care. In Finland 95,6% of the primary health care centers and 95% of the hospital districts used EPR as their primary tool for patient data. Among primary health care centers, the figure was already 93,6% in 2003. Knowing this, one can say that the penetration of EPR is no longer a measure of ICT usage and that new indicators need to be sought.

One new indicator is the exchange of information between health care institutions. In Finland, regional exchange of information has been possible because of the high usage of EPR systems within institutions. Regional exchange of radiological and laboratory data has been one of the first applications, but these days eReferrals and eDischarge letters directly from EPR to EPR are on the increase. These all contribute to the seamless service systems of the patient. The popularity of regional data exchange has resulted in four different widely used data exchange systems. With the patient's consent, the physician instant access to previous patient data from other institutions through a secure connection.

Once the backbone for electronic management of patient data in Finland is ready, the next major challenge is the construction and implementation of the National EPR Archive. The task is not a minor one. There are changes that need to be made in legislature, technology, and ways in conducting daily tasks in health care. A transition period of several years is needed. The greatest challenges may occur in communication between local and regional systems and the national archive. This might require major changes in the current software being used in hospital districts and health care centers. The goal is increased access to electronic personal of health records, both by the physician and the patient.

References

[1]   OECD Reviews of Health Systems – Finland 2005. [cited 2006 Nov 30]. available from: http://www.oecd.org/document/47/0,2340,en_33873108_33873360_35808943_1_1_1_1,00.html
[2]   STAKES; National Research and Development Centre for Welfare and Health – STAKES [cited 2007 Nov 30]. available from: http://www.stakes.fi/EN/index.htm
[3]   Kiviaho K, Winblad I, Reponen J. Terveydenhuollon toimintaprosesseja ja asiointia tukevat atk-sovellukset Suomessa – kartoitus ja käyttöanalyysi.[english summary] FinnTelemedicum. Osaavien keskusten verkoston julkaisuja 8/2004. STAKES, Helsinki, 2005.
[4]   Winblad I, Reponen J, Hämäläinen P, Kangas M. [Abstract in English]. Informaatio- ja kommunikaatioteknologian käyttö Suomen terveydenhuollossa vuonna 2005. Tilanne ja kehityksen suunta. Raportteja 7/2006, Stakes, Helsinki, 2006
[5]   Hämäläinen, P, Reponen, J.Winblad, I. eHealth of Finland, Check point 2006. STAKES reports 1/2007, Helsinki, 2007.
[6]   Reponen J, Niinimäki J, Kumpulainen T, Ilkko E, Karttunen A and Jartti P. Mobile teleradiology with smartphone terminals as a part of a multimedia electronic patient record. In: Lemke HU, Inamura K, Doi K, Vannier MW and Farman AG (Edrs.) *CARS 2005 – Computer Assisted Radiology and Surgery.* Proceedings of the 19th International Congress and Exhibition; Berlin, Germany. Elsevier International Congress Series 1281; 2005. pp. 916-921.
[7]   Reponen J. Radiology as a part of a comprehensive telemedicine and eHealth network. *Int J Circumpolar Health* 63(4) 2004: pp. 429-435.
[8]   Hyppönen H (Edr.) (Abstract in English). Evaluation of the National Electronic Prescribing Pilot II (2005-2006). STAKES, Reports 11/2006. Helsinki, 2006.

eHealth: Combining Health Telematics, Telemedicine, Biomedical Engineering and Bioinformatics to the Edge. Edited by B. Blobel, P. Pharow and M. Nerlich.
IOS Press, 2008

Teleradiology with Satellite Units - Six Years Experience at The Norwegian Radium Hospital

Albrecht REITH and Dag Rune OLSEN [1]

The Norwegian Radium Hospital, University of Oslo, Oslo, Norway

Abstract. Norway has played a leading role in Europe in applying telemedicine in health care services over the past two decades and is still in the forefront of developing telemedicine services both nationally and internationally. Today support for telemedicine comes mainly from the wish to meet the challenges of rising costs in health care. Critical obstacles for implementation of telemedicine techniques may by overcome easier by referring to the experience from other medical centers. A case in point is the six year experience of telemedicine at The Norwegian Radium Hospital, in distributing radiotherapy services to two satellite hospitals hundred kilometers far off. The main lesson learned is: the most serious obstacles are not technological but socio-psychological challenges and that staff up-dating, prior to implementation, is crucial. Case selections, routines, work flows and administrative solutions are described for the daily operations between the main clinic and the satellite units. In conclusion: radiotherapy service by telemedicine is feasible and cost effective. Standardization and quality assurance of radiotherapy at the quality level of a comprehensive cancer center can be offered to a much larger population and may play a role in improved cancer survival outcome.

Keywords: Medical informatics, e-health, telemedicine, radiotherapy, teleradiology, standardization, quality assurance, comprehensive cancer center

Introduction

Norway has played a pioneering role in Europe in applying telemedicine in health care services over the past two decades [1] and is still in the forefront of developing telemedicine services both nationally and internationally [2]. The initiative for telemedicine came from the government which strongly supported telemedicine as an important way of delivering health services and from early on concentrated on a country-wide public health net. In the beginning, the main driving force for telemedicine was the political will to give access to best health service to all citizens in this sparsely populated country characterized by long distances. This challenge was greatest in the North-Norway. Therefore a national research center for telemedicine was located in Tromsø, a university town north of the polar circle. In a recent review,

---

[1] Corresponding Author: Dag Rune Olsen, MD, PhD, Institute for Cancer Research, The Norwegian Radiumhospitalet, Montebello, N 0310, Oslo, Norway; Email: d.r.olsen@medisin.uio.no

the lessons learned from the experiences with telemedicine applications in remote areas have been thoroughly presented [2].

Today, medical services in remote areas are not any longer the main reason for governmental support for telemedicine but rather the wish to meet the challenges of rising costs in health care by exploring new telemedicine techniques in the different disciplines of medicine. This may improve the efficiency as well as the quality of health services. While the potential benefits are obvious, there are also obstacles to extended implementation of telemedicine techniques, both in the medical profession and in the public. There are discussions about medical data protection and - especially within the medical profession - about the reliability and quality of the health services provided by telemedicine. This latter concern may to some extent be motivated by the fear of losing control over local work as well as the fear of loosing jobs. These concerns can be critical obstacles for implementation of telemedicine techniques and have to be taken seriously. Referring to the experience from other medical centers, where telemedicine has been practiced with positive outcome, may be used for reducing these concerns and overcoming the skepticism of the various professional groups. In this context the six year experience of telemedicine at The Norwegian Radium Hospital, in distributing radiotherapy services to hospitals several hundred kilometers far off, may be of general interest.

A tremendous growth in digital information in hospital environment has taken place over the past two decades, and the need for networked digital communications systems has become evident. The conception of digital information system within a hospital environment dates back to the early 1970s; however the lack of basic technology to provide adequate network infrastructure impeded widespread introduction of such systems into clinical practice. During the 1990s the technology matured and digital information handling developed with a tremendous speed, in particular primarily within the field of radiology, but also within other medical disciplines. As such, digital information networking is no longer merely a technological issue, but has also changed the working practice of several medical disciplines.

1. Telemedicine in Radiation Therapy

In the management of cancer, image based diagnostics play a crucial role whereas radiation therapy is a critical component of multi modality therapy in about 50% of all cancer patients. Over the past decades, advances in radiotherapy are to a large extent attributed to technological development, in particular, with respect to imaging and digital technology. Imaging tools have been developed with respect to treatment planning and in treatment verification, as well as for adaptive treatment strategies. The development of digital image information standards, such as DICOM, network protocols and improved connectivity between modalities, have all been critical for the utilization of digital information within a clinical radiotherapy environment. This development, however, doesn't only allow flow of digital information within departments; it also facilitates communication and exchange of digital information between institutions (Figure 1).

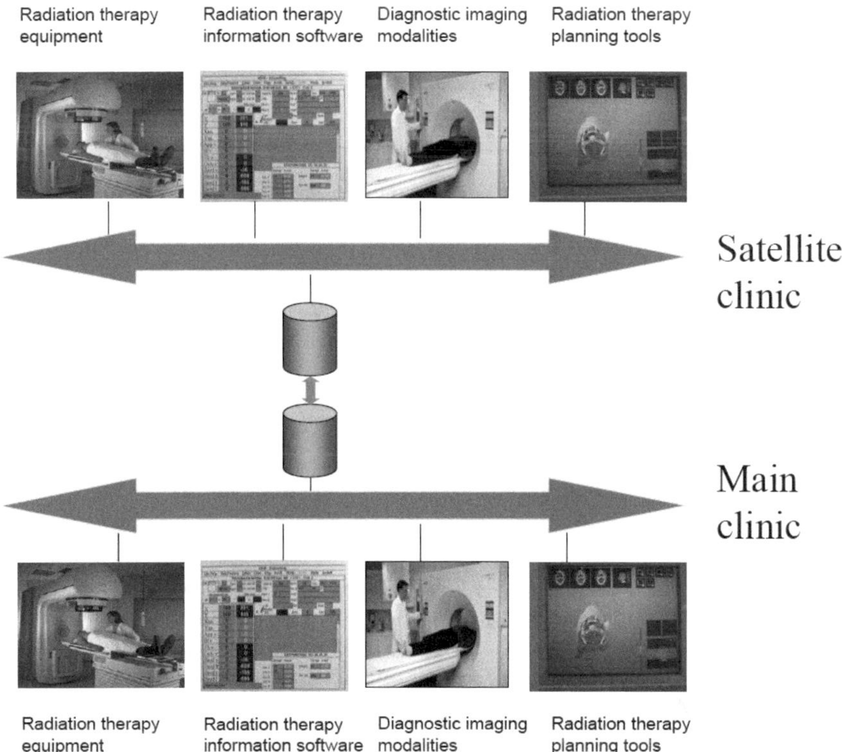

Figure 1. Design of a communication network for digital information transfer within a radiation therapy facility and between radiation therapy clinics, i.e. the main clinic and its satellite units

Telemedicine provides increased access to medical expertise and has been widely adopted in a variety of medical disciplines. Still, radiology is the most common area for telemedicine. Other areas are emerging and have adopted the concept of telemedicine. Initially, telemedicine was regarded merely as a tool for long-distance communication, but has conceptually evolved and the terms "tele-healthcare" and "e-health" have been introduced to include all aspects of communication between medical centers for patient care. Within radiology and radiation therapy digital information, medical images included, have been widely used for many years; in radiation therapy, however, telemedicine, has until recently rarely been implemented on a larger scale [3], [4], [5]. Based on the very nature of radiation therapy, with the vast amount of digital information characteristic for the therapeutic process, one can expect that telemedicine in radiation therapy will become equally important as in radiology in improving the quality and standardization of such procedures. In distributed clinical services, telemedicine may in particular play a critical role. This is not merely restricted to distributed cancer care in rural areas, but also in the provision of high-end radiation therapy, like particle therapy and in therapy of rare cancers [1]. Also telemedicine may facilitate collaboration between institutions in clinical trials and in the quality assurance of such. Telemedicine for cancer patients undergoing radiation therapy facilitates a dialogue between clinical experts on the following issues:

- Identification and delineation of cancerous tissue
- Treatment planning and simulation of individual patients
- Treatment verification of individual patients
- Follow-up and clinical trial management

As a consequence radiotherapy at the quality level of a comprehensive cancer center can be offered to a much larger population and may play a role in improved cancer survival outcome.

In radiation therapy the most evident role of telemedicine can be found in the treatment planning and simulation of individual patients. In this process remote consultation may be of clinical importance in identification and delineation of the cancerous tissue from CT, MR, US and PET images, but also with respect to beam setup and treatment plan evaluation. Identification and appropriate delineation of the cancerous tissue and microscopic disease is probably the most crucial part of the planning process with respect to clinical outcome. At smaller radiation therapy clinics the required expertise may not be available; in such situations telemedicine may be a helpful tool for remote consultations. Ideally, with real-time telemedicine service, identification and delineation on the cancerous tissue, treatment options and treatment plan evaluation can jointly be discussed among physicians of the clinical team, although remotely located. Only few reports on systems dedicated to remote delineation and treatment planning and virtual simulation have been published [5-8]. An alternative to real-time services is the transfer of data between centers for off-line consultation. This alternative is less technology demanding, but does not facilitate the dialogue between the different medical disciplines or members of a clinical team. Also, educational aspects of quality management are best accommodated with real-time telemedicine support. A further development of telemedicine in radiation therapy is follow-up and clinical trial management. Multi-center clinical trials require strict adherence to treatment protocols and telemedicine represent a useful tool in trial management and quality assurance. The German teleradiotherapeutic network for lymphoma trial [5] and the US dose escalation trial for early-stage prostate cancer [7] are excellent examples of such application. Entire sets of treatment data are submitted to a study coordination center including pre-qualification dummy runs from the participating centers. A prerequisite for efficient and consistent data collection is common data formats and network connectivity.

For optimal use of telemedicine, required and demanded services must be matched; in order to evaluate the appropriate level of telemedicine services a functionality classifications has been introduced for radiation therapy [10].

1.1. Level-1

It includes display of radiotherapy related information via teleconferencing which facilitates discussions about identification and delineation of cancerous tissue, treatment options and plan evaluation. Level-1 functionality may be based on video-signal technology and is a low-cost service.

1.2. Level-2

It features digital data transfer between institutions, and limited remote image handling. Remote off-line delineation of cancerous tissue is a typical example of a level-2 service, and requires transfer of complete digital data sets between institutions (Figure 2). There are no unique networking and data storage strategies required for this level of services. However, common standards and protocols must be implemented. High-speed network communication is required for this level of services.

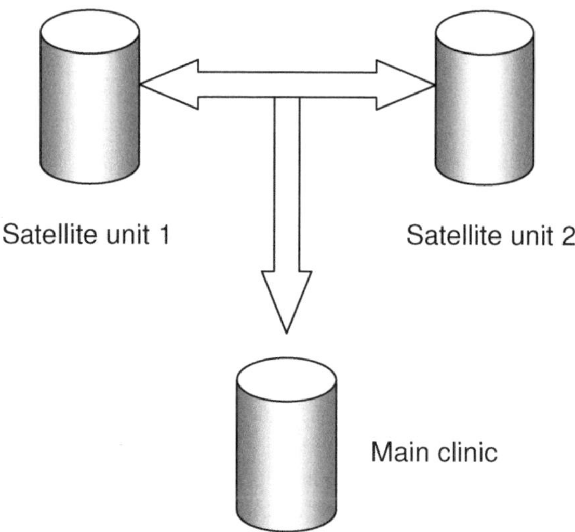

Figure 2. Data transfer flow chart. Radiation therapy data are copied daily from the satellite unit data base to the main clinic's one. In the case of off-line support, in delineation in cancerous tissue and treatment planning, data are transferred from the satellite unit to the main clinic and then back again, on demand

1.3. Level-3

It features real-time services. Direct interaction and discussion may be of particular importance in the identification and delineation of cancerous tissue; probably less so crucial for treatment technique discussions and treatment evaluation. For daily irradiation, treatment data are downloaded from a central data server. At level-3 services, data can be stored remotely and downloaded to the radiation therapy equipment on demand; this requires an absolute reliable communication. High speed network communication is required for this level of services.

Depending on the nature of collaboration and relationship between institutions taking part in a network of telemedicine services level-2 and level-3 applications may raise medico-legal issues with respect to responsibility for treatment of the patient.

2. Current experience

Pioneering institutions in implementing telemedicine, including some functionality for radiation therapy, have been amongst others the Mayo Clinic [11]. The Hokkaido University School of Medicine, developed a dedicated radiation therapy telemedicine system, named THERAPIST, and has over a number of years demonstrated successes in remote simulation of emergency radiotherapy of spinal cord compression [12]. Moreover, Hashimoto and co-workers have shown that remote consulting –where digitally reconstructed radiograms (DRR) and electronic portal images (EPI) are involved - is of value to clinical radiation therapy practice [3].

In a study exploring remote treatment planning, supervision and economics, Norum and co-workers [13] reported on the feasibility of cancer patients undergoing radiation treatment at the University Hospital of North Norway under the supervision of The Norwegian Radium Hospital. Treatment planning systems at the two institutions were connected and videoconferencing units were installed. Both treatment planning and remote simulation procedures were carried out. Cost-minimization analysis demonstrated that remote consultation by telemedicine was highly cost-efficient compared to transferal of the patient to the Norwegian Radium Hospital. Obviously, the conclusion of such cost-effective analysis is highly dependent on local cost structure and has no general validity. However, the study demonstrated that level-1 telemedicine can be established at low cost and with a significant clinical impact.

In 2001 The Norwegian Radium Hospital opened its first radiation therapy satellite unit at Kristiansand followed by a second one in 2002 at Gjøvik. Both satellite units are operated by the main centre, which also has the responsibility for the radiation therapy services. Moreover, the staff at these units is employed by the main clinic. The satellite units were established to provide decentralized radiation therapy, primarily for palliative cancer care and *standard* curative radiation, for e.g. breast cancer (Figure 3). Telemedicine services were established to maintain high clinical quality services at smaller radiation therapy units which cannot have the full range of clinical competence normally found at a comprehensive cancer centre.

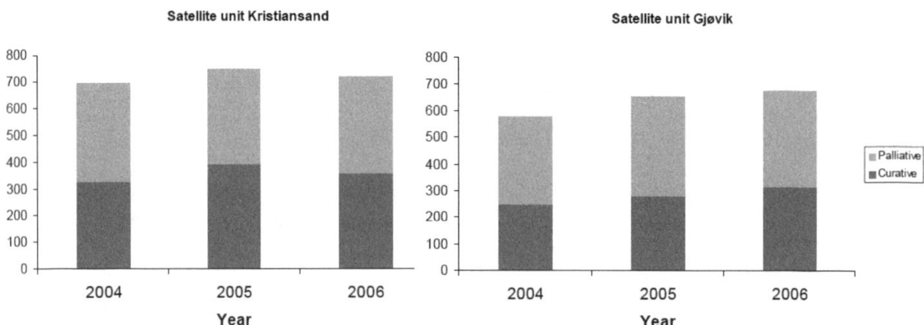

Figure 3. Number of patient treatment series, differentiated between curative and palliative intended radiation therapy, at two satellite units

Both radiation therapy satellite units and the main clinic are equipped with identical software solutions for maximum connectivity and uncomplicated communication and data transfer. Dedicated radiation therapy DICOM-databases are installed at both satellite units as well as the main clinic, and transfer of all radiation therapy data from the satellite units to the main clinic is performed daily - i.e. level-2 applications (Table 1). On a regular basis, i.e. weekly, tumor boards are held with the satellite unit staff involved. These sessions include discussions of treatment plan evaluation and follow up. Also weekly educational sessions involve staff at both the satellite units and the main clinic. Both activities are level-1 services. The system that was developed and installed allows also level-3 services. However, real-time consultations, e.g. regarding delineation of cancerous tissue are rarely performed. To our experience, this is not due to the lack of need for level-3 services, but rather reflects time concern and barriers in using the new technology. Current state telemedicine in radiation therapy represents as such not primarily technological but socio-psychological challenges. Successful implementation of telemedicine in radiation therapy, e.g. in distributed clinical services, require more focus on educating and motivating the staff in utilizing the technology for changing working practice. However, this requires an altered mind set.

Table 1. Frequency of telemedicine services between radiation therapy satellite units and the main clinic

Services	Frequency
Level-1	weekly
Level-2	daily/weekly
Level-3	Rarely

3. Outlook

The experiences of distributing radiotherapy telemedicine services to other hospitals will have importance for handling the merger of the two university hospitals in the health region south, The Norwegian Radium Hospital and the Rikshospitalet. New close co-operations with 2 university hospitals can be foreseen, as 2 of the 5 Norwegian health regions, regions south and east have merged. Generally, the application of telemedicine in radiation diagnostics and therapy – as in other medical branches - *per se* will become important in its self by improving the quality and standardization of radiology procedures with the possibility of clinical outcome. Furthermore, teleradiology can facilitate collaboration between highly specialized centers of excellence with respect to rare medical conditions and also "in the provision of high-end radiation therapy such as proton treatment" [1]. In this context it is of interest that The Norwegian Radium Hospital in 2006 signed an agreement with the University Hospital of Schleswig-Holstein which will build a Particle Center for proton treatment in Kiel. The Kiel particle therapy center will not only serve patients in Northern Germany but also be made available to patients from Scandinavia and the Baltic region. It is foreseen that telemedicine for this leading edge radiation service will play a crucial role for an effective co-operation between the involved medical centers.

There are several lessons from 6 years teleradiology at The Norwegian Radium Hospital and its satellite units:

3.1. General Lessons

- The main problems for implementation of teleradiology are primarily not technological.
- The most serious obstacles are socio-psychological challenges from the staff members involved.
- Therefore successful implementation of telemedicine requires more focus on educating and motivating the staff by e.g. up-dating the personal in utilizing the technology prior to installation.

- CAVE: alter the mind set.

3.2. Specific Lessons

- To overcome problems with interoperability the radiation therapy satellite units and the main clinic are equipped with identical software solutions for maximum connectivity and uncomplicated communication and data transfer.
- For continuous safe data flow, transfer of all radiation therapy data from the satellite units to the main clinic is performed daily.
- Weekly tumor board sessions are held with the satellite unit and main clinic staff including discussions of treatment plan evaluation and follow-up.
- Educational sessions are hold weekly with the staff at the satellite units and the main clinic.
- Real-time consultations, regarding e.g. delineation of cancerous tissue, are rarely used. The reason for this can be time concerns or "mental barriers".

References

[1] Reith A, Olsen DR, Bruland O, Berner A, Risberg B. Information technology in action: the example of Norway. Stud Health Technol Inform; 96:186-9, IOS Press, Amsterdam, 2003.

[2] Hartvigsen G, Johanesen MA, Hasvold P, Bellika JG, Arsand E, Arils E, Gammon D, Pettersen S, Pedersen S. Challenges in ehealth: Lessons learned from 20 years with telemedicine in Tromsø. Stud Health Technol Inform; 129:82-6, IOS Press, Amsterdam, 2007.

[3] Hashimoto S, Shirato H, Kaneko K, Ooshio W, Nishioka T, Miyasaka K. Clinical efficacy of telemedicine in emergency radiotherapy for malignant spinal cord compression. *J Digit Imaging* 2001; 14:124–30.

[4] Smith CL, Chu WK, Enke C. A review of digital image networking technologies for radiation oncology treatment planning. *Med Dosim* 1998; 23:271–7.

[5] Eich HT, Muller RP, Schneeweiss A, Hansemann K, Semrau R, Willich N, Rube C, Sehlen S, Hinkelbein M, Diehl V. Initiation of a teleradiotherapeutic network for patients in German lymphoma studies. *Int J Radiat Oncol Biol Phys* 2004; 58:805–808.

[6] Ntasis E, Maniatis TA, Nikita KS. Secure environment for real-time tele-collaboration on virtual simulation of radiation treatment planning. *Technol Health Care 2003*; 11:41-52.

[7] Huh SJ, Shirato H, Hashimoto S, Shimizu S, Kim DY,Ahn YC, Choi D, Miyasaka K, Mizuno J An integrated service digital network (ISDN)-based international telecommunication between Samsung Medical Center and Hokkaido University using telecommunication helped radiotherapy planning and information system (THERAPIS). *Radiother Oncol* 2000; 56:121–3.

[8] Stitt JA A system of tele-oncology at the University of Wisconsin Hospital and Clinics and regional oncology affiliate institutions. *World Med J* 1998; 97:38–42.

[9] Purdy JA, Harms WB, Michalski J, Cox JD Multi-institutional clinical trials: 3-D conformal radiotherapy quality assurance. Guidelines in an NCI/RTOG study evaluating dose escalation in prostate cancer radiotherapy. *Front Radiat Ther Oncol* 1996; 29:255–63.

[10] Olsen DR, Bruland S, Davis BJ Telemedicine in radiotherapy treatment planning: requirements and applications. *Radiother Oncol* 2000; 54:255–9.

[11] King BF et al. Electronic imaging and clinical implementation: work group approach at Mayo Clinic, Rochester. *J Digital Imaging* 1999; 2:32-6.

[12] Hashimoto S, Shirato H, Nishioka T, Kagei K, Shimizu S, Fujita K, Ogasawara H, Watanabe Y, Miyasaka K Remote verification in radiotherapy using digitally reconstructed radiography (DRR) and portal images: a pilot study. *Int J Radiat Oncol Biol Phys* 2001b; 50:579–85.

[13] Norum J, Bruland OS, Spanne O, Bergmo T, Green T, Olsen DR, Olsen JH, Sjaeng EE, Burkow T. Telemedicine in radiotherapy: a study exploring remote treatment planning, supervision and economics. *J Telemed Telecare*. 2005;11:245-50.

Multidisciplinary and Multilingual
Semantic Interoperability

eHealth: Combining Health Telematics, Telemedicine, Biomedical Engineering and Bioinformatics to the Edge. Edited by B. Blobel, P. Pharow and M. Nerlich.
IOS Press, 2008

219

Establishing and Harmonizing Ontologies in an Interdisciplinary Health Care and Clinical Research Environment

Barry SMITH [a,1] and Mathias BROCHHAUSEN [b]
[a] University at Buffalo, Buffalo, NY, USA
[b] Saarland University, IFOMIS, Saarbrücken, Germany

Abstract. Ontologies are being ever more commonly used in biomedical informatics. The paper provides a survey of some of these uses, and of the relations between ontologies and other terminology resources. In order for ontologies to become truly useful, two objectives must be met. First, ways must be found for the transparent evaluation of ontologies. Second, existing ontologies need to be harmonized. The authors argue that one key foundation for both ontology evaluation and harmonization is the adoption of a realist paradigm in ontology development. For science-based ontologies of the sort which concern us in the eHealth arena, it is reality that provides the common benchmark against which ontologies can be evaluated and aligned within larger frameworks. Given the current multitude of ontologies in the biomedical domain the need for harmonization is becoming ever more urgent. An example of such harmonization within the ACGT project is described, which draws on ontology-based computing as a basis for sharing clinical and laboratory data on cancer research.

Keywords. Ontology, terminology, research

Introduction

This paper aims to provide an overview of some important recent developments in ontological engineering in healthcare and in clinical research. Ontology-based eHealth applications have become ever more popular in recent years, and they are gradually replacing the terminology-based artifacts of an earlier generation. We can in fact distinguish three (overlapping) phases in this development:

1. a phase in which work on terminology and coding schemes was dominated by the influence of library science (with classifications, which often had their origins in earlier printed dictionaries, oriented towards the cataloguing and indexing of published literature),

2. a phase in which such work was dominated by the influence of database design and software technology (with classifications focused on the need to describe and promote access to data, and programmers sometimes making information management decisions for a domain – biomedicine – about which they often had very little understanding), and

---

[1] Corresponding Author: Barry Smith, PhD, Professor, University at Buffalo, 135 Park Hall, North Campus, Buffalo, New York 14260, USA; Email: phismith@buffalo.edu

2.3 The SNOMED initiative

It must be admitted that the attitude of clinical professionals towards ontologies is still somewhat ambivalent. Certainly ontology-based systems are viewed as bringing the promise of intriguing new possibilities in the biomedical informatics and health IT arenas. Such systems are seen as providing the possibility of transforming existing shallow coding schemes such as ICD 9, still used primarily for billing purposes, into more coherent representations of biomedical reality which might be used for purposes of research, for clinical decision support or for the gathering of more useful and more detailed public health statistics. On the other hand however – as Rector *et al.* have pointed out – systems such as those based on description logics can be hard to understand for clinical users [18]. The more formally rigorous the system, the more expensive it is to develop and maintain and the greater the costs incurred in training its users.

The most ambitious initiative to address these problems is currently being mounted by the International Health Terminology Standards Developing Organization [19], which is seeking to establish the SNOMED CT vocabulary as an international master terminology for the entire domain of biomedicine with a description logic backbone. The goal is one of comprehensive coverage of the entire domain of medicine in a multiplicity of languages, starting out from the basis of an English-language vocabulary which already comprehends more than 357,000 concepts and has partial versions in other languages. In addition the SNOMED vocabulary is mapped to other important existing standards, including the widely used ICD classifications of the World Health Organization.

A major advantage of SNOMED CT is the comprehensive reach, which it secures through some 21 hierarchies.

Table 1. SNOMED-CT Hierarchies

Clinical findings	Procedure
Body structure	Anatomical concepts (Body Structure)
Morphologies (Body Structure)	Organism
Physical Force	Substance
Specimen	Social context
Attributes	Context Dependent categories
Physical object	Events
Environments and geographical location	Observable entity
Qualifier value	Staging and Scales
Special concept	Pharmaceutical / biologic product
Record artefact	

2.4 Problems with SNOMED in the Clinical Setting

An issue which has still not been satisfactorily resolved, however, is the degree to which the introduction of sophisticated broad-coverage terminologies such as SNOMED CT into the hospital environment will involve costs in training and implementation which would be so great that they could not be justified by compensating rewards. Billing needs are catered for by simpler terminologies. The rewards of using a more rigorous and comprehensive terminology do indeed promise to be of great significance for example for clinical decision support and for more adequate public health data. By providing common structure and terminology, the SNOMED CT international master vocabulary would go far towards providing a single data source for review and also bring the benefits of less redundant data and easier opportunities for longitudinal studies and meta-analysis and for ensuring consistency of data across the lifetime of the patient and from one healthcare institution to the next. The use of SNOMED CT would allow in addition the use of common tools and techniques, common training and a single validation of data. But the fact that so few healthcare institutions have embraced SNOMED CT for clinical coding seems to suggest that incentives are still missing for the considerable investments which would be needed to harvest these benefits [20].

One additional factor is that SNOMED CT is marked by a number of internal structural problems (for example gaps in the terminology, a lack of compositional structure, shortfalls in consistency from one part of the vocabulary to another) which detract from its appeal to novice users and provide obstacles to its efficient application in coding [11], [21], [22]. In our view it is still the case that too little effort is being invested in attempts to decrease the costs involved in adoption of terminologies such as SNOMED as a basis for clinical coding by improving the degree to which such problems are addressed, and it seems to us that the major existing healthcare terminology resources still lack coherent strategies for incremental improvement.

2.5 Towards Evidence-Based Ontology Development

We believe that at least part of what must be involved in any such strategy is the development of an evidence-based evolutionary methodology for quality assurance of ontologies – a methodology whose application can at one and the same time both enhance the degree to which ontologies constitute a realistic representation of reality and create a more intuitive and more easily maintainable framework for clinical coding The ideal result of the implementation of such a strategy would be a framework which is both biologically accurate and able to supply its users with a view of clinical reality which coheres with their expectations of how this reality should look. Such an outcome would, we believe, not merely save time in coding and raise the accuracy, breadth, and depth of coverage of the results; it would also enhance the degree to which the systems in question can be used by the clinician and researcher for genuinely useful purposes.

We have argued in a number of prior publications [23], [24, [25] that reasoning on the basis of information that comes closer to an adequate picture of reality has the potential to provide the basis for more valuable results, whether in decision support, meta-analysis, or trial management, than reasoning on the basis of representations which confuse features of our data or knowledge with features of the reality on the side of the patient. We will describe below a realism-based project in the domain of post-genomic clinical trials that is designed to yield benefits of just this sort [26].

3. Harmonization and Quality Management in Ontology Development

In the development of the OBO Foundry, and also in some of the more mature initiatives within the framework of the Semantic Web, we can witness a third important trend – in addition to those of *greater realism* and *greater formal rigor* – a trend towards the *harmonization of ontologies* with a view towards ensuring their interoperability. The goal of such harmonization is to bring about a situation in which the coverage of ontologies can be increased in stepwise fashion across ever broader domains of biomedical reality while at the same time preserving the advantages of consistency and of formal rigor [4], [6], [27]. This trend is at the opposite pole from that of SNOMED, which relies on the idea of a single broad-coverage master terminology, in that it seeks to draw in systematic fashion on the benefits of modularity while ensuring extendibility of coverage through interoperation of its separate modules.

3.1 Benefits of Harmonization

Today it is generally agreed that the goal of ontology development should be, not to develop one single ontology covering the entirety of what exists, but rather to find ways in which ontologies covering different domains of reality can be developed in tandem with each other in a way which allows exploitation of the benefits of division of labor and pooling of expertise. Experts in given domains should clearly be the ones to bear the burden of developing and of maintaining the ontologies in those domains. Experience has demonstrated also that experts are willing to invest considerable resources to this end in return for the benefits – analogous to those yielded through participation in the open source software movement [28] – of contributing to the improvement of a valued community resource. But experience suggests also that domain experts need assistance in ontology development in the form of guidelines which tell them which direction to take in their work. This is so especially where ontologies must be created *ab initio*, in areas where the need for controlled vocabularies for data annotation is only now beginning to be acknowledged. Guidance is needed by those new to ontology as to successful methodologies above all to ensure the development of ontologies which will interoperate with those which already exist in neighboring domains.

Such interoperation should also serve to ensure combinability of terms when composite terms need to be formed for specific application purposes. One problematic feature of the SNOMED vocabulary is its non-compositional character, illustrated for example by 'assay for X' terms, such as

- SNOMED 55534003: macrophage migration factor assay,

where the corresponding 'X' term is missing from the vocabulary. SNOMED thereby allows the simple coding of information about *macrophage migration factor assays*, but no correspondingly simple coding of *macrophage migration factors* themselves. The OBO Foundry ontologies, in contrast, embrace a deliberate policy of ensuring compositionality [29]. Indeed compositionality of terms is used as a methodology to support coherent ontology development, as for example in the Foundry's Infectious Disease Ontology (IDO), which provides a repertoire of those basic component terms, such as 'host', 'pathogen', 'vector', which are used in all infectious disease domains, and works with researchers on specific diseases with a need to form specialized ontologies for different combinations of pathogen, host and vector, to create corresponding extensions as far as possible through simple composition [30].

The general strategy, embraced also by the CARO Common Anatomy Reference Ontology [31], is to develop small reference ontologies for well-specified domains and to extend these ontologies to create larger ontology frameworks for specific application purposes by combing terms from different ontologies in what are called 'cross-products' [32]. This strategy contributes to ensuring comparability of the separate ontologies, and therefore also to guaranteeing alignment of the data annotated in their terms. It serves at the same time, again, to provide common guidelines for the developers of the specialized ontologies and to allow the lessons learned by early adopters of the strategy to be passed on to their successors as the guidelines become incrementally refined. [33].

The OBO Foundry is a systematic realization of this strategy. Following the model of the Gene Ontology, ontologies are created for specific domains on the basis of standards which have been accepted in advance by separate groups of ontology developers because they are designed to secure interoperability of their separate ontologies. The Foundry thereby provides an evolving suite of orthogonal basic science ontologies for rigorous annotation of different kinds of experimental data. At the same time it provides rules for the creation of cross-product terms on the basis of terms from its constituent ontologies joined together via relations formally defined in the Foundry's Relation Ontology (RO) [34]. These rules are applied as a means of removing the arbitrariness involved in the informal cut-and-paste strategies for term-composition embraced by more traditional terminologies. On the one hand orthogonality of the source ontologies goes a long way to ensuring a unique choice for constituent terms where complex term formation is needed; on the other hand the formal definitions of the RO help to ensure unambiguous meaning of the results of this combination. Because all complex terms are required to be defined as cross-products of more basic terms, compositionality, with associated benefits for automatic reasoning, is ensured.

By providing regimented sources and templates for term composition the Foundry is, we believe, helping to avoid the bottlenecks currently created for example in the case of SNOMED CT development, where each new term must be approved for inclusion in the ontology, through a multi-stage committee process, on the basis of intuitive rules rather than of formal principles.

3.2 Harmonization Efforts in Pre-Existing Systems

Independently of the success of either the OBO Foundry initiative or of SNOMED CT's efforts towards international standardization, it is already clear that in developing ontology-based applications in the biomedical field, account must be taken of a large number of pre-existing terminologies, controlled vocabularies and ontologies, some of which – such as MedDRA, ICDx, LOINC, OMIM, and other constituent vocabularies of the UMLS Meta-thesaurus [35] – already have the status of de facto standards. Increasingly it is becoming clear that it will be necessary to achieve progressive integration of such representations, too, and to this end strategies must be found to bring about an incremental, evidence-based, process of harmonization. This will need to be achieved, in part at least, on the one hand by ensuring internal formal coherence of each representation, and on the other hand by maximizing their conformity with the results of on-going scientific research, ideally as this is documented within external gold standard reference ontologies such as those proposed within the Foundry framework. Unfortunately the need for such radical harmonization has still not been generally recognized, though small steps in the necessary direction can be witnessed.

3.3 Challenges to harmonization

The different ontologies, terminologies and other means of knowledge representation in the biomedical domain are often governed by different attitudes towards reality, towards the representation of reality, and towards the most effective practical use of representations in data management. The resultant multiplicity of approaches poses severe challenges to harmonization.

A key challenge is that of preserving coherence as the reach of the ontologies becomes ever further extended and the ontologies themselves become ever more complex. Ways will need to be found to ensure that this extended reach and complexity does not act to the detriment of what has already been achieved within given healthcare institutions or disciplinary communities. The introduction of ontology-based technology or of global resources such as SNOMED CT should not lead to a corruption or dilution of quality standards already established, and it should not lead to already working terminological solutions developed to meet specific local needs becoming overwhelmed by the needs of conformity with larger frameworks. To achieve this end within the OBO Foundry, techniques are being delivered to create slimmed-down versions or 'views' of larger ontologies designed to achieve specific local purposes while ensuring consistency with the larger framework [36], [37].

The harmonization of ontologies must be to some degree centrally organized through directives which enjoy consensus support and are clearly documented in such a way as to address the needs of a variety of different types of audience and to secure their willingness to participate. But if harmonization is not to bring negative consequences it must be effected in a stepwise fashion, with careful precautions to ensure that existing solutions are not jeopardized.

4. Utilizing Upper Level Ontologies for Harmonization put this Earlier with Stuff on Harmonization

Providing an upper level overarching ontology framework for reality representation is a basic feature of harmonization. According to the Standard Upper Ontology (SUO) working group of IEEE:

- An upper ontology is limited to concepts that are meta, generic, abstract and philosophical, and therefore are general enough to address (at a high level) a broad range of domain areas. Concepts specific to given domains will not be included; however, this standard will provide a structure and a set of general concepts upon which domain ontologies (e.g. medical, financial, engineering, etc.) could be constructed [38].

Upper level ontologies can provide not merely basic categories ensuring good ontology organization but also a set of tested principles that can be re-used by others in the development of specific domain ontologies. The Basic Formal Ontology (BFO), which serves as upper level kernel of OBO Foundry ontologies, rests on a basic distinction between continuants and occurrents. The former are entities in reality that endure (continue to exist) through time. They persist self-identically even while undergoing changes of various sorts. The latter *occur*, which means that they have, in addition to their spatial dimensions, also a fourth, a temporal dimension. Occurrents (for example processes) unfold through a period of time in such a way that they can be divided into temporal parts or phases. They have a beginning, a middle, and an end [7]. Continuants, in contrast (for example organisms), exist in full at any time at which they exist at all, while at the same time gaining and losing parts in the course of development and growth.

Using an upper level ontology can foster harmonization by providing a uniform and coherent approach to reality representation at the topmost level of organization. It is at the lower levels, however, that we will find those terms which predominate in practical uses of the ontology. General criteria of the sort embodied in an upper level ontology provide useful tools when organizing these lower level terms [39].

An upper ontology thus stands to domain ontology in roughly the same relation as mathematics to physics. We need to prove mathematical theorems only once, and we can thereafter use these theorems over and over again in different physical theories. Similarly, a major advantage of an upper level ontology is its status as a tested resource, whose re-use prevents time-consuming re-development of those meta-level structures which are needed by domain scientists to organize their ontology resources, but which embody principles of which these domain scientists will likely have an imperfect grasp.

5. Methodologies in Ontology Development

5.1 What does 'Ontology' mean?

We hold that the hypothesis of realism is fundamental to the realization of the goal of evidence-based harmonization in ontology development, and that the still widely popular 'conceptualist' alternatives to this hypothesis in fact constitute obstacles to success in its achievement because the conceptualist can point to no benchmark against which such success could be measured.

The conceptualist view, still popular in knowledge engineering and AI circles, sees ontologies as representations of what are called 'concepts', which means, roughly, units of knowledge (or of meaning) in the mind of human beings [36]. The definitions of Gruber [40] and Studer *et al.* [41] are concept-based definitions of ontology in this sense. Here, in contrast, we propose the following definition:

- An ontology is a representation of the universals or classes in reality and of the relations existing between these universals or classes.

Universals are the real invariants or patterns in the world apprehended by the specific sciences. The relation between universals and particulars is one of *instantiation*. Universals are multiply instantiated: they exist at different places and times in the different particulars which instantiate them [7]. Universals are designated by general terms in ontologies such as 'dog' or 'cell' or 'oophorectomy' or 'diabetes'. 'Dog' is the name of a universal which is instantiated by my dog Fido and by your dog Rover. There are however also general terms which do not designate universals, such as 'dog owned by the Emporer' or 'patients with diabetes in the Homburg University Hospital'.

In these terms we can propose the following specification of the relation between universals and what, in Semantic Web circles, are called 'classes'. In our idiolect a *class* is a collection of all and only those particulars to which a given general term applies. Where the general term in question refers to a universal, then the corresponding class, called the *extension* of the universal, comprehends all and only those particulars which as a matter of fact instantiate the corresponding universal [42].

Our realist view is based on a distinction between three levels of reality:

1. the ideas, thoughts in our minds which form representations of specific portions of reality,
2. those representational artifacts (including ontologies, textbooks, and so forth) which we develop to make these mental representations concretely accessible to others,
3. reality itself, which serves as the target of these mental and physical artifacts.

We believe that success in ontology development depends on keeping clear the distinction between these three levels [42] and on recognizing that the reality which our representations are developed to represent exists independently of these representations themselves. Only in relatively rare cases (for example in the ontology of psychiatry), is this reality inside our heads, but even there it is possible to keep the three levels clearly distinct.

5.2 Methods of Ontology Development

A realist paradigm in ontology development brings the need to foster the creation of gold standard ontologies which reflect current scientific understanding and serve both as models of good practice and also as benchmarks against which the correctness of other ontologies can be gauged. Such gold standard ontologies, the Foundational Model of Anatomy [43] is our paradigm example, should be not merely in good order as they stand as representations of their selected domain of reality; they should also employ state-of-the-art practices in order to ensure that they are well-maintained and updated as knowledge advances.

Such gold standard ontologies must, we believe, be developed and maintained by experts in the corresponding domains. Techniques of ontology development via natural language processing (NLP) as applied for example to textbook literature sources produce results which still fall far short of the necessary formal rigor and scientific accuracy. Such techniques would, if they could be successfully developed, bring tremendous benefits in the biomedical domain, where ontologies and other terminology resources may be very large and may need to be updated rapidly in response to large-scale changes in our underlying scientific knowledge. Increasingly, therefore, we anticipate that NLP tools will provide valuable assistance to ontology-based research. We do not, however, anticipate that such tools will themselves be capable of being used in the creation of ontologies which can serve in the role of gold standard along the lines described. Indeed we believe that gold standard ontologies will themselves provide an indispensable presupposition to their successful application to other purposes.

6. Ontology based clinical research initiatives

6.1 The ACGT Project

Recent years have seen a number of initiatives resting on the use of ontologies to facilitate cross-linkage of clinical research activities among institutions and communities of researchers. One such initiative financed by the European Union within its 6th Framework Programme is the Advancing Clinico-Genomic Trials on Cancer (ACGT) project. The goal of this project is to enable the rapid sharing of data gained in both clinical trials and associated genomic studies. In order to meet this goal ACGT is providing a GRID structure designed to transmit the data between different groups of users in real time according to need, with data integration being achieved by means of an ontology-based mediator [44].

The ontology-related efforts of the ACGT project provide an example of one large-scale effort to create new ontologies useful to clinical research, and it provides a valuable testbed for learning lessons about successful and non-successful strategies for their integration with existing clinically relevant ontology resources.

When considering the development of an ontology-based information-sharing system for the cancer domain, the National Cancer Institute Thesaurus (NCIT) is a terminology resource of obvious importance. Yet, there are a number of drawbacks preventing the use of the NCIT itself as ontology for the ACGT project, in part because its formal resources are too meager for our purposes, with only a fraction of NCIT terms being supplied with the formal definitions of the sort required by its official description logic framework. The NCIT contains only one relation, namely the subtype relation (*is_a*), as contrasted with the plurality of formally defined relations included, for example, within the OBO Relation Ontology. Further, the NCIT (like the UMLS source vocabularies from which it is derived) is marked by a number of problems in its internal structure and coverage [45, 46], including problems in the treatment of *is_a*. A small example can be found in its treatment of 'Organism', which includes among its subtypes for example 'Other Organism Groupings', so that we have

- Other Organism Groupings *is_a* Organism [14].

6.2 The ACGT Master Ontology

In light of such problems the ACGT consortium developed its own Master Ontology (MO) to address the goal of data integration for the domains of clinical studies, genomic research, and clinical cancer management and care. The ontology was constructed in modular fashion, with Clinical Trial and Patient Management Ontology modules designed to be reused for different clinical domains. The ontology has thus far been developed manually, in order to secure the high standards of knowledge representation outlined in the foregoing.

One basic principle of ontology development is that ontologies include only what is general (classes, universals), and thus not particulars (instances, tokens). Hence the ACGT MO does not include real world instances but only universals. It also embraces principles of good practice designed ensure a proper treatment of the *is_a* relation. First it insists on a formal rule according to which

- A is_a B if and only if all instances of A are also instances of B.

This rule guarantees the transitivity of the is_a relation (so that from A is_a B and B is_a C, we can infer A is_a C) and thus allows application to the corresponding statements a simple but nonetheless very useful kind of reasoning. The rule can also be used to ensure a coherent structure of the backbone is_a hierarchy (taxonomy) by ruling out those informal is_a relations still used in a number of terminology resources, as for example in SNOMED:

- cow is_a class mammalian,
- kingdom animalia is_a organism, and so on.

Second ACGT MO embraces the rule of single inheritance, designed to guarantee that the backbone *is_a* hierarchy of the ontology should be a genuine hierarchy in the sense that each child term should have at most one single parent, according to the rule:

- if A is_a B and B is_a C, then A and C are identical.

The central aim is to avoid the sorts of polysemy (*'is_a* overloading'), and associated errors, that often results where multiple inheritance is allowed. This rule is designed also to support the sort of modularity of ontologies, and associated engineering benefits, captured in Alan Rector's project of normalization [47]. As Rector points out, the restriction to single inheritance in the hierarchy asserted within the ontology is perfectly compatible with use of the ontology to infer a poly-hierarchy as required. In Rector's view, managing a large body of complex definitions becomes easier using a single inheritance hierarchy. This it is easier to make changes in a simple hierarchy when changes are needed. There are also human factors. Experience has shown that people make mistakes with when they have the freedom to deviate from the principle of single inheritance.

The basic principles of the development of the ACGT MO have been derived directly from BFO. The ACGT MO is aligned with OBO Foundry ontologies such as the FMA [48] and GO. It also incorporates slightly modified versions of existing medical classifications such as the TNM system [49] in ways designed to enhance their interoperability with other ontologies in the system.

6.3 Clinical Trial Management and Ontology Harmonization within the ACGT Project

The central goal of the ACGT project is to put clinicians in the driver's seat, thus ensuring that all project efforts are in the service of patient care. The ACGT MO has been developed in close collaboration with clinicians utilizing existing Clinical Report Forms (CRFs) to gather documentation on the universals and classes in their respective target domains. All versions of the ontology have been reviewed by clinical partners who have proposed changes and extensions according to need. In this process the problem of handling an ontology with more than 1300 classes became apparent. This led to the decision that ACGT should aim to provide tools to view the ontology in user-friendly ways. The basis for these efforts is a clinical view of the ACGT MO (resting, as it were, on the full ontology running behind the scenes), a view based on tracking the workflows common in clinical practice thereby encapsulating the clinician's approach to a medical problem.

A group of IT specialists, clinicians and ontologists in ACGT has proposed the development of a novel ontology-based system to administer clinical trials [26] called ObTiMA (for Ontology-based Trial Management for ACGT). ObTiMA allows each clinical trial administrator to create automatically an ontology-based Clinical Data Management System [50] tailored to the needs of each given trial. One core intended functionality of ObTiMA, currently in its test phase, is an ontology-based tool for the generation of clinical report forms called CRF Creator. The idea here is that instead of mapping the data in existing clinical databases to external ontologies, the data that is collected will be classified in terms of the ontology from the very start. ObTiMA will support the clinician in both planning and management of clinical trials. In addition, it is planned to serve as a tool for the maintenance of the ACGT MO itself, in a fashion designed to ensure just the kind of tight connection between ontology and empirical investigation that is the key to evidence-based ontology development. As trial administrators propose new terms to be submitted for review by the ontology's curators, this provides a way in which advances in biomedical knowledge can become automatically incorporated into the system and so made available to all its users distributed across a plurality of diverse institutions. It also brings about updates of clinical report form templates in such a way that at least certain aspects of legacy data generated in terms of earlier versions of the ontology can become updated automatically.

7. Conclusion

The need for ontology harmonization, based on principles-based ontology evaluation, is now accepted in a number of influential ontology circles. But these efforts need to be still more intensively pursued. The potential users of ontology-based tools in the eHealth domain still need to be convinced that such tools will be not only easy to use but also useful in their work. Ontology development and evaluation efforts must therefore always rest on close collaboration with the intended users.

The successful ontologies in the biomedical domain all work in the same way [6]. Researchers working in a given domain have data; they need to make this data available for semantic search and algorithmic processing; and to achieve this end they take steps to create a consensus-based ontology for annotating (describing) their data, working with ontologists who help them to ensure that their ontology can interoperate with ontologies already created for neighboring domains. Experience suggests that the most reliable way to create an ontology for such purposes is on the basis of a collaboration between experienced ontologists working to explicit, tested guidelines with domain expects working to address real data annotation needs.

References

[1]   http://www.nlm.nih.gov/mesh.
[2]   http://www.hl7.org.
[3]   Smith B, Ceusters B. HL7 RIM: An Incoherent Standard. In: Hasman A, Haux R, van der Lei J, De Clercq E, Roger-France F (Edrs.) *Ubiquity: Technology for Better Health in Aging Societies,* pp. 133–138. Series Studies in Health Technology and Informatics, Vol. 124. IOS Press, Amsterdam, 2006.
[4]   http://www.geneontology.org.
[5]   http://obofoundry.org.
[6]   Smith B, Ashburner M, Rosse C, et al. The OBO Foundry: Coordinated evolution of ontologies to support biomedical data integration, *Nature Biotechnology*; 25(11) 2007: pp. 1251-1255.
[7]   Grenon P, Smith B, Goldberg. Biodynamic Ontology: Applying BFO in the Biomedical Domain. In: Pisanelli DM (ed.): *Ontologies in Medicine,* pp. 20-38. IOS Press, Amsterdam, 2004.
[8]   http://www.snomed.org/snomedct.
[9]   Ceusters W, Spackman KA, Smith B. Would SNOMED CT benefit from Realism-Based Ontology Evolution? In Teich JM, Suermondt J, Hripcsak C. (Edrs.), American Medical Informatics Association 2007 Annual Symposium Proceedings, *Biomedical and Health Informatics: From Foundations to Applications to Policy,* pp. 105-109. Chicago IL, 2007.
[10]   Cimino JJ. Desiderata for controlled medical vocabularies in the Twenty-First Century. *Methods Inf Med*; 37(4–5) (1998): 394–403.
[11]   Bodenreider O, Smith B, Burgun A. The ontology-epistemology divide: A case study in medical terminology. FOIS (Formal Ontology and Information Systems) 2004: 185-95.
[12]   http://www.w3.org/2001/sw/hcls/.
[13]   http://www.opengalen.org/
[14]   http://nciterms.nci.nih.gov/NCIBrowser/Dictionary.do.
[15]   http://www.geneontology.org/GO.format.shtml.
[16]   http://www.berkeleybop.org/obo-conv.cgi.

[17] Ruttenberg A, Clark T, Bug W, et al. Advancing translational research with the Semantic Web. *BMC Bioinformatics*, 8 (2007).

[18] Rector AL, Zanstra PE, Solomon WD, Rogers JE, Baud R et al. Reconciling Users Needs and Formal Requirement: Issues in Developing Re-Usable Ontology for Medicine. *IEEE Transactions on Information Technology in BioMedicine* 2(4) 1999: pp. 229-242.

[19] http://www.ihtsdo.org/.

[20] www.hiww.org/smcs2006/talks/Rector.ppt.

[21] Ceusters W, Smith B, Kumar A, et al. Ontology-based error detection in SNOMED-CT®. *Proc Medinfo 2004*: 482-6. IOS Press, Amsterdam, 2004.

[22] Ceusters W, Smith B, Kumar A, et al. Mistakes in medical ontologies: Where do they come from and how can they be detected? *Studies in Health Technology and Informatics;* 102: 145-64. IOS Press, Amsterdam, 2004.

[23] Köhler J, Munn K, Rüegg A, et al. (2006) Quality control for terms and definitions in ontologies and taxonomies. *BMC Bioinformatics*;7:212-20.

[24] Smith B, Ceusters W. An ontology-based methodology for the migration of medical terminologies to Electronic Health Records. *Proc AMIA Symp 2005*: pp. 704-708.

[25] Rosse C, Kumar A, Mejino JLV, et al. A strategy for improving and integrating biomedical ontologies. *Proc AMIA Symp 2005*: pp. 639–643.

[26] Weiler G, Brochhausen M, Graf N, Hoppe A, Schera F, Kiefer S. Ontology Based Data Management Systems for Post-Genomic Clinical Trials within an European Grid Infrastructure for Cancer Research. *29th IEEE EMBS Annual International Conference, Lyon.* (in press)

[27] Ceusters W. Towards a Realism-Based Metric for Quality Assurance in Ontology Matching. In: Bennett B, Fellbaum C (eds) Formal Ontology in Information Systems. Proceedings of FOIS-2006, pp. 321-332. Amsterdam, 2006.

[28] Webber S. The Success of Open Source,: Harvard University Press, Cambridge, MA, 2004.

[29] Mungall CJ. Obol: integrating language and meaning in bio-ontologies. *Comparative and Functional Genomics* 5, 6-7 2004: pp. 509-520.

[30] http://www.bioontology.org/wiki/index.php/Infectious_Disease_Ontology.

[31] Haendel, M, et al. CARO: the Common Anatomy Reference Ontology. In: Burger et al. (eds): *Anatomy Ontologies for Bioinformatics*, Springer, New York. (in press)

[32] Hill DP, Blake JA, Richardson JE, Ringwald M. Extension and integration of the Gene Ontology (GO): Combining GO vocabularies with external vocabularies. *Genome Res.* 12 2002: pp. 1982-1991.

[33] http://sourceforge.net/mailarchive/forum.php?forum_name=obo-crossproduct.

[34] http://obofoundry.org/ro.

[35] www.nlm.nih.gov/pubs/factsheets/umlsmeta.html.

[36] http://www.geneontology.org/GO.slims.shtml.

[37] Detwiler LT, Brinkley JF. Custom Views of Reference Ontologies. *Proceedings, American Medical Informatics Association Fall Symposium*, 909. Bethesda, MD, 2006.

[38] http://suo.ieee.org.

[39] Smith B. From Concepts to Clinical Reality: An Essay on the Benchmarking of Biomedical Terminologies. *Journal of Biomedical Informatics* 39(3) 2006: pp. 288-298.

[40] Gruber TR. A Translation Approach to Portable Ontologies. *Knowledge Acquisition*, 5 1993: pp. 199-220.

[41] Studer R, Benjamins VR, Fensel D. Knowledge Engineering: Principles and Methods *Data & Knowledge Engineering*, 25(1-2) 1998: pp. 161-198.

[42] Smith B, Kusnierczyk W, Schober D, Ceusters W. Towards a Reference Terminology for Ontological Research and Development in the Biomedical Domain. *KR-MED 2006.*

[43] Rosse C, Mejino JLF. The Foundational Model of Anatomy ontology. In: Burger A et al. (eds.): *Anatomy Ontologies for Bioinformatics.* Springer, New York. (in press)

[44] Tsiknakis M, Brochhausen M, Nabrzyski J, Pucaski L, Potamias G, Desmedt C, Kafetzopoulos D. A semantic grid infrastructure enabling integrated access and analysis of multilevel biomedical data in support of post-genomic clinical trials on Cancer. *IEEE Transactions on Information Technology in Biomedicine*, (Special issue on Bio-Grids). (in print)

[45] Ceusters W, Smith B, Goldberg L. A Terminological and Ontological Analysis of the NCI Thesaurus. *Methods of Information in Medicine* 44 2005: pp. 213-220.

[46] Kumar A, Smith B. Oncology Ontology in the NCI Thesaurus. *Artificial Intelligence in Medicine Europe* (AIME 2005). Lecture Notes in Computer Science 3581 2005: pp. 213-220.

[47] Rector A. Modularisation of Domain Ontologies Implemented in Description Logics and related formalisms including OWL. *K-CAP'03*, pp. 121-128. October 23-25, 2003, Sanibel Island, Florida, USA, 2003.

[48] http://sig.biostr.washington.edu/projects/fm.

[49] Wittekind C, Meyer IIJ, Bootz F. TNM. Klassifikation maligner Tumoren. 6. Aufl., Springer, Heidelberg, 2005.

[50] Graf N, Weiler G, Brochhausen M, Schera F, Hoppe A, Tsiknakis M, Kiefer S. The Importance of an Ontology Based Clinical Data Management System (OCDMS) for Clinico-Genomic Trials in ACGT (Advancing Clinico-Genomic Trials on Cancer), November 1-3, SIOP Mumbai, Mumbai, 2007.

eHealth: Combining Health Telematics, Telemedicine, Biomedical Engineering and Bioinformatics to the Edge. Edited by B. Blobel, P. Pharow and M. Nerlich.
IOS Press, 2008

Multilingual Documentation and Classification

Kevin DONNELLY [1]
College of American Pathologists / SNOMED® Terminology Solutions, Northfield, Illinois, USA

Abstract. Health care providers around the world have used classification systems for decades as a basis for documentation, communications, statistical reporting, reimbursement and research. In more recent years machine-readable medical terminologies have taken on greater importance with the adoption of electronic health records and the need for greater granularity of data in clinical systems. Use of a clinical terminology harmonised with classifications, implemented within a clinical information system, will enable the delivery of many patient health benefits including electronic clinical decision support, disease screening and enhanced patient safety. In order to be usable these systems must be translated into the language of use, without losing meaning. It is evident that today one system cannot meet all requirements which call for collaboration and harmonisation in order to achieve true interoperability on a multilingual basis.

Keywords. Classification, multilinguality, SNOMED, ICD

Introduction

Clinicians and information technology specialists have made steady progress toward developing fully electronic health information systems, in hospitals and health systems. National healthcare IT systems are now being implemented in countries such as the UK, Canada, Denmark, the United States and Australia. Classification systems have been in use in these countries for many years. The most commonly recognized classification system is the International Classification of Diseases (ICD) from the World Health Organisation, which in its tenth edition (ICD-10). Various efforts have been undertaken in the development of terminologies around the world with significant advancements in the United States and the United Kingdom, which have lead to the development of The Systematized Nomenclature of Medicine (SNOMED) whose current version is SNOMED Clinical Terms® (SNOMED CT®). While several classifications and terminologies exist, this paper references SNOMED CT and the ICD family due to their prevalence around the world.

Most healthcare systems around the world continue to rely on paper based medical records. If medical professionals are to adopt electronic medical records then it is important that classifications and terminologies are translated into local languages. While ICD-10 is available in the 6 official languages of the WHO, it has also been

---

[1] Corresponding Author: Kevin Donelly, Vice President and General Manager, SNOMED® Terminology Solutions, College of American Pathologists, 325 Waukegan Road, Northfield, Il 60093, USA; Email: *kdonnel@cap.org* ; URL: http://www.snomed.org

translated into numerous other languages. The base language of SNOMED CT is English with a US and a UK version. The growing international collaboration in medicine adds additional needs for translation. The increasingly widespread practice of people moving between nations and continents, for example for vacation, economic or political reasons, and the emerging momentum for the implementation of electronic healthcare records, means that there will be a greater need for the sharing and exchange of citizens' electronic healthcare records between nations. This can only be achieved if there are common international standards in terminologies and classifications underpinning healthcare systems.

Practical consideration must also be given to the intended purpose and use of classifications and terminologies. Historically classifications have been utilized for secondary uses such as epidemiological reporting, quality measurements and other statistical and research purposes. Coding has primarily occurred retrospectively by skilled health information management professionals. Terminologies have been primarily used in electronic data capture activities as part of the patient care process. Clinicians record data at the point of care with the data being captured in a structured format for storage, retrieval and aggregation.

1. Growing demand for Health Information Technology

Information Technology has become a central theme in healthcare agendas throughout the world. Whether the driving force is patient care, cost containment, public health, integration of proteomics and genomics into clinical practice, or myriad other issues, the conclusion has been reached that significant advances cannot be made without the use of Health Information Technology (HIT). Our existing system of paper-based records will no longer work. Managing and controlling the costs of healthcare have become a necessity for patients, providers, third-party payers and governments, who are increasingly looking to information technology to provide answers and solutions. Massive amounts of money are being budgeted and spent on Health IT (HIT), and particularly on systems to implement electronic health records (EHR). Overall, the total expenditure on HIT has doubled from $15 billion worth of goods and services in 1997 to over $30 billion in 2006 [1]. The overall interest in this area is clear, as evidenced by global activity on health information technology.

While these projects are largely focused on the unique requirements of each country, there are broader opportunities that are demanding international solutions that consolidate competing, and often contradictory, healthcare standards to simplify implementation and provide interoperability among national healthcare systems. One instance is the European Union, which is in the process of defining its healthcare policies for the coming decades and will require systems and standards that operate seamlessly and accurately across borders.

The free movement of persons is one of the four fundamental rights for citizens of the EU, and gives citizens the opportunity to live, work, establish a business, and study in all EU Member States. Health policy makers must ensure that healthcare is available for EU citizens who move and are on the move. The Danish citizen on holiday in France must have access to care at least equal to that in Denmark and of equal quality and economy. They must provide emergency services for people travelling on short-term stays for tourism non-emergency services for those residing mid-term or long-term. How can this be accomplished without an electronic record with a clinical terminology and classifications able to be translated from Danish to French with meaning retained?

On a national or international basis, effective use of classifications and standardized clinical terminology makes healthcare knowledge more usable and accessible. Core terminology enables a consistent way of capturing, sharing and aggregating health data across specialties, healthcare settings and sites of care. It is difficult, if not impossible, to drive significant improvements in nations' health outcomes, costs and quality without a standardized clinical terminology. At the same time classifications play a key role in the provision of patient care and thus must work in harmony with terminology. The increasingly widespread practice of people moving between nations and continents, and the emerging momentum for the implementation of electronic healthcare records, means that there will be a greater need for the sharing and exchange of citizens' electronic healthcare records between nations. This can only be achieved if there are common international standards underpinning healthcare systems with multilingual accommodations.

Multiple practitioners can share important patient information, trigger effective treatment guidelines, and improve patient outcomes with the assurance that, descriptions of diagnoses and treatments are represented consistently across all health care providers. Clinical care, decision support, and research, in addition to patient safety initiatives, rely on the same information: diseases, treatments, aetiologies, clinical findings, therapies, procedures and outcomes all become digitised. To foster efficiency, users can record data just once, at the level of specificity they choose, and then search it repeatedly for knowledge support, statistical reporting, outcomes measurement, evidence-based medicine, performance data and cost analysis.

This means that, at a national level, governments will be able to extract key statistical data to provide information for areas such as disease surveillance to assess trends in the health of a nation; provide facilities to manage public health outbreaks, natural disasters and bio terrorism.

2. Unique roles and uses for terminologies and classifications

The International Classification of Diseases, ICD, traces its roots back to the 1700's as a statical means for classification of deaths. Currently ICD is on its 10th revision and used in numerous countries around the world for statistical comparisons. The World Health Organisation coordinates activities with member states around the world to maintain and guide the development of ICD. ICD-10 is organized into 21 chapters. Chapters cover areas such as; certain infections and parasitic diseases, neoplasms, and external causes of morbidity and mortality. The basic ICD is a single list of three alphanumeric character codes, organised by category, from A00 to Z99. The first letter in the code is associated with the chapter from which it is derived.

Classifications organize complex sets of data such as a visit by a patient to their general practitioner. Classifications deal with a specific area of medicine such as disease with the ICD family, or procedures or domains such as nursing or laboratory medicine. Classification by their inherent structure can then be grouped into various categories and applied to specific use cases for activities such as reimbursement and quality measurement. Their use around the world makes them a critical component of the delivery of healthcare around the world.

SNOMED CT traces its roots back to 1964, when the College of American Pathologists (CAP) developed its first terminology, the Systematized Nomenclature of Pathology (SNOP), which provided pathologists with a clear and consistent set of terms and codes for use in storing and retrieving medical data. The first version of SNOP contained about 11,000 terms and set a new standard for medical terminologies.

Over the next 40 years, the CAP continued to improve and expand its healthcare terminologies, providing the framework for clear and accessible medical records. In 1974, the scope of SNOP was expanded into the Systematized Nomenclature of Medicine (SNOMED), including a broad array of terms encompassing the full range of medical specialties and healthcare environments. SNOMED continued to expand and its next major watershed event was in 1999 with the creation of SNOMED RT (Reference Terms), this fifth major revision of the CAP's healthcare terminologies as was the first to be released in electronic form only and included more than ten times the content of the original SNOP.

SNOMED CT is designed for use in software applications like the electronic patient record, decision support systems, and to support the electronic communication of information between different clinical applications.

At the core of SNOMED CT is the concept, which contains representations of over 300,000 healthcare-related concepts. Each concept is identified by a unique ConceptId and is distributed as a row in the Concepts Table. Each Concept includes alternative identifiers of the same concept using:

- The five-character code used in Clinical Terms Version 3 (and earlier Read Codes versions).
- The six to eight-character code used in SNOMED International. Role of top-level concepts

The top-level of the subtype hierarchy contains Concepts that represent broad semantic types. These include the following.

Table 1. Subtype Hierarchy Concepts

Attribute	Physical force
Body structure	Physical object
Context-dependent category	Procedure
Environments and geographical locations	Qualifier value
Event	Social context
Clinical Finding	Specimen
Observable entity	Staging and scales
Organism	Substance
Pharmaceutical / biologic product	Special concept

A Concept can have more than one super type parent. However, each Concept is a subtype descendant of one and only one top-level Concept. Thus a Concept that is a "disease" cannot also be a "procedure". In Figure 1 there are three distinct routes between the Concept "bacterial pneumonia" and the root concept. However, all of these routes converge at or below the top-level Concept "disease".

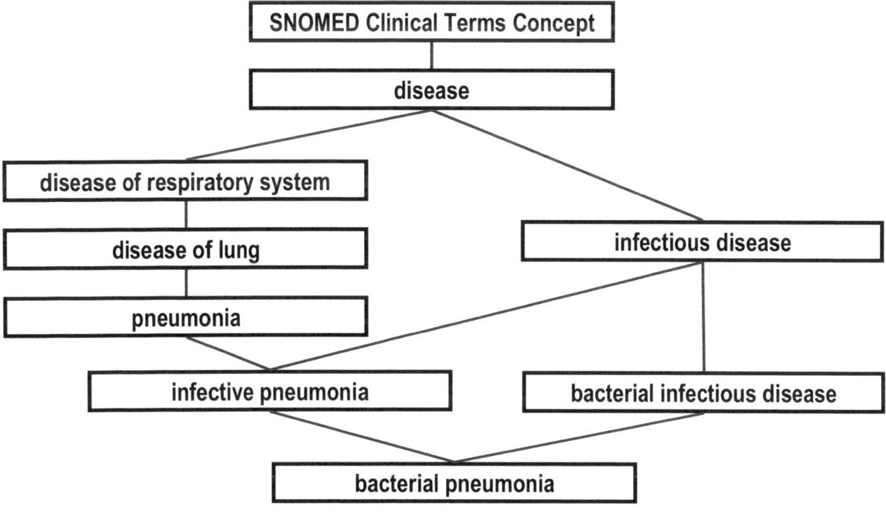

Figure 1. Concept Hierarchies

The next fundamental element of SNOMED CT is the description. A Description associates a human-readable term with a Concept that it describes. A Concept may be associated with multiple alternative Descriptions that represent the Preferred Term, Synonyms, or Fully Specified Name for the Concept in a particular language or dialect. A Description may be a preferred name in one language and a synonym in another. This is indicated by references to the Description from an appropriate Language Subset. Each Description is identified by a unique DescriptionId and is distributed as a row in the Descriptions.

The final fundamental element of SNOMED CT is the relationship. Relationships represent an association between two Concepts. Each Relationship is identified by a unique RelationshipId and is distributed as a row in the Relationships Table. A Relationship contains identifiers of two logically associated Concepts and the identifier of another Concept that indicates the Relationship Type by which they are associated.

- For example, a Relationship may assert that "arthritis" (first related concept) "is a" (relationship type) "joint disorder" (second related concept).

A Relationship may itself be represented in a hierarchical structure called a role hierarchy.

- For example, Direct Device and Indirect Device are both subtypes in the Procedure Device role hierarchy.
- Concepts can have relationships defined with Direct Device, Indirect Device, or Procedure Device.
- Data retrieval can be constructed to recognize the role hierarchy membership and collect all concepts with descendants of Procedure Device.

Table 2. Tabular view of the "is a" relationships for an example concept[2]

Super types of **bacterial pneumonia**				
bacterial pneumonia *is a* **bacterial infectious disease**				
	bacterial infectious disease *is a* **infectious disease**			
		infectious disease *is a* **disease**		
			disease *is a* **SNOMED Clinical Terms Concept**	
bacterial pneumonia *is a* **infective pneumonia**				
	infective pneumonia *is a* **pneumonia**			
		pneumonia *is a* **disease of lung**		
			disease of lung *is a* **disease of respiratory system**	
				disease of respiratory system *is a* **disease**
				disease *is a* **SNOMED Clinical Terms Concept**
	infective pneumonia *is a* **infectious disease**			
		infectious disease *is a* **disease**		
			disease *is a* **SNOMED Clinical Terms Concept**	

The design of SNOMED CT adds unique numeric identifiers, includes links to legacy codes, supports a sustainable migration and maintenance strategy, permits adaptability for national purposes, and fosters alignment with other terminologies and standards such as HL7, XML, LOINC, and DICOM. SNOMED CT delivers on a promise of standardized quality clinical terminology that is required for effective collection of clinical data, its retrieval, aggregation and re-use as well as the sharing, linking and exchanging of medical information.

3. Convergence of terminologies and classifications

Together, terminologies, such as SNOMED-CT, and classification systems, such as ICD-9 and ICD-10, are the foundation required for semantic interoperability that allows for the effective use of healthcare data across various systems, organisations and national borders. National healthcare IT system transformations in countries such as the UK, Canada, Denmark, the United States, and Australia have recognized this requirement. Each country has its own unique set of local, regional, national and international classifications and terminologies to deal with. Figure 2 depicts an example from the United States where various terminologies and classifications for drugs, devices, procedures, professions and domains.

A terminology with the depth and breadth of SNOMED CT can be used as a core terminology for complex national systems as exemplified by that of the United States While SNOMED CT can be used as the means of data capture in the electronic health record, it needs to tie to the various other terminologies and classifications.

---

[2] Note that the Relationships shown in the table and diagram are not the definitive released Relationships of these Concepts. They have been simplified to illustrate particular points in the text.

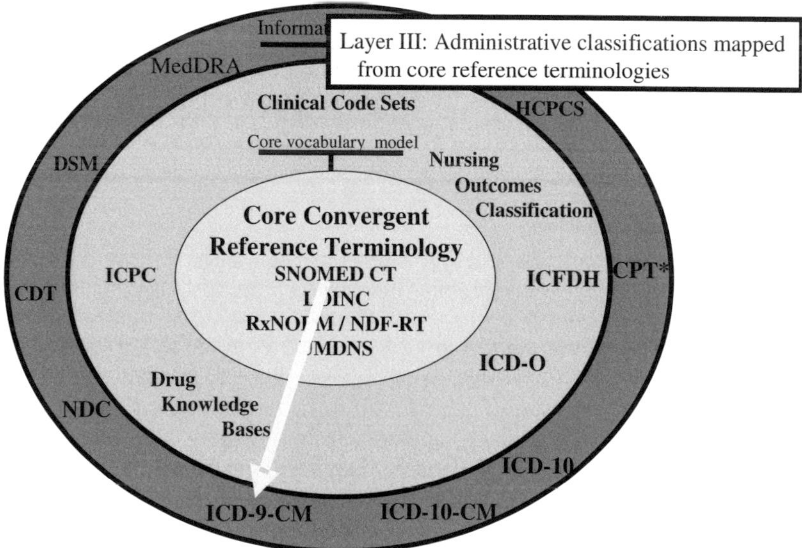

Figure 2. US Integrated Terminology Model

Numerous methods have been used to coordinate between SNOMED CT and other terminologies. Driven by a philosophy of "code once, use many times", if clinical care is recorded in a patient record using SNOMED CT, mapping tables can be used to identify the related code(s) in another scheme, such as billing/ reimbursement.

While mappings are always subject to human review and consistency with local policies and practices, another part of the vision is to automate as much of the mapping process as possible using a rule-based approach. Every map must have an articulated use case that defines its audience, purpose, and methods. Mappings and integrations link SNOMED CT with other terminologies and classifications so that healthcare data collected for one purpose can be used for another purpose, and ease in the migration to newer systems.

4. Harmonisation

While tools and techniques such as mapping are practical ways to enable the interaction of terminologies and classifications, more is needed. Classifications and terminologies and their underlying intellectual property are owned and maintained by various organisations. Efforts must be launched to engage interaction between these organisations in order to develop a strategy for harmonisation of activities in order to support specific use cases.

The International Health Terminology Standards Development Organisation (IHTSDO) has designed harmonisation into its governance principles and organisation.

The IHTSDO will create harmonisation boards with other standards and classification organisation. These boards would work together with other organisations involved in the ownership, maintenance and support of terminologies and classifications in order to develop the best methods for working together and meeting the requirements of complex medical systems around the world.

5. Translation Considerations

Translation in medicine takes on greater challenges then those of a typical translation. Typically it requires teams of professional medical translators, linguists and editors who work together to ensure that meaning is retained from the target language. At the same time commercial grade quality assurance processes and translation tools are used to achieve maximum accuracy of representation in target languages. In the case of SNOMED CT translations, clinical validators from a variety of medical specialties, representing each country in which the target language release will be used, review the work of the translation team. Localisations specific to dialectal variations of each language would be prepared as needed. In order to perform effective translations, clear rules, guidelines and standards must be established and agreed upon prior to undertaking the task. These same principles will need to be considered in undertaking harmonisation efforts, where multilingual representations are expected, with respect to the method being utilized for harmonisation.

6. Conclusion

The use of health information technology to solve the issues facing healthcare organisations around the world is growing. Classifications and terminologies are required if ambitious objectives are to be met. The most efficient way to meet these objectives is to use existing terminologies and classifications for the purpose that they were originally designed for. One classification or one terminology today will not satisfy all needs. Working together healthcare organisations of all sizes, scope and purpose can fulfil the aims of health information technology if their approaches are properly harmonised. The use of clinical information systems will enable the delivery of many patient health benefits including electronic clinical decision support, disease screening and enhanced patient safety.

Effective use of classifications and terminologies enable effective secondary use of the clinical data for performance management and the evaluation of resources to patient outcomes without the need for time consuming and costly separate data collection. The net result is the opportunity for better healthcare for all.

Acknowledgement

© 2002-2007 SNOMED CT – The International Health Terminology Standards Development Organisation (IHTSDO). All rights reserved. SNOMED CT® was originally created by The College of American Pathologists. "SNOMED" and "SNOMED CT" are registered trademarks of the IHTSDO. SNOMED CT has been created by combining SNOMED RT and a computer based nomenclature and classification known as Clinical Terms Version 3, formerly known as Read Codes Version 3, which was created on behalf of the UK Department of Health and is Crown copyright.

References

[1]   Johnston D, Pan E, and Middleton B. *Finding the Value in Healthcare Information Technologies* (2002)

*eHealth: Combining Health Telematics, Telemedicine, Biomedical Engineering and
Bioinformatics to the Edge. Edited by B. Blobel, P. Pharow and M. Nerlich.
IOS Press, 2008*

eHealth Interoperability

W. Ed HAMMOND [1]

*Department of Community and Family Medicine, Duke University
Medical Center, Durham, North Carolina, USA*

Abstract. For improving quality and safety of patient's care, for keeping the costs
of health services, but also for successfully managing public health communication
and cooperation between all stakeholders is inevitable. Such interoperability can
be provided at different levels from simple data exchange up to business
interoperability. The paper introduces those interoperability levels and
international standards specifying and facilitating them. In that context, the
expression of business requirements by domain analysis models or story boards as
well as by functional models of the core applications enabling interoperability like
EHR systems have been tackled. The role of decision support systems and
infrastructural services has been considered as well.

Keywords. Interoperability, EHR, standards, HL7

Introduction

The evolution of information technology in health care can be measured by the
introduction of new words into the vocabulary of the field. Interoperability is one of
those words. It represents the concept of bringing data together from the perspective of
a single patient as well as being able to perform aggregated data analyses across
patients. In the paper documentation world, a patient typically had many medical
records, even in a single institution. In the Duke Medical Center, each clinical
department would have its own patient documentation, and in many cases divisions
would have their own records in addition. For example, the dialysis unit kept its own
records in addition to the record kept by the department of radiology. As a result,
patients always had to repeat demographic and reimbursement data as well as provide a
past history from memory. Therefore, documentation, including a list of active
medications, was rarely complete and became the source of medical errors and higher
costs of tests due to duplication of tests. Even with the advent of electronic storage of
patient documentation, data could not be combined as a result of no standard
terminology, no standard collection of data, and no common formats. Attempts, at
Duke, to implement a disease registry for diabetics or to create an institutional wide
problem list were met with failure.

Globally, pressures from governments, auditors, performance evaluators, and
patients demanded better and more effective care. Publications from the Institute of
Medicine beginning in 1991 with *The Computer-based Patient Record: An Essential*

---

[1] Corresponding Author: William Ed Hammond, Ph.D., Professor Emeritus, Department of Community
and Family Medicine, Duke University Medical Center, Box 2914, 27710 Durham, NC, USA; Email:
hammo001@mc.duke.edu

Technology for Health Care [1], an increased emphasis was placed on the computerization and sharing of patient data. When the revision of this book completed in 1997 [2], the authors found that very little had changed and two chapters were added as part of the revision that mostly brought the technology up-to-date. In 2000, *To Err is Human: Building a Safer Health System* [3] captured government and public opinion with startling figures of the number of preventable deaths due to medical errors. A companion book, *Crossing the Quality Chasm: A New Health System for the 21st Century* [4] and a Rand study [5] on quality increased concerns that the U.S. health system was broken. In the U.S., only 54% of patients received appropriate and adequate care. The focus now was on documentation of care and the use of that documentation to insure complete, appropriate and effective care. Medical errors, particularly medication errors, required a complete medication history, complete list of allergies, and knowledge of the interaction of drugs among other things. In 2004, the IOM publication *Patient Safety: Achieving a New Standard for Care* [6] clearly make the case that national and even global standards were a necessity to permit the aggregation and sharing of patient data.

Increasing costs of care put additional pressure of enabling systems that would provide complete, high quality data at the points and time of care. Further, the old practice of collecting data independently for multiple purposes no longer would be affordable. Reusable data and secondary uses of data became demanded characteristics for IT systems. Clinical Trials and other research, reimbursement, reporting requirements, education, and patient care shared common needs. In most countries, and particularly the U.S., IT systems were all different and uncoordinated. The most commonly used terminology was a local dialect, and attempts to share data even within the same institution required expensive mapping, contain errors, and loss of information.

In the U.S. in 2002, President Bush declared a national goal for every resident to have a personal electronic health record within 10 years. This theme was repeated frequently over the next few years and echoed by the Secretary of Health and Human Services, Tommy Thompson, and by his successor, Secretary Michael Leavitt. The American Healthcare Information Community and the Office of the National Coordinator for Health Information Technology were established to lead the country in realizing that goal. The theme became interoperability must be achieved in health care information system, and standards were necessary for that to happen.

1. What is Interoperability?

Interoperability has not been uniquely defined by the health informatics community. Loosely speaking, interoperability means that we can bring data together from any source, merge or aggregate that data retaining and understanding its meaning, purpose and use. The Institute of Electronic and Electrical Engineers defined interoperability in 1991 as "… the ability of two or more systems or components to exchange information and use the information that has been exchanged" [7]. The definition is reasonable if only the technical requirements of interoperability are considered. The National Alliance for Health Information Technology (NAHIT) defines interoperability as "… the ability of different information technology systems, software applications, and networks to communicate, to exchange data accurately, effectively and consistently, and to use the information that has been exchanged" [8]. NAHIT goes further and defines level of interoperability from a level 0 which essentially is not interoperable to a level 4 which is true interoperability. Perhaps a more accurate term for these levels is data sharing. Anything less than true interoperability has information loss, is subject to errors, adds to the cost of data exchange, and is rarely in synchronization.

Interoperability includes many facets for dada management – technical, political, business, legal, social and organizational. The first and foremost requirement is that of understanding the elements that make up the interchange – *semantic interoperability*. If the data exchanged does not represent a clear and unambiguous component in which both meaning and circumstance is understood, then interoperability cannot be obtained. The Biblical story of the Tower of Babel [9] in which God confused the language of the whole world resulting in the inability to continue to work together to build the tower to heaven. Health care is in much the same situation. The second requirement for interoperability is the ability to exchange information including the ability to accurately identify the person involved so the data can be merged and the support of common functionality – *functional interoperability*. Finally, even if true semantic and functional interoperability exists, there must be business rules that define when and what will be interchanged – *business interoperability*. In addition, rules of privacy and confidentiality must be satisfied. In an operational sense, the business rules among the participants must include a willingness to exchange the data complying with basic business rules, satisfying an agreed upon time response and availability. Any gap or remiss in data sharing threatens the integrity of the entire system.

2. Understanding the Underlying Infrastructure for Interoperability

An infrastructure must be established to support the necessary exchange of data among unrelated and independent parties to the exchange of data. The general model for data interchange and health care interoperability generally is based regional health data interchange areas, sometimes referred to as a Regional Health Information Organization (RHIO), in which a person's data or pointers to that data is brought together and functions as an individual's essential Electronic Health Record (EHR). Two models currently exist: the centralized model in which data is collected from the various sites of care and aggregated as the EHR. The second model is a federated model in which the data is retained at each site of care and is aggregated and exchanged as needed. Pointers to the different sites are kept in a central database. The later seems only to serve a purpose of control of data and has many disadvantages. A centralized model provides better service, better security of data, better reliability and a more effective use of resources. Further, the regional approach better serves a higher level model of a National Healthcare Information Network. Regional systems may be accessed for integrated analyses, centralized reporting, health surveillance and other public health functions.

There are a number of approaches in which an understanding of what is required is determined. Story boards and use cases are commonly used from which the requirements of an interoperable healthcare system maybe be ascertained. Both the AHIC and the Healthcare Informatics Standards Planning Panel (HITSP) in the U.S. have created use cases to help what standards are required for interoperability. Currently those use cases include biosurveillance; consumer empowerment; EHR: lab result reporting and emergency responder; quality; and medication management. The value of these very general use cases in designing interoperable systems remains to be seen. The challenge is to build interoperable systems that provide integrated functions instead of focusing on, for example, an emergency department (ED). The system that serves an ED must support a core set of functions inherent in all EHRS as well as other special functions unique to an ED. Data for a patient arriving in an ED must come for the patient's EHR. The data from the ED encounter must flow into the patient's EHR. However, use case are extremely useful in understand what data elements are required and for what purposes as well as the exchange of those elements among participants in the patient's care. Story boards help identify the actors and the roles those actors play.

Another useful tool that actually is built from use cases and story boards are domain analysis diagrams (DAM) and activity diagrams (AD). The DAM merges use cases into work flow and data flow presentations. The DAM helps understand decision points, trigger events and data interchanges as well as functional requirements.

3. Semantic Interoperability

Semantic interoperability starts with atomic data elements which are the basic components that are fundamental in the expression of concepts to be documented and communicated as part of the healthcare and related processes. In present systems, data elements are poorly and ambiguously defined and vary in data type, name and other characteristics. Simple questions such as "Have or do you smoke?" may be interpreted many ways. What constitutes unstable angina? Yet clinical research and patient care are based on these ambiguities. The names of these data elements are the most confusing of all. There are over 200 identified "controlled" terminologies in use as well as many local and synonym variants in terms. Duke University Medical Center has over 60 different terminologies in use throughout the institution. Terms lack common definitions, names, structures, units, and form, defying any merger of data. The National Library of Medicine has created the Unified Medical Language System (UMLS) in which many of these terminologies are mapped into a single coding system. However, errors in mapping, redundant terms, mixed business and licensing rules and other business constraints prevent UMLS from becoming an integrated medical terminology.

We even have several terms, sometimes interchangeable, that we use for the set of names of data elements: vocabulary, terminology, classification, nomenclature, and most recently ontology. Health Level Seven has initiated an effort to bring together representations of all clinical specialty groups to use a common process, common rules and a common syntax to define a master set of data elements with a defined set of attributes. Each atomic data element would have a unique and unambiguous definition, a unique name, a unique code, a data type, units, a permitted value set, and other attributes as required. This master data element repository would be mirrored around the world and would be available at no charge. The underlying rule would be that all documentation of care would use only terms that were included in the master data set repository, complying with the explicit meaning. Ideally, the names would become the universal terminology, but could be mapped into existing terminologies. So-called minimum data sets for defined business purposes would be derived from the master repository. In the absence of such a master repository, the healthcare community is faced with the use of at least 10 controlled terminologies. Leading this list are SNOMED-CT, LOINC, RxNorm, ICD 9 and ICD 10, CPT, ICPC, and MedDRA.

A Reference Information Model serves to provide a common model for classes and relationship among classes to build common structures. The HL7 RIM is currently the model most widely used. The RIM also serves to permit the defining of syntactic structures and the binding of data elements to the classes. A second and different model is defined in the CEN standard EN 13606 Health informatics – EHR communication.

Few data elements exist in atomic form. For example, the very common measure of blood pressure should include a systolic pressure, a diastolic pressure, the patient position when the pressure was recorded, which arm was used, cuff size, and method used. Interoperability requires a defined syntax for these compound data elements, a unique number and certain attributes that are similar to the atomic elements. These compound structures are called archetypes by CEN and templates by HL7. More complex data structures may also be defined such as person's names, addresses, e-mail addresses, telephone numbers, etc. from an administrative perspective. In HL7, these administrative structures are called Common Message Element Types (CMETs). From a medical perspective, complex elements might include an asthma workup, a well baby workup, a TB screen or an admission profile. Things now become a bit fuzzy in defining these structures. HL7, for example, may call these structures a clinical statement or a template. Semantic interoperability will require the merger of these various structures into a common structure with a common syntax and include a common naming and numbering scheme. These more complicated data element structures should also be stored in a master repository and be available globally at no cost to users. All of these data structures need to have persistence once approved, must be maintained, and must be able to be updated continuously. Further, anyone in the world should be able to propose a data structure subject to submission rules and a vetting process by experts.

The next level of data structure is the document standardization. Perhaps the most widely used document standard globally is the HL7 Clinical Document Architecture (CDA) Standard [10, 11]. The CDA is used for claims attachments, discharge summaries, infectious disease reports, patient summaries, referrals, and other similar reports. The CDA includes a header containing document number, sender identification, receiver identification, document name, data and time stamp. In release one, the body of the document is unstructured. In Release 2, the body may be structured using a schema to define the content. Release 2, yet to be released permits defined structure down to the data element. At the moment, competition exists between the HL7 CDA and ASTM International's Continuity of Care Record (CCR) [12, 13]. HL7 and ASTM have created a compromise standard that blends the content of the CCR into the CDA – called the Continuity of Care Document [14]. This standard has been endorsed by the Electronic Health Record Vendor Association (EHRVA).

4. Functional Interoperability

4.1 Messaging Standards

Messaging is moving data from point A to point B. In itself, it only requires a common, known communication protocol and a shared syntax for sending and receiving data. Exchanging data between a sender and receiver was one of the first applications in the use of IT for health care. Examples include reporting laboratory results, reporting the admission or discharge of a patient, sending a claim for payment, or sending a prescription to a pharmacy. The requirement of interoperability, however, goes far beyond those simple requirements. Unfortunately, even after 40 years of performing these tasks, we still have problems obtaining interoperability. The problems that prevent success for interoperability lies in both methodology and in the fact that several disparate groups must come together to solve the full spectrum of problems.

Functional interoperability usually begins with messaging. Questions are what data is transmitted when. Most of the scenarios we use to define what must be done in data exchange are often more hypothetical than real. While transmitting complete, lifelong EHRs when a person moves to a new location has value and happens to about 10% of the population annually, may not be an adequate business case to justify the expense of creating an infrastructure framework to justify the time and expense. A greater challenge is providing the needed component data at the right time and place. Examples include a patient referred to another facility for a particular treatment or a patient seen in an emergency room for a specific acute problem. Functional interoperability requires defining these trigger events, defining the data to be exchanged, and dealing with corrections, additions and updates over the time of interest.

Although exchanging all kinds of data could be easily accomplished with one kind of standard, several domain specific standards exist for the exchange of data. The most widely implemented general clinical data messaging standard is the HL7 v2.x series of data transport standard. This standard, first defined in 1987 and having evolved to the current version 2.6 is used in over 95% of the hospitals in the U.S. as well as other countries.

Version 2.x standards are based on messages whose content is based on specific trigger events. The format is a message consisting of segments which in turn consist of data fields made of components made of elements. Fields are separated by delimiters. The model for v2.x is implicit and was defined by experienced individuals who knew what data they needed to exchange when. Version 2.x is used when both the sender and receiver are known, and conformance agreements can be put into place. If the receiver was not known, v2.x cannot provide interoperability. Version 2.x standards have the advantage of easy understanding and implementation. The disadvantage is in the high degree of optionality and consequently ambiguity. Later versions of v2.x use XML syntax to take advantage of XML tools.

To solve the problems of interoperability for v2.x, HL7 began a new approach for an interoperable Version 3 standard based on the Reference Information Model. Version 3.0 is based on a core structured content that includes a prescribed set of data types, data elements, vocabulary, templates and clinical statements. This approach provides an interoperable conceptual foundation that is semantically interoperable and uses an abstract design methodology. This version uses XML syntax where the tags reflect the data model.

The Clinical Data Architecture HL7 standard is also based on the RIM and can itself be used for the transport of data. ASTM's CCR standard can also be used for clinical data transport as can the CCD discussed previously. The DICOM standard is used for transporting images of any form; the National Council for Prescription Drug Programs has created a suite of medication standards including the SCRIPT standard for prescription data; ASC X12(N) has created Electronic Data Interchange standards for reimbursement; IEEE has standards for medical devices and home care sensors; and OASIS standards for the exchange of business information. The Integrating the Healthcare Environment (IHE), a collaborative effort with the Radiological Society of North America and the Healthcare Information and Management Systems Society, working with various clinical groups, provides profiles for end-to-end requirements from the above sets of standards. A typical application will require expertise in all of these standards. The required expertise is further extended when one includes ISO and CEN standards.

4.2 Decision Support Standards

The requirements for decision support applications and knowledge management as part of an EHR system has long been postulated. The lack of semantic interoperability has prevented wide spread application of clinical decision support systems (CDSS). HL7 has a technical committee that has created standards for knowledge representation, logic structures for decision rules, clinical guidelines and disease management protocols. Specific standards include the Arden Syntax, GELLO, Guideline Interchange Format (GLIF), and the Infobutton. ASTM has a guideline standard Guidelines Elements Model (GEM). HL7 also has ongoing work based on a virtual EHR that drives decision support algorithms.

4.3 EHR Functional Standards

In spite of its importance, there is no consistent, agreed-on definition of the Electronic Health Record, or what are its different flavors such as an Electronic Medical Record, a Population Health Record, a Summary Health Record, and a Personal Health Record. Part of that definition, however, is what functions or capabilities must exist in an EHR system for it to meet a minimum set of requirements. HL7 has created a standard, the Electronic Health Record – Functional Model that became a normative standard in February 2007. This standard defines functionalities in 3 categories: direct care (care management, clinical decision support, and operations communications and management); supportive (clinical support, measurement analysis, research and reports, and administrative and financial); and information infra-structure (security, health record information and management, unique identity, registry and directory services, health informatics and terminology standards, interoperability standards, business rules management, and workflow management). The HL7 EHR-FM standard has been used by the Certification Commission for Health Information Technology for define requirements for certification of EHR vendors.

Other standards required for functional interoperability include functional standards for regional healthcare information organizations (RHIOs and HIEs) and National Healthcare Information Networks. Other standards include developing functional profiles for different sites, EHR content standards, and structure and architectural standards.

A related set of standards include identification standards for persons, providers, facilities, and employers. Actually, interoperability would be considerably easier if all objects, actors and attributes were assigned a unique and universal identification number. The pilot testing of ePrescribing in the U.S. in 2005 found that medication records from different sources could not be combined for an individual person with acceptable accuracy in the absence of a unique Person Identification Number.

4.4 Other requirements

Several other issues must be addressed to obtain true interoperability. There are a number of issues in privacy, security and confidentiality that must be solved. Strategies that permit patient control of data must be interoperable across sites sharing data. The person's wishes must be preserved across all of the sites sharing and using the information. Policies for opt-in and opt-out need to be standardized. Rules and methods for de-identification of data must be defined and enforced. Security standards include access control, authentication, authorization, non-repudiation, encryption, digital signature and access logs.

We need standards document registries with documents assigned a universal code and name. When any mapping is required, it needs to be done once and made available globally. We need standard clinical trials registries, a standard process for identifying candidates for clinical trials. We need a standard for forms and a standard way of asking questions on forms.

5. Business Interoperability

Even with perfect semantic and functional interoperability, additional business agreements must be defined and standards created to permit the sharing of specific data for specific events. If we were to create a global registry of data elements for health care, included complex and compound elements with unique codes and documents with unique codes and every site only used elements as defined in the site, it would be easy to define electronically and in real time business agreements for the exchange of data. For example, a nursing home could create a profile that would define what data elements should accompany the transfer of a patient from the hospital to the nursing home. Reimbursement claim requirements could be driven by algorithmic specification of data depending on problem and events. Research protocols would be a specification of data elements from the patient care process.

6. Conclusions

Reaching true and total interoperability is such an overwhelming requirement that it cannot be done in one step. We do need to make steps that are large enough to have value but are small enough to be doable in a reasonable period of time. Even so, there are semantic issues, stakeholder issues, functional issues, business issues, and operational issues that must be solved. The report from the President's Commission on Systemic Interoperability [15] suggests a focus on a medication record. Another straight-forward but doable task might be to create an interoperable environment in which laboratory results may be sent from commercial laboratories, shared among health care facilities, and merged into a single patient record. The ROI should be more than sufficient in higher quality care, safer care, and reduction in unnecessary repeat testing.

To move ahead, we need to make decisions and selections from existing standards, identify any existing gaps and create the required standards, strongly push adoption and implementation of systems using standards. Reference [16] includes a more detailed discussion of additional requirements for interoperability, barriers to achieving interoperability, and some necessary steps.

References

[1]   Institute of Medicine. Dick RS, Steen EB, and Detmer DE (Edrs.) *The Computer-Based Patient Record: An Essential Technology for Health Care.* National Academy Press, Washington DC, 1991.

[2]   Institute of Medicine. Dick RS, Steen EB, and Detmer DE (Edrs.) *The Computer-Based Patient Record: An Essential Technology for Health Care.* National Academy Press, Washington DC, 1997.

[3]   Institute of Medicine. Kohn LT, Corrigan JM, and Donaldson MS (Edrs.) *To Err Is Human: Building a Safer Health System.* National Academy Press, Washington DC, 2000.

[4]   Institute of Medicine. *Crossing The Quality Chasm: A New Health System for the 21st Century.* National Academy Press, Washington DC, 2001.

[5]   McGlynn EA, et al. The Quality of Health Care Delivered to Adults in the United States. NEJM 2003; 348:26.

[6]   Institute of Medicine. Aspden P, Corrigan JM, Wolcott J, and Erickson SM (Edrs.) *Patient Safety: Achieving A New Standard For Care.* National Academy of Science, Washington DC, 2004.

[7]   Institute of Electrical and Electronic Engineers. *IEEE Standard Computer Dictionary: A Compilation of IEEE Standard Computer Glossaries.* New York, NY, 1991.

[8]   The National Alliance for Health Information Technology, "What is Interoperability?" 2006. available at http://www.nahit.org/cms/index.php?option=com_content&task=view&id=186&Itemid=195 (accessed 31 October 2007).

[9]   *Holy Bible.* Genesis: 11:1-9.

[10] Health Level Seven, Inc. HL7 Clinical Document Architecture, Release 2.0. available at http://www. hl7.org (accessed 31 October 31, 2007).

[11] Dolin RH, et al. The HL7 Clinical Document Architecture. J AM Med Inform Assoc 2001:8:552-569.

[12] ASTM International, ASTM E 2369 Standard Specification for Continuity of Care Record (CCR). 2005. Referenced ASTM standards, available at www.astm.org.

[13] Ferranti JM, Musser RC, Kawamoto K, and Hammond WE. The Clinical Document Architecture and the Continuity of Care Record: A Critical Analysis. J AM Med Inform Assoc 2006; 3:245-252.

[14] Health Level Seven, Inc. HL7 Continuity of Care Document, Release 1.0. available at http//www.hl7.org. (accessed 31 October 2007).

[15] Commission on Systemic Interoperability. *Ending the Document Game: Connecting and Transforming Your Healthcare Through Information Technology.* U.S Government Printing Office, Washington, DC, 2005. available at http://www.EndingTheDocumentGame.gov (accessed 31 October 20070.

[16] Hammond WE. Solving the Interoperability Dilemma. In: Merritt D (Edr.) *Paper Kills: Transforming Health and Healthcare with Information Technology.* CHT Press, 2007.

Changes in Medical Documentation over the Last Five Decades

Joachim DUDECK [1]
Institute of Medical Informatics, University of Giessen, Germany

Abstract. In medical documentation, standardized coding schemes are used to facilitate sharing, transformation and reusability of data. First, classification systems coding schemes have been introduced. While classification systems are mainly used for statistical purposes, individual care documentation moves towards the use of nomenclatures coding schemes. The paper presents an overview of the development of coding schemes. Different coding schemes serve different purposes. Multiaxial schemes are the way of choice for comprehensively documenting complex care processes. There is a movement from mono-hierarchical classification systems to concept-based, multi-purpose and multi-hierarchical terminologies.

Keywords. Medical documentation, coding schemes, classification, nomenclature

Introduction

Medical documentation is concerned with the recording and storing of medical data from different sources in standardized formats to facilitate sharing, portability and reusabiltity of data and to support patient care and medical research. In Medical Documentation, data are almost always represented by standardized codes out of nationally or internationally accepted coding schemes. The coding schemes are generated under different goals,

- to categorize data from similar objects in one class and to provide each class with an appropriate code (classification system)
- to identify each independent and unique object with a distinct code (nomenclature or sometimes also called terminology)

Classification systems are mainly used for statistical purposes, applications and evaluations when the behavior of the classes of similar objects and not the objects itself are of interest and investigated. Nomenclatures or sometimes also called terminologies are applied when the behavior of the single object should be distinctly described or investigated. Classification systems have been the mainly used coding schemes in the 20th century. But one can see that Medical Documentation is moving towards the more frequently application of Nomenclatures in the upcoming 21st century mainly due to the increased application of Electronic Health Records and related systems. The historical changes in Medical Documentation are therefore mainly changes in the applied classification systems and nomenclatures.

---

[1] Corresponding Author: Joachim Dudeck, MD, PhD, Professor Emeritus, Goethestr. 5, 35423 Lich, Germany; Email: Joachim.W.Dudeck@informatik.med.uni giessen.de

It is not possible to describe the development of all systems which are currently in use. For each medical domain we have now nearly always more than one coding scheme. Those coding schemas have been almost always developed and are maintained by different institutions. This impedes the interoperability which is required by modern eHealth applications to a very large extent. In the following paper a short overview over the development of coding schemes for Medical documentation in the last century should be presented and some aspects of the future in the current century should be given.

1. Classification Systems

In the last century, classification systems have been the mostly used coding schemas in Medical Documentation. Classification systems are generated by assigning similar objects to one class. But similarity can be seen under different aspects. Classes can be defined by diseases which are common in hospitals or physicians offices, by diseases which mainly occur as causes of death or by diseases which have surgical treatment or by the cost of diseases etc. Dependent on the chosen similarity, different classification systems will result which assign objects to quite distinct classes.

In the beginning of modern international Medical Documentation diseases which represented causes of death have been of main interest. The first internationally accepted medical classification system, the "International Classification of diseases (ICD)", established in the last years of the 19th century and introduced in the beginning of the 20th century was not a "classification of diseases" but a "classification of causes of death" [1]. In 1900 the first revision of the original list of diagnosis was adopted as ICD1 and it was decided to update this version every ten years. Up to the fifth version the ICD was still a classification of the causes of death.

Already in the thirties the interest in coding of diseases in hospitals increased, in particular in the English speaking countries. In US, Canada, UK lists of causes of diseases and injuries have been developed and used in parallel to the ICD. These two branches of medical classification systems have been brought together in ICD6, which was published in 1949 and which was now called "International Classification of Diseases, Injuries, and Causes of Death" [2]. But ICD6 and also ICD7, which include only minor modifications were not real applicable in the clinical environment. Too many diagnoses which were distinct from the clinical point of view were still assigned to the same ICD class so that the codes could not be distinguished. Several national developments of classification systems have therefore been initiated at that time to improve and facilitate the application of coding schemes in hospitals and physicians offices [3].

Initiated by the German Society of Medical Documentation and Statistics (GMDS), in Germany the "Klinischer Diagnoseschlüssel (KDS)" was developed by Immich [4]. Immich recognized that the one dimensional code of the ICD did require too many compromises. He therefore introduced a two dimensional coding scheme whereby the first two digits described the topographic location and the third and fourth digit the nosological class of the disease. The Pancreas i.e. had the topographic digits 68, carcinoma the nosological digits 51-53, Pancreas Carcinoma received the code 6851. With this approach constructs like the dagger and asterisk classification could be avoided. It was therefore proposed and discussed for a long time to introduce this multi dimensional notation also in ICD10. The KDS was in use in German hospitals until the end of the eighties. Unfortunately, it was not maintained continuously and became therefore obsolete in particular as soon as ICD10 was available.

In the UK a similar situation occurred about ten years later in particular in the environment of physicians' offices due to the restrictions even of the already available ICD8, but also due to some requirements of the data processing systems [5]. A strictly hierarchical structured classification system was designed by Read. The first version of the Read codes consisted of four characters, where the first character was a letter, while the others were digits in strictly hierarchical order (Figure 1).

<pre>
G....   is circulatory system diseases
G3...   is ischaemic heart disease
G30..   is acute MI
G300.   is acute anterolateral infarct
</pre>

Figure 1. Structure of Read Codes Version 1

Version 2 of Read Codes extended the code to five characters. The Read code was frequently used in the UK. At the beginning of the nineties, a new version, Read codes version 3, was introduced which followed a concept oriented approach.

In parallel to these developments, the ICD was extended and improved. The seventh revision had only minor modifications. Even the eight revision left the basic structure of the ICD unchanged, but included a large number of additional specifications. A more comprehensive modification was carried out in the 9th revision in which the so called dagger (†) and asterisk (*) coding was introduced which allowed the parallel coding of a general disease and its manifestation. ICD9 was extended in the US to the five digits ICD9-CM (Clinical Modification).

2. Introduction of Nomenclatures

Several other developments of coding schemes have been accomplished at this very fertile period as far as Medical Documentation is concerned. The development of the ICD was initiated by Pathologists. But there were no coding schema available for describing the findings of Pathologists at the table and in the microscope. In pathology, findings are always evaluated under different aspects, the location the material comes from, the morphology of the tissue, the etiology of the disease, and often the disorders in functionality. It is not possible to combine these different aspects in a one dimensional classification. Therefore a multidimensional nomenclature was defined, called the "Systematized Nomenclature of Pathology (SNOP)" to classify the finding according to its Topography, Morphology, Etiology and Function which was mainly used by Pathologists [6].

After the successful acceptance, SNOP was extended by three additional dimensions (diagnosis, procedure, occupation) for application in Medicine, the "Systematized Nomenclature of Medicine (SNOMED)". The goal of these two nomenclatures was to describe each pathologic finding or disease distinctly by components of the related axes. Figure 2 shows the designation of codes in classification systems and in nomenclatures. The axis codes in the nomenclature are assigned at the application. This process is called post-coordination.

ICD9 Classification		**SNOMED Nomenclature**		
Acute appendicitis	=	Appendix	+	acute inflammation
540		T-59200		M-4100
Staphylococcal pneumonia	= Lung	+ inflammation	+ staphylococcus	
482.4	T-28000	M-40000	L-24800	

Figure2. Classification and Nomenclature - In the classification, the disease is assigned to one class with a related code. In the SNOMED nomenclature, the disease is regarded from different point of views represented by the relevant axes of the nomenclature. The combination of axis codes describes the disease. Since the axis codes are assigned at application, this process is called post-coordination

Several versions up to SNOMED III have been delivered with modified axes and sets of new codes. It was expected that diseases could be described more precisely by this approach. But the axes codes had always to be assigned at the application. This post-coordinated assignation of codes is a time consuming process. SNOMED was therefore not very well accepted and only very rarely applied in medicine. In contrary, SNOP has been used more frequently by pathologists, in particular in the description of malign tumors.

Malign tumors had been primarily described by localization and dignity codes in the ICD only. A first classification of Morphology was published at the beginning of the fifties by the American Cancer Society [7]. In the seventies the classification of malign tumors in ICD8 was combined with the tumors codes in the Morphology axis of SNOP in ICD-O. In combination with ICD10, ICD-O is now available in the 3rd Version. ICD-O is worldwide used in particular by cancer registries.

ICD-O describes the tumor itself but not the tumor stadium. For this purpose the TNM classification was developed by Denoix at the UICC already in the fifties, and was worldwide accepted in the eighties as standard of Tumor staging [8].

In particular in the development of reimbursement classifications the interest in coding of procedures also increased in the seventies. SNOMED contained already a procedure axis. The International Classification of Procedures in Medicine (ICPM) was primarily developed by the WHO and used in ICD9-CM as Volume 3 in the seventies and eighties. Several national versions have now been published, in Germany several chapters are used as the official procedure classification OPS which is annually adapted to new requirements of the DRGs.

Whereas terminology systems have been nearly exclusively used for medical and administrative purposes, a classification was required to introduce a new approach for the reimbursement of hospitals at the beginning of the eighties. For this task information on diagnosis and procedures had to be combined in a new classification system. Related to ICD9-CM and including volume 3 (procedure), a completely new classification system was initiated, the now also in several national versions worldwide used system of "Diagnose Related Groups (DRGs)" [9].

Figure 3 shows the development of the most important classification systems and nomenclatures up to the end of the eighties. Medical documentation was still dominated by the use of ICD9 (ICD9-CM in US), Read Codes in UK, ICD-O and TNM. The DRGs were introduced in the US.

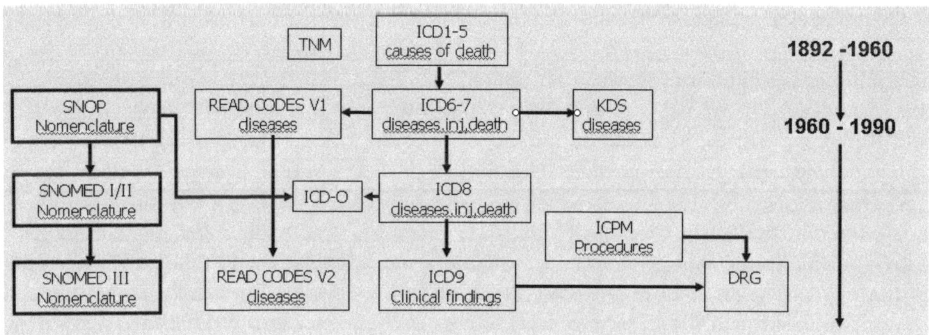

Figure 3. Development of classification systems and nomenclatures in medicine up to the end of the eighties

3. Data Dictionaries in Hospital Information Systems

In the eighties and nineties, several hospital information systems have been implemented which tried to provide comprehensive services including knowledge based functions for improving patient care. This opened completely new perspectives on medical documentation. Collected and stored medical data were now extensively used not only for statistical and administrative purposes but for supporting patient care. It became apparent, that comprehensive approaches including knowledge functions require comprehensive data standards. In those systems so called data dictionaries have been developed and introduced locally. The first system was the HELP system in Salt Lake City [10] with the PTXT Data Dictionary. PTXT was a mono-hierarchical dictionary, but it provided already the same structure of codes for diagnosis, procedures, drugs, laboratory data etc. Each item had to be declared in the PTXT data dictionary before it could be used in the HELP system.

Several other systems have been developed in the following years: the MED at Columbia, the GMDD in Giessen [11, 12], and others. They became multi-hierarchical, the content was extended. The experiences gained and collected during the application of Medical Data Dictionaries were combined and abstracted in the very fundamental paper of Cimino [13] which influenced the development of terminologies in the last decade to a very large extent. Cimino defined "desiderata" i.e. features and properties that are required in vocabularies in the 21st century. The vocabularies should be international and multi-purpose oriented. Their design should contain the following features:

>comprehensive content, concept-based, uniqueness, formal definitions, concept permanence, multiple hierarchies, meaningless concept identifiers, multiple granularities, context specific information, handling of synonyms, easy adaptability to new developments in Medicine, composition - decomposition, avoiding of NOS.

The most important progress has been the concept-orientation. Concepts are understood as a collection of names identical in meaning which describe distinct objects at a specified level of abstraction. Between concepts, relationships can be defined in multiple hierarchies. Hierarchy is one construct within those vocabularies but it is no longer the leading construct as it is in classification systems.

4. Developments after 1990

The Cimino concept was broadly accepted. SNOMED and READ Codes moved into this direction. On the basis of SNOMED III, the concept-oriented version SNOMED RT (Reference Terms) was developed. Also the Read Code version 3 became concept-oriented. The College of American Pathologists and the National Health Service in the UK decided therefore to combine these two approaches into one common solution, SNOMED CT (Clinical Terms). SNOMED CT was maintained by the College of American Pathologists for nearly a decade. To extend the international basis of SNOMED CT, the International Health Terminology Standard Development Organization (IHTSDO) has been founded in 2007 which is now supported by nine countries.

SNOMED CT is currently the only terminology which fulfils all the features required in the paper of Cimino [13]. Nevertheless it needs international acceptance.

Also in the nineties, another terminology was developed which provides a comprehensive set of codes to describe uniquely laboratory and technical procedures and in particular their results, the LOINC (Logical Observation Identifiers Names and Codes) terminology [14]. LOINC is now worldwide accepted as the leading terminology in particular of results of clinical investigations.

ICD10 has been extended towards clinical data. It is now called "International Classification of diseases and related health problems". It contains not only diagnosis but also symptoms, signs and health problems. It is now a clinical classification but is still organized in the old hierarchical structure. ICD10 is sufficient for statistical, administrative and reimbursement purposes but it does not meet the increasing needs in particular of Electronic Health Records.

5. Medication Terminologies

Standardized recording of medications received an increasing interest in the last decade. The documentation of prescription and in particular the monitoring of prescriptions by knowledge based functions is an important issue in improving the delivery of patient care. Several terminology data bases have been developed in the nineties to support this effort but unfortunately in different ways and independent of each other.

The ATC classification was already used in the Nordic Countries in the eighties. In 1996 it was accepted by the WHO as an international standard. ATC tries to describe the drug by the treated anatomic structure (A), the pharmaceutical and therapeutical (T) and the chemical (C) properties. Also the daily dosage can be defined [15].

In the US RXNorm is now the dominating standard for describing medications. RXNorm is concept-oriented and follows the Cimino Desiderata to a great extend. It is also compatible to SNOMED CT [16].

In SNOMED CT a comprehensive concept for drug representation has been implemented based on the "Dictionary of Medicines and Medical Devices (dm+d)" of the NHS [17]. It is structured according to the generic names of drugs. Brand names have to be added by national extensions [18].

A completely different development was carried out at MedDRA, the Medical Dictionary for Regulatory Activities. MedDRA was developed and is maintained by the International Conference on Harmonization (ICH). MedDRA supports the registration of medical products and contains besides diagnoses, symptoms, drugs, in particular side affects investigated during the registration process. It can be considered as a multiaxial nomenclature, but is not real compatible with the other developments in the nineties [19].

6. Current Situation

Figure 4 gives a comprehensive overview of the most important developments in classification systems and nomenclatures in the last and in the beginning of this century. During the last three decades, several medical terminologies and classification systems have been developed. In this paper only a few of them and their relationships could be described. It could be seen, that the integration and the experiences gained with data dictionaries in hospital information systems have influenced the development of medical terminologies in particular in the last ten years. One can see a distinct movement from mono-hierarchical classification systems to concept-based, multipurpose and multi-hierarchical terminologies. This development supports the increasing applications of Electronic Health Record systems while classification systems are almost always not meeting the demands of the health records.

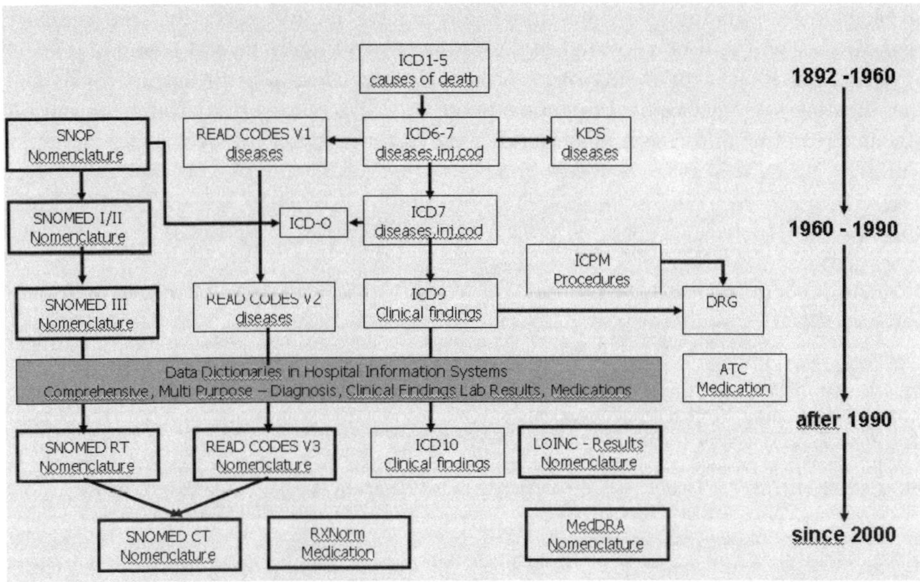

Figure 4. Overview of the main development streams in medical classification systems and nomenclatures. The developments of the last decade has been influenced by the experiences gained with data dictionaries in hospital information systems

On the other side there are now for nearly every medical domain more than one applicable terminology system. Each system has its own notation. This reduces the interoperability, increases the cost of maintenance and training of skilled personal to a large extend. After these decades of expansion of medical terminologies it seems now useful and necessary to consider seriously harmonization processes to map at least different terminologies into each other. IHTSDO has already established a forum for harmonization boards in its Management Board, which already runs harmonization efforts with other terminology boards.

But mapping of several terminology systems might be the first step only. It is understandable from history that the described development did occur. But is it in the long run really necessary to stay with nearly one hundred classification systems and nomenclatures in Medicine? [20, 21] This question is currently probably difficult to answer. But there has already been a comparable process with operating systems in computers. Even twenty years ago nobody would have believed that we sometimes can stay successfully with two operating systems only, Windows and Unix. But it happened. Why couldn't the same occur with terminology systems. It would probably need some more years.

Having this in mind, AMIA together with AHIMA has formed a Terminology and Classification Policy Task Force in 2006 which investigated carefully the actual status of terminologies and classification systems [20]. In its final report the task force describes the current situation as ineffective, as a chaos which requires immediate action It proposes the "formation of a Centralized Terminology Authority" for making actively progress in the harmonization process. This seems to be necessary since it will be difficult to infiltrate effectively the introverted kingdoms of the terminology and classification system developers. But this will be necessary for guarantying acceptance of Medical Terminologies in the future. Or can we really expect that the ordinary medical user will still be prepared in the future to work with several terminologies in the same area resp. with twenty or even more different notations of terminologies and classification system. Medical documentation will be accepted in the long run only if we can streamline this currently "chaotic" area. But it will be hard work.

References

[1]   Knibbs GH. The International Classification of Disease and Causes of Death and its revision. *Medical Journal of Australia*, 1929, 1:2-12.

[2]   History of the development of the ICD, http://www.who.int/classifications/icd/en/HistoryOfICD.pdf accessed 071204

[3]   Manual of the international statistical classification of diseases, injuries, and causes of death. Sixth revision. Geneva, World Health Organization, 1949

[4]   Immich, H. *Klinischer Diagnoseschlüssel*. 1966 Stuttgart

[5]   Information in practice, http://www.bmj.com/cgi/content/full/325/7372/1090 accessed 07-12-18

[6]   College of American Pathologists. *Systematized Nomenclature of Pathology*. Chicago Ill., 1965.

[7]   American Cancer Society. *Manual of Tumor Nomenclature and Coding*. New York NY, 1951.

[8]   http://www.uicc.org/ accessed 07-12-20

[9]   Diagnosis related groups (DRGs) and the Medicare Program: Implications for Medical Terminology, http://govinfo.library.unt.edu/ota/Ota_4/DATA/1983/8306.PDF accessed 07-12-23

[10] Warner HR, Olmsted CM, Rutherford BD. HELP-a program for medical decision-making. *Comput and Biomed Res*. 1972 Feb;5(1):65-74

[11] Cimino JJ. From data to knowledge through concept-oriented terminologies: Experiences with the Medical Entities Dictionary, *JAMIA* 7 (3) (2000) 288-297

[12] Huff SM, Cimino JJ. Medical data dictionaries and their use in Medical Information System Development. In: Prokosch HU, Dudeck J (Edrs.) *Hospital Information Systems*, pp. 53-75. Springer, Berlin, 1995.

[13] Cimino JJ. Desiderata for Controlled Medical Vocabularies in the Twenty-first Century. *Meth. Inf. Med*. 1998: 37: 394-403

[14] Regenstrief Institute. LOINC. http://www.regenstrief.org/medinformatics/loinc..accessed 07-12-22

[15] WHO Collaborating Centre for Drug Statistics Methodology, The ATC Classification - Structure and Principles, http://www.whocc.no/atcddd/ accessed 07-12-22

[16] National Library of Medicine, RXNorm Overview, http://www.nlm.nih.gov/research/umls/rxnorm/overview.html accessed 07-12-22

[17] NHS, Dictionary of Medicines and Medical Devices, http://www.dmd.nhs.uk/about accessed 07-12-21

[18] College of American Pathologists, SNOMED CT User Guide January 2007 http://www.ihtsdo.org/fileadmin/user_upload/Docs_01/Technical_Docs/snomed_ct_user_guide.pdf accessed 07-12-22

[19] Health Canada, Medical Dictionary for Regulatory Activities (MedDRA), http://www.hc-sc.gc.ca/dhp-mps/medeff/advers-react-neg/fs-if/meddrafs_fd_e.html accessed 07-12-22

[20] AMIA/AHIMA. Healthcare Terminologies and Classifications: An Action Agenda for the United States http://www.amia.org/inside/initiatives/docs/terminologiesandclassifications.pdf accessed 07-12-22

[21] Richeson RL, Krischer J. Data Standards in Clinical Research: Gaps, Overlaps, Challenges, and Future Directions. *JAMIA* 2007, 14:687-696

List of Authors

Charalampos Aslanidis, PhD
Institute of Clinical Chemistry and Laboratory Medicine
University of Regensburg, Medical Faculty
Franz-Josef-Strauss Allee 11
D-93042 Regensburg, Germany
Email: aslanidis@klinik.uni-regensburg.de

Andrew Balas, MD, PhD, Professor
Dean, College of Health Sciences
Old Dominion University
Norfolk, VA 23529, USA
Email: abalas@odu.edu

Marion J. Ball, PhD, Professor Emerita
Johns Hopkins University School of Nursing
Baltimore, Maryland, USA
ED Fellow, IBM Center for Healthcare Management
IBM Research
5706 Coley Court, Baltimore, MD 21210, U.S.A.
Email: marionball@us.ibm.com

Bernd Blobel, PhD, Associate Professor
Head, eHealth Competence Center
University of Regensburg, Medical Faculty
Franz-Josef-Strauss-Allee 11
93053 Regensburg
Germany
Email: bernd.blobel@klinik.uni-regensburg.de

Mathias Brochhausen, PhD
Institute for Philosophy, IFOMIS
Saarland University
P.O. Box 15 11 50
D-66041 Saarbrücken, Germany
Email: mathias.brochhausen@ifomis.uni-saarland.de

Melinda Y. Costin, MD, PhD, Adjunct Professor
Johns Hopkins. University School of Nursing
Baylor Information Services
Baylor Health Care System
Dallas, Texas, USA

Christian Dierks, MD, Ph.D., LL.D., Professor
Dierks+Bohle, Attns. Berlin
Walter-Benjamin-Platz 6
D-10629 Berlin
Email: dierks@db-law.de

Kevin Donnelly, Vice President and General Manager
SNOMED® Terminology Solutions
College of American Pathologists
325 Waukegan Road
Northfield, Il. 60093, USA
Email: kdonnel@cap.org

Joachim W. Dudeck, MD, PhD, Professor Emeritus
Goethestr. 5
35423 Lich, Germany
Email: Joachim.W.Dudeck@informatik.med.uni-giessen.de

Päivi Hämäläinen, PhD, Associate Professor
National Research and Development Centre for Welfare and Health
(STAKES)
P.O. Box 220, Lintulahdenkuja 4
FI-00531 Helsinki, Finland
Email: paivi.hamalainen@stakes.fi

William Ed Hammond, PhD, Professor Emeritus
Department of Community and Family Medicine
Duke University Medical Center
Box 2914, 27710 Durham, NC, USA
Email: hammo001@mc.duke.edu

Reinhold Haux, PhD, Professor
Peter-Reichertz-Institut für Medizinische Informatik
TU Braunschweig
Mühlenpfordtstraße 23
38106 Braunschweig
Germany
Email: r.haux@tu-bs.de

Ilias Iakovidis, PhD
Deputy Head of Unit, ICT for Health Unit, DG INFSO
European Commission
B-1049 Brussels, Belgium
Email: Ilias.Iakovidis@ec.europa.eu

Sokratis Katsikas, PhD, Professor
University of Piraeus
Dept. of Technology Education & Digital Systems
150 Androutsou St.
18532 Piraeus, Greece
Email: ska@unipi.gr

Karsten Klein
InterComponentWare AG
Industriestraße 41
69190 Walldorf (Baden), Germany
Email: karsten.klein@icw.de

Eike-Henner W. Kluge, PhD, Professor
Department of Philosophy
University of Victoria, Canada
Email: ekluge@uvic.ca

Gerhard Knorr, Ministerialdirigent Dr.
Head of the Hospital Department
Bavarian State Ministry of Labour and Social Affairs, Family and
Women
Munich, Bavaria, Germany
Email: Gerhard.Knorr@stmas.bayern.de

Sabine Koch, PhD, Associate Professor
Centre for eHealth, Uppsala University, Sweden, and
Department of Learning, Informatics, Management and Ethics
Karolinska Institute, Stockholm, Sweden
Email: sabine.koch@ehealth.uu.se

Santosh Krishna, PhD, EdS, Assistant Professor
Department of Community Health, Division of Biostatistics
School of Public Health, Saint Louis University
3545 Lafayette Ave.
St. Louis, MO 63104, USA
Email: KrishnaS@slu.edu

S. Yunkap Kwankam, PhD, Professor
e-Health Coordinator, Department of Knowledge Management and
Sharing
World Health Organization
20, Avenue Appia
Geneva 27, Switzerland
Email: kwankamy@who.int

Christoph Lehmann, MD, PhD, Associate Professor
Johns Hopkins University School of Medicine
Baltimore, Maryland, USA
Email: clehmann@jhmi.edu

Gerhard Liebisch, PhD
Institute of Clinical Chemistry and Laboratory Medicine
University of Regensburg, Medical Faculty
Franz-Josef-Strauss Allee 11
D-93042 Regensburg, Germany
Email: gerhard.liebisch@klinik.uni-regensburg.de

Thomas Liebscher, PhD
InterComponentWare AG
Industriestraße 41
69190 Walldorf (Baden), Germany
Email: Thomas.Liebscher@icw.de

Javier Lopez, PhD, Professor
University of Malaga, Spain
Computer Science Department
E.T.S. Ingenieria Informatica
Campus de Teatinos
University of Malaga
29071-Malaga, Spain
Email: jlm@lcc.uma.es

Nancy Lorenzi, PhD, Professor
Dept. of Biomedical Informatics
Vanderbilt University Medical Center
2209 Garland Avenue
Nashville, TN 37232-8340, USA
Email: nancy.lorenzi@Vanderbilt.Edu

George Mihalas, PhD, Professor
Victor Babes University of Medicine and Pharmacy
Eftimie Murgu Sq 2
Timisoara 300041, Romania
Email: mihalas@umft.ro.

Kotaro Minato, PhD
Graduate School of Information Science
Nara Institute of Science and Technology
Takayama 8916-5, Ikoma
Nara 630-0192, Japan

Peter J. Murray, MD, PhD
IMIA Interim Vice President for Strategic Planning Implementation
Centre for Health Informatics R@D CHIRAD
Coachman's Cottage, Nocton Hall
Nocton, Lincoln, United Kingdom
Email: peter@chirad.net

Megumi Nakao, PhD
Graduate School of Information Science
Nara Institute of Science and Technology
Takayama 8916-5, Ikoma
Nara 630-0192, Japan
Email: meg@is.naist.jp

Dag Rune Olsen, MD, PhD
Institute for Cancer Research
The Norwegian Radiumhospitalet
Montebello
Oslo, Norway
Email: d.r.olsen@medisin.uio.no

Evelyn Orsó, PhD
Institute of Clinical Chemistry and Laboratory Medicine
University of Regensburg, Medical Faculty
Franz-Josef-Strauss Allee 11
D-93042 Regensburg, Germany
Email: evelyn.orso@klinik.uni-regensburg.de

Günther Pernul, PhD, Professor
Institute for Business Informatics
University of Regensburg
Universitätstrasse 31
93053 Regensburg, Germany
Email: guenther.pernul@wiwi.uni-regensburg.de

Octavian Purcarea, MD, PhD
ICT for Health Unit, DG INFSO
European Commission
B-1049 Brussels, Belgium
Email: octavian.purcarea@ec.europa.eu

Erich R. Reinhardt, PhD, Professor
Member of the Board of Siemens AG
President and CEO of Siemens Medical Solutions
Siemens Medical Solutions
Henkestraße 127
91052 Erlangen, Germany
Email: erich.reinhardt@siemens.com

Albrecht Reith, MD, PhD, Professor
The Norwegian Radiumhospitalet
Montebello
Oslo, Norway
Email: albrecht.reith@labmed.uio.no

Jarmo Reponen, MD, PhD, Professor
FinnTelemedicum, University of Oulu
c/o KTTYL, P.O.Box 5000
FIN-90014 Oulu, Finland
Email: jarmo.reponen@oulu.fi.

Tetsuo Sato, PhD
Graduate School of Information Science
Nara Institute of Science and Technology
Takayama 8916-5, Ikoma
Nara 630-0192, Japan

Barry Smith, PhD, Professor
University at Buffalo
135 Park Hall, North Campus
Buffalo, New York 14260, USA
Email: phismith@buffalo.edu

Gerd Schmitz, MD, PhD, Professor
Institute of Clinical Chemistry and Laboratory Medicine
University of Regensburg, Medical Faculty
Franz-Josef-Strauss Allee 11
D-93042 Regensburg, Germany
Email: gerd.schmitz@klinik.uni-regensburg.de

Tadao Sugiura, PhD, Associate Professor
Graduate School of Information Science
Nara Institute of Science and Technology
Takayama 8916-5, Ikoma, Nara 630-0192, Japan
Email: sugiura@is.naist.jp

Hiroshi Tanaka, MD, PhD, Professor
Director General, University Center for Information Medicine
Tokyo Medical and Dental University
Koyasu Building, 1-5-45 Yushima Bunkyo-ku
Tokyo 113-8510, Japan
Email: tanaka@cim.tmd.ac.jp

Tsigeweini A. Tessema, MD, PhD
College of Health Sciences
Old Dominion University
Norfolk, VA 23529, USA
Email: ttessema@odu.edu

Ilkka Winblad, PhD, Associate Professor
FinnTelemedicum, University of Oulu
c/o KTTYL, P.O.Box 5000
FIN-90014 Oulu, Finland
Email: ilkka.winblad@oulu.fi

Astrid C. Wolf
InterComponentWare AG
Industriestraße 41
69190 Walldorf (Baden), Germany
Email: Astrid.Wolf@icw.de

Oliver Ziebold
InterComponentWare AG
Industriestraße 41
69190 Walldorf (Baden), Germany
Email: Oliver.Ziebold@icw.de

Jana Zvárová, PhD, Professor
Charles University Prague
European Center for Medical Informatics, Statistics and Epidemiology
Pod Vodarenskou vezi 2
182 07 Prague 8, Czech Republic
Email: jana.zvarova@euromise.cz

eHealth: Combining Health Telematics, Telemedicine, Biomedical Engineering and Bioinformatics to the Edge. Edited by B. Blobel, P. Pharow and M. Nerlich.
IOS Press, 2008

Author Index